Inflammation and pregnancy

Inflammation and pregnancy

Edited by

Donald M Peebles MD MRCOG
Reader/Honorary Consultant in Obstetrics
Department of Obstetrics and Gynaecology
University College London
London
UK

and

Leslie Myatt PhD
Professor of Obstetrics and Gynecology
University of Cincinnati College of Medicine
Cincinnati, OH
USA

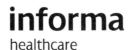

First published in 2006 by Informa Healthcare, Telephone House, 69-77 Paul Street, London EC2A 4LQ, UK.

Simultaneously published in the USA by Informa Healthcare, 52 Vanderbilt Avenue, 7th Floor, New York, NY 10017, USA.

Informa Healthcare is a trading division of Informa UK Ltd. Registered Office: 37–41 Mortimer Street, London W1T 3JH, UK. Registered in England and Wales number 1072954.

A CIP record for this book is available from the British Library.

Library of Congress Cataloging-in-Publication Data available on application

ISBN-13: 9781842142721

Orders may be sent to: Informa Healthcare, Sheepen Place, Colchester, Essex CO3 3LP, UK
Telephone: +44 (0)20 7017 5540
Email: CSDhealthcarebooks@informa.com
Website: http://informahealthcarebooks.com/

For corporate sales please contact: CorporateBooksIHC@informa.com
For foreign rights please contact: RightsIHC@informa.com
For reprint permissions please contact: PermissionsIHC@informa.com

Contents

CONTENTS

Contributors

Mandish K Dhanjal BSc MRCP MRCOG
Consultant Obstetrician and Gynaecologist
Queen Charlotte's and Chelsea Hospital
London
UK
and
Honorary Senior Lecturer
Division of Surgery, Oncology, Reproductive Biology and
Anaesthetics
Imperial College
London
UK

David Edwards FMedSci
Professor
Institute of Reproductive and Developmental Biology
Imperial College
London
UK

Jimmy Espinoza MD
Perinatology Research Branch NICHD, NIH, DHHS
Bethesda, MD and Detroit, MI
USA
and
Department of Obstetrics and Gynecology
Wayne State University
Detroit, MI
USA

Stephen J Fortunato MD
The Perinatal Research Center of The Women's Health
Research and Education Foundation
Nashville, TN
USA

Ricardo Gomez MD
Center for Perinatal Diagnosis and Research (CEDIP)
Hospital Dr. Sotero del Rio
Puente Alto
Chile

Luís F Gonçalves MD
Head, Prenatal Diagnosis Unit
Perinatology Research Branch NICHD, NIH, DHHS
Bethesda, MD and Detroit, MI
USA
and
Assistant Professor of Obstetrics and Gynecology
Wayne State University
Detroit, MI
USA

Larry J Guilbert PhD
Department of Medical Microbiology and Immunology
University of Alberta
Edmonton
Canada
and
Perinatal Research Centre
University of Alberta
Edmonton
Canada

Denise G Hemmings PhD
Department of Obstetrics and Gynecology
University of Alberta
Edmonton
Canada
and
Perinatal Research Centre
University of Alberta
Edmonton
Canada

Joan S Hunt PhD
Department of Anatomy and Cell Biology
University of Kansas Medical Center
Kansas City, KS
USA

Alan H Jobe MD PhD
Professor of Pediatrics
Department of Pediatrics and Pulmonary Biology
Cincinnati Children's Hospital Medical Center
University of Cincinnati
Cincinnati, OH
USA

Jeffrey A Keelan PhD
Senior Lecturer
Liggins Institute and Department of Pharmacology and
Clinical Pharmacology
University of Auckland
Auckland
New Zealand

Juan Pedro Kusanovic MD
Research Associate
Perinatology Research Branch NICHD, NIH, DHHS
Wayne State University School of Medicine
Detroit, MI
USA

Susan Laird PhD
Principal Lecturer
Biomedical Research Centre
Sheffield Hallam University
Sheffield
UK

Tin-Chiu Li MD PhD FRCOG MRCP
Consultant Obstetrician and Gynecologist and
Honorary Professor of Reproductive Medicine and Surgery
Sheffield Teaching Hospitals
Sheffield
UK

Ramsey H McIntire PhD
Department of Anatomy and Cell Biology
University of Kansas Medical Center
Kansas City, KS
USA

Ramkumar Menon MS
The Perinatal Research Center of The Women's Health
Research and Education Foundation
Nashville, TN
USA

Murray D Mitchell DPhil DSc FRSNZ
Professor
Liggins Institute and Department of Pharmacology and
Clinical Pharmacology
University of Auckland
Auckland
New Zealand
and
National Research Centre for Growth and Development
Auckland
New Zealand

Timothy JM Moss PhD
Senior Research Fellow
School of Women's and Infants' Health
The University of Western Australia
Perth, WA
Australia

Leslie Myatt PhD
Professor of Obstetrics and Gynecology
University of Cincinnati College of Medicine
Cincinnati, OH
USA

Catherine Nelson-Piercy MA FRCP
Consultant Obstetric Physician
St Thomas' Hospital and Queen Charlotte's and Chelsea
Hospital
London
UK

Donald M Peebles MD MRCOG
Reader / Honorary Consultant in Obstetrics
Department of Obstetrics and Gynaecology
University College London
London
UK

Lucilla Poston PhD FRCOG
Professor of Maternal and Fetal Health
Maternal and Fetal Research Unit
Division of Reproductive Health, Endocrinology and
Development
King's College London
London
UK

Siobhan Quenby BSc MBBS MD MRCOG
School of Reproductive and Developmental Medicine
University of Liverpool
Liverpool Women's Hospital
Liverpool
UK

Maarten Raijmakers PhD
Maternal and Fetal Research Unit
Division of Reproductive Health, Endocrinology and
Development
King's College London
London
UK
and
Department of Clinical Chemistry
Máxima Medical Centre
Veldhoven
The Netherlands

Chris WG Redman BChir FRCP FRCOG
Professor of Obstetric Medicine
Nuffield Department of Obstetrics and Gynaecology
John Radcliffe Hospital
Oxford
UK

Roberto Romero MD
Perinatology Research Branch NICHD, NIH, DHHS
Bethesda, MD and Detroit, MI
USA

Ian L Sargent PhD
Nuffield Department of Obstetrics and Gynaecology
John Radcliffe Hospital
Oxford
UK

Susern Tan MBBS MRCP
Division of Surgery, Oncology, Reproductive Sciences and
Anaesthetics
Imperial College London
London
UK

Mark A Turner
School of Reproductive and Developmental Medicine
University of Liverpool
Liverpool Women's Hospital
Liverpool
UK

Gill Vince
School of Clinical Laboratory Sciences
University of Liverpool
Liverpool
UK

Preface

Most medical books deal with a specific disease or organ; this book is different in that it focuses on a basic biologic process, inflammation, and its role in pregnancy. There are many reasons why this is an important and topical subject. Inflammation is a Janus-like process. Appropriate regulation of inflammation underlies establishment of a normal pregnancy and is integral to normal parturition. Conversely, it has become clear over recent years that inflammation is also a major component of the most serious obstetric complications such as miscarriage, pre-eclampsia and preterm labor. Similarly, many of the neonatal complications associated with prematurity, such as lung and brain injury, are now thought to be a consequence of a 'fetal inflammatory response' to the factors underlying preterm labor. New cellular and molecular techniques have allowed major advances in our understanding of the components of the inflammatory pathway and clinical experience from other fields of medicine, such as rheumatology, have shown how these advances can lead to immunemodulating therapies that can improve patient outcome.

Our purpose in collating this book was to provide a definitive text that would cover basic immunology and then review ways in which components of the immune response contribute to both normal and abnormal pregnancy. The result is a collection of chapters by clinicians and scientists from around the world who have two things in common – an international scientific reputation and a deep-rooted interest in inflammation and pregnancy. The chapters themselves cover a wide range of topics, from molecular mechanisms, such as those responsible for embryo implantation, to the clinical management of auto-immune diseases that may be influenced by pregnancy. Some themes emerge: many processes are common to all the conditions discussed and there isn't a chapter that doesn't mention pro-inflammatory cytokines such as interleukin-1 or tumor necrosis factor alpha. At the same time one becomes aware of the many different research strategies and interests that can arise from study of the single process of inflammation; this may be partly due to the complex and sometimes contradictory nature of the influence that inflammation has on disease processes, e.g why does inflammation improve lung maturation and early function but lead to bronchopulmonary dysplasia in the long term?

We are extremely grateful to the authors who put by so much time to produce this book at a time when many institutions do not acknowledge this type of academic output. We think that the result will be a helpful source of information and inspiration for those caring for women and their babies as well as scientists wishing to become involved in this complex but rewarding area.

Donald M Peebles
Leslie Myatt

1. Inflammatory cells and cytokine production

Joan S Hunt and Ramsey H McIntire

Joan S Hunt and Ramsey H McIntire

Joan S Hunt and Ramsey H McIntire

INTRODUCTION

Inflammation associated with disruption of the uterine epithelium and implantation of the blastocyst in the uterus has immediate consequences that promote fertility, alerting the mother that pregnancy is imminent. Thereafter, inflammation, particularly that stimulated by infections, is highly undesirable. It wrecks havoc on the delicate balance of immune cells and immune-associated molecules that are in place to protect semiallogeneic pregnancy.

Prior to pregnancy, the uterus is a site of mucosal immunity with the same basic characteristics as respiratory and gastrointestinal mucosa. Immune cells capable of developing specific, acquired immunity for the mother are abundant and their products are readily channeled into patterns consistent with initiation of an immune response should infection or invasion by microorganisms occur. Concurrently with implantation, dramatic changes take place in the leukocyte subpopulations resident in the uterus. Immune cells programmed for antigen-specific, acquired immunity are essentially eliminated and are replaced by cells of the natural, innate immune system exhibiting immunosuppressive properties.

Infections of the fetal membranes and ultimately the fetus itself are common in pregnancy and frequently result in preterm labor and delivery. Infections drive proliferation of the maternal and fetal immune cells, which are normally in a mode consistent with protection of the embryo/fetus from maternal cell-mediated immunity, into inflammatory patterns. These cells and their host of cell-destroying inflammation-associated cytokines such as tumor necrosis factor-α (TNF-α) and other products are extremely dangerous to the fetus, overriding the normal anti-inflammatory environment of the pregnant uterus and causing intrinsic damage to fetal cells. In this chapter, the cells and cytokines known to characterize the cycling and pregnant human uterus are described and the conditions that lead to changes are pinpointed.

THE CYCLING HUMAN UTERUS

Lymphoid aggregates containing antigen-specific T and B lymphocytes constitute a major aspect of host defense in the human endometrium. The endometrium also hosts cells of the innate immune system such as macrophages and their close relatives, dendritic cells, as well as natural killer (NK) cells.[1,2] As the cycle reaches its conclusion, mast cells are prominent.[3] Unlike the other leukocytes, which normally function in host defense, the mast cells appear to have a critical role in driving menstruation.[4–6] Leukocyte subset proportions in the cycling endometrium depend in large part on levels of female sex hormones. For example, studies in mice have shown that estrogens stimulate an influx of leukocytes into the uterus during the estrus phase that include eosinophils and macrophages but not antigen-specific T and B cells,[7] and human NK cell populations depend on progesterone for maintenance and proliferation in situ.[8,9]

Pregnancy introduces a new organ, the placenta, which is also a site of synthesis of chemokines. The chemoattractive ligands produced in decidua and placentas that may influence the changes are shown in Table 1.1.[10–15] One ligand, CCL5/RANTES, is produced only in decidua and two ligands, CCL21/6 Ckine/SLC and CXCL1, are found only in placentas, but most of the ligands have been identified in both maternal and fetal compartments. Leukocytes are common sources of the chemokines, and some have been identified in extravillous cytotrophoblast cells, but villous cytotrophoblast cells, which are secluded behind syncytiotrophoblast, rarely exhibit the ligands.

Table 1.1 Chemokines in the decidua and villous placenta by cell type

Ligands	Decidua			Villous placenta		
	Leukocytes	Stromal cells	xvCTB	Macrophages	Stromal cells	vCTB
CCL2/MCP-1	+	+/0	0	+	0	0
CCL3MIP-1α	+	+	+	+	+	0
CCL5/RANTES	0	+	0	0	0	0
CCL7/MCP-3	0	+/0	0	0	+	0
CCL14/HCC-1	0	+	+	0	+	0
CCL21/6Ckine/SLC	0	0	0	0	+/0	0
CXCL1	0	0	0	0	+	0
CXCL6/GCP-2	0	+/0	+	0	+/0	0
CXCL8/IL-8	+	+	0	+	+	+
CXCL10/IP-10	0	+	0	0	+/0	+/0
CXCL11/ITAC	+/0	+	0	0	+	0
CXCL12/SDF-1	+/0	0	+	0	+/0	0
CXCL14/BRAK	0	+/0	0	+/0	0	0
CX3CL1/fractalkine	0	+	0	0	+	0

+, detected; 0, not detected; +/− inconsistent results;
xvCTB, extravillous cytotrophoblast cells; vCTB, villous cytotrophoblast cells.
Summarized from References 10–15. Reprinted from Reference 18 with permission of Elsevier Inc.

MATERNAL IMMUNE RESPONSES TO FERTILIZATION AND IMPLANTATION IN UNCOMPLICATED PREGNANCIES

PREIMPLANTATION EVENTS

Signaling of imminent pregnancy to mothers is very likely to be a function of the preimplantation embryo, but whether these signals are immunological is as yet poorly understood in humans. In ruminants, an interferon (IFN-τ) delivers signals to decidual cells that may or may not include immune cells,[16] whereas in mice, transforming growth factor-β1 (TGF-β1) in the male ejaculate appears to have an important role in programming maternal immunological receptivity to the implanting blastocyst.[17]

Preimplantation human embryos express human chorionic gonadotropin (hCG) as well as a soluble isoform of HLA-G; both have been postulated to signal the onset of implantation and pregnancy, as noted in a recent review.[18] Of particular current interest to assisted reproductive technology, low levels of soluble HLA-G are associated with poor implantation potential of in-vitro cultured embryos,[19] but whether this relates to signaling to the mother's immune system is not known. Applying information gained in a mouse model to human pregnancy is invariably risky, but evidence that TGF-β1 is abundant in the human placenta[20] and may be a product of human decidual macrophages stimulated by soluble HLA-G[21] supports the idea that this multifunctional cytokine could act as a critical immunomodulatory cytokine in human pregnancy.

IMPLANTATION AND THE MATERNAL IMMUNE RESPONSE

Normal early implantation has an inflammatory component, but ongoing pregnancy has its own hallmarks, as discussed below. Because of the inherent difficulties in obtaining and studying early implantation in women, much of the information that is available has been generated by studies in mice. Concurrent with invasion of the uterine epithelium by the blastocyst, a T helper type 1 (Th1)-type reaction takes place. The Th1-type reaction is characterized by an influx of leukocytes and synthesis of an array of inflammatory molecules such as interleukin-1 (IL-1).[22] This initial inflammatory response may comprise an informative signal to the mother to prepare for the cohabiting embryo.

Although there could be more than one explanation for inflammation in this setting, most reproductive biologists would agree that simple tissue destruction due to disruption of the epithelial and stromal cells of the endometrium is likely to be the major trigger. Nonetheless, reproductive immunologists have proposed that implantation-associated inflammation might be an immune recognition response. In humans, intervals to pregnancy are lengthier when mothers and fathers are genetically similar,[23] and genetic similarity would reduce the possibility of an immune-based inflammatory response. The practice of immunizing potential mothers with their husband's or third-party leukocytes is based on this idea but has been shown in double-blind studies not to be a useful technique and may even be dangerous.[24] Because of poor pregnancy outcomes and the potential for transmission of pathogenic microorganisms, the practice is prohibited in the United States by the Food and Drug Administration (FDA) except under approved experimental protocols.

Studies in mice have suggested that implantation situations where mothers and their embryos/fetuses fail to erect appropriate barriers to protect the fetuses can lead to fetal destruction. Molecules that have been implicated are:

- an apoptosis-inducing member of the TNF family of ligands, Fas ligand[25]
- Crry, a regulatory protein on trophoblast cells that protects against complement-mediated immune destruction[26]
- indoleamine 2,3-dioxygenase (IDO).[27]

Of these, the first two have received support from studies on genetically deficient mice,[25,26] whereas loss of pregnancy is not a feature of IDO knockout mice.[28] Yet at this point the most convincing evidence supporting the idea that lack of these immunological barriers may compromise human pregnancy remains indirect; for example, individuals lacking all three of the human complement regulatory proteins are unknown. Lack of direct evidence may be the result of multiple, overlapping protective mechanisms; when a genetic deficiency prevents mothers from synthesizing either human leukocyte antigen HLA-G1 or HLA-G5, pregnancy still goes forward. It has been postulated that these mothers synthesize other HLA-G isoform(s) with similar functions that compensate for their deficiencies.[29]

REPROGRAMMING FOR PREGNANCY

The pregnant uterus and placenta are immune privileged sites wherein acquired immunity is highly restricted. Several decades of experimentation have revealed that both the mother and her embryo/fetus cooperate to create an appropriate immunological environment for fetal growth and development, as outlined recently.[18,30] The changes are generally believed to be necessary for the maintenance of semiallogeneic pregnancy, where the mother and baby are genetically different. In this situation, maternal immune cell attack on the fetus would be a major risk if countermeasures were not concurrently developed.

Destructive maternal immune responses to paternal antigens expressed by embryonic tissues are extremely limited, a finding that is in itself surprising given basic immunological principles of graft rejection. However, when dissected, it becomes clear that although there are certainly instances of destructive immunity, the targets are invariably cells derived from the inner cell mass rather than the trophoblast layer. Immunogenic, paternally derived antigens on fetal cells derived from the inner cell mass include the rhesus (Rh) antigen on fetal erythrocytes, which can stimulate erythroblastosis, and leukocyte and platelet antigens, which can stimulate severe immune reactions and ultimately loss of the fetus if untreated. By contrast, the trophoblast cell layer that surrounds and encompasses the embryo from the blastocyst stage onwards appears usually not to be the target of cytotoxic immune cells/molecules. Phospholipid antibodies that could interfere with placental structure and/or function via effects on trophoblast cells may be notable exceptions.[31]

The danger theory

Although there are no simple explanations to the question of how tolerance to fetal tissues is generated or maintained, one particularly interesting idea is that the mother senses no danger. This proposal from P Matzinger is termed the 'danger' model of immunity.[32] It suggests that immune responses are not initiated by foreignness of an antigen to the host but rather by the capacity of the foreign antigen to create damage. Presumably, the mother would not view trophoblast cell antigens as dangerous, although danger would most certainly be sensed if the antigens arose from pathogenic microorganisms. One infamous bacterial antigen is lipopolysaccharide (LPS), which stimulates macrophage inflammatory cytokines via binding to an LPS receptor, CD14, thus endangering the delicate cytokine balance in the pregnant uterus.

The placenta as programmer: role of the trophoblast cell

One generally accepted idea is that maternal tolerance is a function of pregnancy-associated changes in the uterine environment. Recently, experimental evidence has accumulated in support of the idea that this critical re-programming is driven by products of the fetal placenta and its associated membranes. The concept that placental trophoblast cells bear the major responsibility for protecting the embryo/fetus from maternal immune rejection due to recognition of 'foreign' paternal antigens on trophoblast cells has taken firm hold.[18,30]

Novel pathways for signaling tolerance to the mother by the placenta and fetal membranes include but are not restricted to:

- directing migration of maternal leukocytes
- controlling trophoblast cell expression of the molecules that normally mediate graft rejection (HLAs)
- expressing high levels of proteins that inhibit antigen presentation (B7) and/or have immunosuppressive properties
- producing molecules that can kill activated lymphocytes (TNF superfamily of ligands)
- displaying proteins that protect against cytotoxic antibodies.

ALTERATIONS IN UTERINE IMMUNE CELL SUBPOPULATIONS DURING NORMAL PREGNANCY

One major strategy for avoiding maternal immune rejection of the fetus is replacement of antigen-specific leukocytes in the uterus with leukocytes of the natural immune system. The pregnant uterus is characterized by high numbers of NK cells and macrophages, and lesser numbers of dendritic cells and regulatory T cells (T_{reg}).[18] Products of the fetus that may influence changes in leukocyte populations and densities include monocyte inflammatory protein-1α (MIP-1α, CCL3), which has been identified as a major product of cytotrophoblast cells capable of attracting monocytes and NK cells into the human uterus[12] and IL-8, which influences neutrophil and other leukocyte populations.[10]

The leukocytes generating natural immunity in pregnancy exhibit functional profiles that differ significantly from those exhibited by the same subsets of leukocytes in the cycling uterus; the cells are environmentally programmed into an anti-inflammatory mode that is consistent with tolerance to fetal antigens.[18,33] Programming events that might be overcome by danger signals such as products of infectious microorganisms are discussed below.

NK cells

NK cells are abundant in the decidua during the first two trimesters of pregnancy, constituting 20–40% of the decidual stromal cells, then declining abruptly in the final trimester.[8,9,34] Human uterine NK cells (uNK) are small cells of the lymphoid lineage that contain distinct granules and express a pattern of cell surface markers, CD56[bright]CD16[−], which distinguishes them from NK cells in the blood, most of which are CD56[dim]CD16[+]. NK cells normally serve an immune surveillance function, killing infected and abnormal cells, but this is not true of uNK cells. Despite having reservoirs of killer molecules such as granzymes and TNF-α in their granules,[35] uNK cells do not kill their normal target cells. The uNK cells are producers of both Th1-type cytokines such as IFN-γ that are associated with inflammation and cell activation, and Th2-type cytokines such as TGF-β that drive the immune system into anti-inflammatory pathways.[36] Although NK cells are known for their surveillance function, recognizing and destroying both infected and aberrant host cells, this appears not to occur in human decidua. Failure to attack is believed to be due to controlled expression of HLA and delivery of inhibitory rather than stimulatory signals to the uNK by migrating cytotrophoblast cells.[37] Despite considerable experimentation, the role(s) these cells play in pregnancy remain unclear.[38,39] Two popular ideas for which experimental support has been developed in the mouse are that the uNK cells participate in modification of maternal vasculature via production of IFN-γ and promote placental growth and development.[40]

Macrophages

In contrast to the fluctuating levels of decidual NK cells, macrophages are a constant feature of the decidua, averaging 15–20% of the human decidual stromal cells.[41–43] These multipurpose cells are frequently located close to invading cytotrophoblast cells, and are adjacent to the uterine glandular epithelium and proximal to uterine blood vessels. They are proposed to be critical to host defense, uterine homeostasis, and local immune modulation.[33,41–45] The human decidual macrophages are activated, as evidenced by their expression of HLA class II, CD11c, and CD86 antigens,[18] and could therefore present microbial or other exogenous antigens to T lymphocytes if such cells were nearby. Yet this avenue to acquired immunity is probably closed; decidual macrophage cytokine profiles indicate that the cells are programmed into an immune suppressive mode, producing powerful immunoinhibitory cytokines such as IL-10 and TGF-β1.[21,46] Decidual macrophages have been reported to express B7-H1,[47] an inhibitory member of the B7 family of costimulatory molecules, as well as ILT3, DC-SIGN, MS-1 and factor 13,[18] all of which are markers associated with immune evasion and activation of macrophages into a suppressive profile.

Dendritic cells

Dendritic cells, a powerful type of antigen presenting cell, are found in small numbers in the decidua.[18,48] These may be either CD83[+] mature dendritic cells, which represent approximately 1% of decidual stromal cells,[49] or CD83[−] immature macrophage/dendritic cells. Mature CD83[+] decidual dendritic cells exhibit an immunosuppressive phenotype.[50] These cells secrete less IL-12, a promoter of T-cell activation, than monocyte-derived dendritic cells, and induce Th2-producing T cells when co-cultured with naïve CD4[+] T cells. Immature (CD83[−]) dendritic cells induce T-cell anergy.

T lymphocytes

T lymphocytes constitute only about 10% of the decidual leukocytes.[18] Of the CD3[+] subpopulation, most are CD8[+], i.e. of the cytotoxic T-cell group, but some are mucosal T cells bearing TcRγ/δ and others are CD4[+] helper T lymphocytes. Among the CD3[+]CD4[+] T cells are regulatory T cells (T_{reg}) exhibiting CD4[+]CD25[+].[51] The cells, whose proliferation is stimulated by estrogen,[52] constitute approximately 14% of CD4[+] cells in early decidua,[51] and so, altogether, constitute only a small fraction of decidual leukocytes. The decidual T_{reg} cells are similar to those in other locations, expressing intracellular cytotoxic T-lymphocyte antigen-4 (CTLA-4), GITR, and OX40, all of which are markers for this subset.[51] T_{reg} cells are powerful negative regulators of immunity. These cells are responsible in large part for maintaining peripheral tolerance when reactive T-cell clones have arisen de novo against self-antigens or have escaped from thymic selection.[53–55] The cells produce both IL-10 and TGF-β1, now identified as two major immunosuppressive cytokines at the maternal–fetal interface.

OTHER CRITICAL IMMUNOLOGICAL FEATURES OF THE MATERNAL–FETAL INTERFACE

A crucial point in considering mechanisms for protection of the fetal semiallograft is that many overlapping strategies are in place. These are most notable in human pregnancies, where a single fetus is the rule.

Restricted HLA

A major, perhaps the major, mechanism of protection of fetal trophoblast cells in the placenta and its membranes is restricted expression of the cell surface antigens that normally stimulate graft rejection, i.e. HLA-A, -B (class Ia antigens), and -D (class II antigens). This subject has been extensively studied and recently reviewed.[19] In brief, trophoblast cells exhibit mainly molecules from the HLA class I gene family that have few alleles, the cells produce both membrane and soluble isoforms of the same molecules, all of which have immunoinhibitory properties, and the trophoblast cells do not express HLA class II antigens. There are exceptions to this, but the outcome of encounters between HLA class I-expressing trophoblast cells and immune cells is redirection of the immune cell functions into immunosuppressive pathways.[19] Interestingly, one major trophoblast cell class Ib antigen, HLA-G, has major deletions and substitutions in its regulatory regions that preclude dramatic enhancement of expression by the usual HLA class I enhancer, IFN-γ, a topic that has been recently reviewed.[19]

Soluble molecules

Well-documented strategies for avoiding graft rejection in pregnancy include production of soluble molecules that have immunosuppressive properties such as steroid hormones, prostaglandins, and cytokines. Pregnancy in mice was first termed a Th2-type phenomenon by Wegmann and coworkers.[56] In the immune system, T lymphocytes can be roughly categorized into cytotoxic T lymphocytes (CTLs) and T helper (Th) cells. Th cells can be further stratified into Th1 cells, which produce inflammatory cytokines, and Th2 cells, which produce anti-inflammatory cytokines and promote B-lymphocyte development. Although appealing in its simplicity, the concept of a Th2 bias in pregnancy is better defined in mice than in women, where many Th1-type cytokines such as IFN-γ and TNF-α have important roles in homeostasis of the pregnant uterus and placenta, as illustrated in a report showing that IFN-γ must be appropriately regulated or preeclampsia ensues.[57]

TGF-β1 is one of the group of anti-inflammatory cytokines that are generally believed to serve as critical countermeasures to graft rejection in pregnancy. In mice, TGF-β1 is delivered in the ejaculate, where it modulates initial maternal responses to implantation;[17] in rats, the cytokine is synthesized in diverse uterine cells;[58] and in women, TGF-β1 is synthesized in placentas[20] and may be produced in uterine macrophages as a consequence of encounter with placental HLA-G5 or HLA-G6, two of the soluble isoforms of HLA-G.[21] TGF-β1, together with IL-10, another powerful lymphocyte inhibiting agent that is produced by uterine NK cells and macrophages,[59] serves to prevent massive infiltration of leukocytes and killer activation of those that are resident in the uterus. In this effort, immunosuppressive cytokines in the uterus are critically aided by progesterone and prostaglandin E_2, both of which are highly immunosuppressive.

Cell surface molecules

Trophoblast cells express several apoptosis-inducing molecules, most of which are members of the TNF superfamily of ligands. These do not harm trophoblast cells, which have effective strategies for protection from their own potentially destructive cytokines but may help defend against activated T lymphocytes with specificity for trophoblast cell antigens. Recent studies have shown that the syncytial trophoblast layer also expresses a molecule, B7H1, that hinders development of cytotoxic lymphocytes.[47] Trophoblast cells protect themselves from attack by cytotoxic maternal antibodies by expressing extraordinarily high densities of three different regulatory proteins that interfere with killing by antibody plus complement.[60] The placenta, in fact, is a source of molecules that promote maternal antibody production by synthesizing B-lymphocyte-supporting, non-apoptosis-inducing molecules of the TNF superfamily of ligands.[61] Thus, antibody production is enhanced, neonatal FcR (Fc receptor) on syncytiotrophoblast transports needed antibody into the fetal blood circulation, and cytotoxic antibodies are turned away by the complement regulatory proteins.

INFLAMMATION IN PREGNANCY

Even though specific conditions in mothers such as high temperatures, a short cervix, and inadequate immune systems may lead to miscarriage, infections are the primary cause. Infections cause heightened inflammation in the pregnant uterus as a consequence of the ability of some organisms to overcome normal maternal–fetal mechanisms for maintaining the pregnant uterus as an immunosuppressive environment.[62–64] As described above, the pregnant uterus is a site where support of embryonic development is preferred to maintenance of host defense. Cells of the innate immune system predominate, and resident as well as incoming hematopoietic cells are programmed for anti-inflammatory rather than inflammatory responses. This contrasts sharply to the cycling uterus where various antimicrobials, including defensins, are abundant.[65] As a result, infections are less vigorously controlled in the pregnant than in the cycling uterus, with infection-associated preterm labor an unfortunate consequence.

Figure 1.1 is taken from an early review by Hunt[62] which proposed that the uteroplacental macrophage, as a site of synthesis of both inflammatory and anti-inflammatory molecules, occupies a central role in infected and normal pregnancies. Much has been learned since this article was published in 1989, including the fact that IFN-γ and LPS have separate and distinct pathways for regulating cytokine production in this lineage. A more contemporary view is shown in Figure 1.2, where a product of the placenta, HLA-G, drives uterine macrophages into an alternative activation pathway where anti-inflammatory cytokines such as TGF-β1 are produced. LPS-carrying bacteria counter and may overcome the signals from the placenta and drive the uterine macrophages into a pathway where production of inflammatory cytokines such as TNF-α is preferred. Thus, the delicately balanced cytokine network that facilitates semiallogeneic pregnancy is constantly at risk.

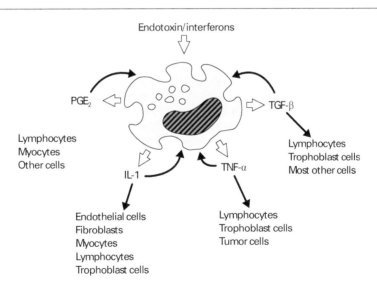

Figure 1.1 A schematic drawing offering the concept that macrophages in the uterus targeted by IFN-γ and/or endotoxin (LPS), produce both inflammatory and anti-inflammatory molecules that have paracrine and autocrine effects. (Redrawn from Hunt.[62])

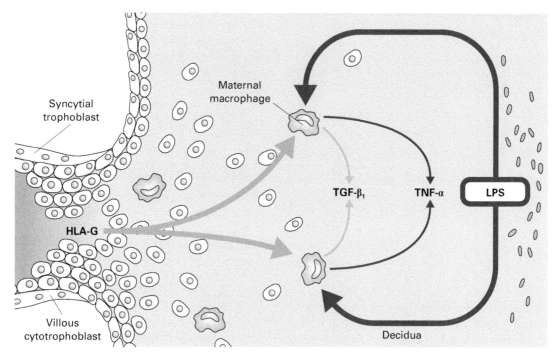

Figure 1.2 A simplified, contemporary view of targeting of uterine macrophages by an immunosuppressive placental product, HLA-G, or an activating product of bacteria, LPS. The former drives production of an anti-inflammatory cytokine, TGF-β1, and the latter drives production of inflammary cytokines such as TNF-α. Not shown are placental products such as progesterone that have anti-inflammatory properties and other conditions of pregnancy such as trauma or viral infections that have inflammatory effects.

Premature rupture of the membranes

Infections may either precede or accompany premature rupture of the membranes. Simhan and Canavan[66] have recently reported that preterm premature rupture of the membranes (pPROM) accounts for one-third of all preterm births and affects 120 000 pregnancies in the United States each year. In their studies, 25–40% of amniotic fluids obtained by transabdominal amniocentesis yielded positive cultures and most of these patients did not give evidence of clinical chorioamnionitis. Bibby and Stewart[67] report that preterm births account for 47% of all neonatal deaths. Gomez et al[68] have suggested that this decision is made by the mother in accordance with pathways initiated in the host and may have survival value. Premature rupture of the membranes (PROM) with chorioamnionitis is also a serious problem. As discussed below, infections are not limited to maternal tissues; the placenta may also be a target.

Causative organisms

Although most bacterial and viral infections cause no damage to the embryo or fetus, some, such as *Rubella*, are notoriously destructive, and a few account for miscarriage. Microorganisms implicated in pregnancy interruption include *Ureaplasma urealyticum*, cytomegalovirus, *Listeria monocytogenes*, parvovirus B19, and the bacterial vaginosis organisms *Gardnerella* and *Mycoplasma*. Organisms causing peridontal disease and high levels of circulating inflammation-associated cytokines have also been implicated in miscarriage.[69] Other organisms arise from the urogenital and gastrointestinal tracts, and many of these abundantly express the dangerous LPS cell wall component.[70]

Mechanisms of damage

The scientific literature contains an abundance of evidence that inflammation overcomes the normal immunological environment of the pregnant uterus. One dramatic change is replacement of the predominant, long-lived innate immune cells with short-lived inflammatory cells, primarily neutrophils, attracted by IL-8. The microorganisms replicate rapidly in the environment of high nutrition, alter the components, and decrease the supply of nutrients to the embryo/fetus.

A second major pathway by which LPS-bearing and other organisms cause damage is via stimulation of resident immune cells, particularly the macrophages, through their specific pattern recognition receptors, the toll-like receptors (TLRs). Although all of the TLRs may be important in the non-pregnant and pregnant female reproductive tract, TLR-4 is of particular interest as it is the recognition structure for LPS and is present only in the cervix, endometrium, and uterine tubes, being absent in vagina and ectocervix.[71] Thus, TLR-4 may play a role in host defense against ascending infections. An unfortunate consequence of TLR-4 activation is that uterine cells are driven away from their normal anti-inflammatory (alternative activation) mode into inflammation-associated pathways. Studies on uterine and placental macrophages as well as trophoblast cells have shown that TLRs able to effect activation are present on these cells.[72–74] Hagberg et al[75] report that the amniotic fluid of 50% of the women with pPROM has elevated IL-6 and IL-8. Early in the investigation of the decidual macrophage, the ability of infections by microorganisms bearing LPS to stimulate production of inflammation-related cytokines such as TNF-α was proposed (see Figure 1.1) and this has turned out to be the case. In chorioamnionitis, for example, TNF-α, as well as IL-6 and IL-8, is highly abundant. Romero et al have carefully charted the appearance of these molecules in maternal blood and amniotic fluid and developed associations among cytokine levels, infection and preterm labor/delivery.[76]

Placental inflammation

Redline has recently reviewed placental inflammation and the damage done by infections.[77] The placenta organ is heavily populated with macrophages, which, early in pregnancy, are called Hofbauer cells. Although the placental macrophages only gradually develop the capability to produce abundant cytokines, the cells express HLA class II antigens during the second trimester[78] and may therefore program T lymphocytes. Term placental macrophages are fully capable of synthesizing inflammatory cytokines such as TNF-α.[79] It has been proposed that TNF-α production by placental macrophages assists in parturition, but infection may accelerate the process. As viewed by Redline, placental inflammation is caused by either microorganisms or by host responses to non-replicating antigens and can cause multiple injuries, including loss of placental function, induction of preterm labor and preterm birth, release of inflammatory mediators that then damage fetal organs, and infections of the fetus itself.[77] Regarding damage to the fetus, IL-18 appears to correlate with brain injury in preterm infants.[70]

POTENTIAL INTERVENTIONS

Overwhelming infections are difficult to control. The most commonly used medications to avoid preterm delivery are antibiotics to inhibit replication of pathogens[76,80] and the corticosteroids, which are capable of programming immune cells. Regarding antibiotics, Kenyon et al[80] have recently reviewed antibiotics for preterm rupture of the membranes, and have concluded that the administration of antibiotics after PROM is associated with a delay in delivery and reduced maternal as well as neonatal morbidity. They advised avoidance of amoxicillin/clavulanate because of the increased risk of neonatal necrotizing enterocolitis.

As for steroidal hormones, some, including estrogens, promote rather than retard inflammation. Estrogens enhance the rate of transcription of the *IFN-γ* gene,[81] a major proinflammatory cytokine. Its functional opposite, progesterone, is the major environmental factor that drives uterine leukocytes in an anti-inflammatory mode. This powerful hormone has many unique characteristics, not the least of which is its ability to mimic the actions of corticosteroids such as dexamethasone,[82] which reduce inflammation. In a manner similar to corticosteroids, progesterone has a calming effect on immune cells, reducing their production of inflammation-associated cytokines and programming the cells into anti-inflammatory pathways. It is therefore not surprising that when additional anti-inflammatory power is needed, physicians employ glucocorticoids and, recently, progesterone itself to rescue pregnancy.

PERSPECTIVES

Preterm birth due to infection and inflammation is widely recognized as a major health problem.[69,77] Much of the damage and loss of life is due to activation of an extensive network of inflammatory cytokines. Temporal patterns of uteroplacental cytokine production have been difficult to map in human pregnancies, but associations of inflammatory cytokines with pregnancy loss is well documented and recent discoveries indicate that allelic differences programming higher or lower responses such as those in the TNF-α alleles could play a role. Efforts are now being made in many departments of obstetrics and gynecology to determine whether a cytokine gene profile might be established that would assist in predicting inflammatory responses in women.

Progress has been made in understanding the underlying causes of interruption of pregnancy, but strategies for preventing and/or controlling undesirable outcomes, although improved in some locales, remain less than satisfactory. This is due in large part to the multiple underlying causes and the difficulties associated with treating various conditions while simultaneously avoiding harm to the embryo/fetus. Therapies targeted to specific conditions, particularly those involved in inflammation such as the TLRs,[70] would clearly be of value.

REFERENCES

1. Jones RK, Bulmer JN, Searle RF. Phenotypic and functional studies of leukocytes in human endometrium and endometriosis. Hum Reprod Update 1998; 4:702–709.
2. Searle RF, Jones RK, Bulmer JN. Phenotypic analysis and proliferative responses of human endometrial granulated lymphocytes during the menstrual cycle. Biol Reprod 1999; 60:871–878.
3. Jeziorska M, Salamonsen LA, Woolley DE. Mast cell and eosinophil distribution and activation in human endometrium throughout the menstrual cycle. Biol Reprod 1995; 53:312–320.
4. Zhang J, Nie G, Jian W, Woolley DE, Salamonsen LA. Mast cell regulation of human endometrial matrix metalloproteinases: a mechanism underlying menstruation. Biol Reprod 1998 59:693–703.
5. Salamonsen LA, Lathbury, LJ. Endometrial leukocytes and menstruation. Hum Reprod Update 2000; 6:16–27.
6. Salamonsen LA, Zhang J, Brasted M. Leukocyte networks and human endometrial remodeling. J Reprod Immunol 2002; 57:95–108.
7. Miller L, Hunt JS. Sex steroid hormones and macrophage function. Life Sci 1996; 59:1–14.
8. Moffett-King A. Natural killer cells and pregnancy. Nat Rev Immunol 2002; 2:656–663.
9. Trundley A, Moffett A. Human uterine leukocytes and pregnancy. Tissue Antigens 2004; 63:1–12.
10. Saito S, Kasahara T, Sakakura S et al. Detection and localization of interleukin-8 mRNA and protein in human placenta and decidual tissues. J Reprod Immunol 1994; 27:161–172.
11. Garcia-Velasco JA, Arici A. Chemokines and human reproduction. Fertil Steril 1999; 71:983–993.
12. Drake PM, Gunn M, Charo IF et al. Human placental cytotrophoblasts attract monocytes and CD56^{bright} natural killer cells via the actions of monocyte inflammatory protein 1α. J Exp Med 2001; 193:1199–1212.
13. Red-Horse K, Drake PM, Gunn MD, Fisher SJ. Chemokine ligand and receptor expression in the pregnant uterus: reciprocal patterns in complementary cell subsets suggest functional roles. Am J Pathol 2001; 159:2199–2213.
14. Kayisli UA, Mahutte NG, Arici A. Uterine chemokines in reproductive physiology and pathology. Am J Reprod Immunol 2002; 47:213–221.
15. Drake PM, Red-Horse K, Fisher SJ. Reciprocal chemokine receptor and ligand expression in the human placenta: implications for cytotrophoblast differentiation. Dev Dyn 2004; 229:877–885.
16. Spencer TE, Bazer FW. Conceptus signals for establishment and maintenance of pregnancy. Reprod Biol Endocrinol 2004; 2:49.
17. Robertson SA, Mau VJ, Hudson SN, Tremellen KP. Cytokine-leukocyte networks and the establishment of pregnancy. Am J Reprod Immunol 1997; 37:438–442.
18. Hunt JS, McIntire RH, Petroff MG. Immunobiology of human pregnancy. In: Knobil and Neill's Physiology of Reproduction. Volume 2. Third edition. (Knobil E, Neill JD, eds). San Diego: Elsevier; 2006: 2759–2785.
19. Hunt JS, Petroff MG, McIntire RH, Ober C. HLA-G and immune tolerance in pregnancy. FASEB J 2005; 19:681–693.
20. Lysiak JJ, Hunt J, Pringle GA, Lala PK. Localization of transforming growth factor β and its natural inhibitor decorin in the human placenta and decidua throughout gestation. Placenta 1995; 16:221–231.
21. McIntire RH, Morales PJ, Petroff MG et al. Recombinant HLA-G5 and -G6 drive U937 myelomonocytic cell production of TGF-β1. J Leukocyte Biol 2005; 76:1220–1228.

22. McMaster MT, Newton RC, Dey SK, Andrews GK. Activation and distribution of inflammatory cells in the mouse uterus during the preimplantation period. J Immunol 1992; 148:1699–1705.

23. Ober C. Studies of HLA, fertility and mate choice in a human isolate. Hum Reprod Update 1999; 5:103–107.

24. Ober C, Karrison T, Odem RR et al. Mononuclear-cell immunisation in prevention of recurrent miscarriages: a randomised trial. Lancet 1999; 354:365–369.

25. Hunt JS, Vassmer D, Ferguson TA, Miller L. Fas ligand is positioned in mouse uterus and placenta to prevent trafficking of activated leukocytes between the mother and the conceptus. J Immunol 1997; 158:4122–4128.

26. Xu C, Mao D, Holers VM et al. A critical role for murine complement receptor crry in fetomaternal tolerance. Science 2000; 287:498–501.

27. Munn DH, Zhou M, Attwood JT et al. Prevention of allogeneic fetal rejection by tryptophan catabolism. Science 1998; 281:1191–1193.

28. Baban B, Chandler P, McCool D et al. Indoleamine 2,3-dioxygenase expression is restricted to fetal trophoblast giant cells during murine gestation and is maternal genome specific. J Reprod Immunol 2004; 61:67–77.

29. Ober C, Aldrich C, Rosinsky B et al. HLA-G1 protein expression is not essential for fetal survival. Placenta 1998; 19:127–132.

30. Kammerer U, von Wolff M, Markert UR. Immunology of human endometrium. Immunobiol 2004; 209:569–574.

31. Rai R, Regan L. Antiphospholipid antibodies, infertility and recurrent miscarriage. Curr Opin Obstet Gynecol 1997; 9:279–282.

32. Matzinger P. Tolerance, danger, and the extended family. Annu Rev Immunol 1994; 12:991–1045.

33. Hunt JS, Robertson SA. Uterine macrophages and environmental programming for pregnancy success. J Reprod Immunol 1996; 32:1–25.

34. Starkey PM, Sargent IL, Redman CW. Cell populations in human early pregnancy decidua: characterization and isolation of large granular lymphocytes by flow cytometry. Immunology 1988; 65:129–134.

35. Parr EL, Chen H-L, Parr MB, Hunt JS. Synthesis and granular localization of tumor necrosis factor-alpha in activated NK cells in the pregnant mouse uterus. J Reprod Immunol 1995; 28:31–40.

36. Eriksson M, Meadows SK, Wira CR, Sentman CL. Unique phenotype of human uterine NK cells and their regulation by TGF-β. J Leukoc Biol 2004; 76:667–675.

37. King A, Allan DS, Bowen M, Powis SJ. HLA-E is expressed on trophoblast and interacts with CD94/NKG2 receptors on decidual NK cells. Eur J Immunol 2000; 30:1623–1631.

38. Croy BA, He H, Esadeg S, et al. Uterine natural killer cells: insights into their cellular and molecular biology from mouse modeling. Reproduction 2003; 126:149–160.

39. Bulmer JN, Lash GE. Human uterine natural killer cells: a reappraisal. Mol Immunol 2005; 42:511–521.

40. Ashkar AA, Di Santo JP, Croy BA. Interferon γ contributes to initiation of uterine vascular modification, decidual integrity, and uterine natural killer cell maturation during normal murine pregnancy. J Exp Med 2000; 192:259–269.

41. Bulmer JN, Pace D, Ritson A. Immunoregulatory cells in human decidua: morphology, immunohistochemistry and function. Reprod Nutr Dev 1988; 28:1599–1613.

42. Hunt JS. Current topic: the role of macrophages in the uterine response to pregnancy. Placenta 1990; 11:467–475.

43. Vince GS, Starkey PM, Jackson MC, Sargent IL. Flow cytometric characterisation of cell populations in human pregnancy decidua and isolation of decidual macrophages. J Immunol Methods 1990; 132:181–189.

44. Hunt JS. Immunologically relevant cells in the uterus. Biol Reprod 1994; 50:461–466.

45. Hunt JS, Petroff MG, Burnett TG. Uterine leukocytes: key players in pregnancy. Semin Cell Dev Biol 2000; 11:127–137.

46. Heikkinen J, Mottonen M, Komi J, Alanen A. Phenotypic characterization of human decidual macrophages. Clin Exp Immunol 2003; 131:498–505.

47. Petroff MG, Chen L, Phillips TA, Azzola D. B7 family molecules are favorably positioned at the human maternal–fetal interface. Biol Reprod 2003; 68:1496–1504.

48. Gardner L, Moffett A. Dendritic cells in the human decidua. Biol Reprod 2003; 69:438–446.

49. Kammerer U, Schoppet M, McLellan AD et al. Human decidua contains potent immunostimulatory CD83(+) dendritic cells. Am J Pathol 2000; 157:159–169.

50. Miyazaki S, Tsuda H, Sakai M, Hori S et al. Predominance of Th2-promoting dendritic cells in early human pregnancy decidua. J Leukoc Biol 2003; 74:514–522.

51. Heikkinen J, Mottonen M, Alanen A, Lassila O. Phenotypic characterization of regulatory T cells in the human decidua. Clin Exp Immunol 2004; 136:373–378.

52. Polanczyk MJ, Carson BD, Subramanian S et al. Cutting edge: estrogen drives expansion of the CD4$^+$CD25$^+$ regulatory T cell compartment. J Immunol 2004; 173:2227–2230.

53. Itoh M, Takahashi T, Sakaguchi N et al. Thymus and autoimmunity: production of CD25$^+$CD4$^+$ naturally anergic and suppressive T cells as a key function of the thymus in maintaining immunologic self-tolerance. J Immunol 1999; 162:5317–5326.

54. Sakaguchi S. Regulatory T cells: key controllers of immunologic self-tolerance. Cell 2000; 101:455–458.

55. Read S, Powrie F. CD4 (+) regulatory T cells. Curr Opin Immunol 2001; 13:644–649.

56. Wegmann TG, Lin H, Guilbert L, Mosmann TR. Bidirectional cytokine interactions in the maternal–fetal relationship: is successful pregnancy a Th2 phenomenon? Immunol Today 1993; 14:353–356.

57. Banerjee S, Smallwood A, Moorhead J et al. Placental expression of IFNγ and its receptor IFNγR2 fail to switch from early hypoxic to late normotensive development in preeclampsia. J Clin Endocrinol Metab 2005; 90:944–952.

58. Chen H-L, Yelavarthi KK, Hu X-L, Hunt JS. Identification of transforming growth factor-β1 mRNA in virgin and pregnant rats by in situ hybridization. J Reprod Immunol 1993; 25:221–233.

59. Heikkinen J, Mottonen M, Komi J et al. Phenotypic characterization of human decidual macrophages. Clin Exp Immunol 2003; 131:498.

60. Hsi B-L, Hunt JS, Atkinson JP. Detection of complement regulatory proteins on subpopulations of human trophoblast. J Reprod Immunol 1991; 19:209–223.

61. Phillips TA, Ni J, Hunt JS. Cell-specific expression of B lymphocyte-(APRIL, BLyS) and Th2- (CD30L/CD153) promoting tumor necrosis factor superfamily ligands in human placentas. J Leukocyte Biol 2003; 74:81–87.

62. Hunt JS. Cytokine networks in the uteroplacental unit: macrophages as pivotal regulatory cells. J Reprod Immunol 1989; 16:1–17.

63. Gomez R, Ghezzi F, Romero R et al. Premature labor and intra-amniotic infection. Clinical aspects and role of cytokines in diagnosis and pathophysiology. Clin Perinatol 1995; 22:281–342.

64. Ruiz RJ, Fullerton J, Dudley DJ. The interrelationship of maternal stress, endocrine factors and inflammation on gestational length. Obstet Gynecol Surv 2003; 58:415–428.

65. King AE, Critchley HO, Kelly RW. Innate immune defences in the human endometrium. Reprod Biol Endocrinol 2003; 1:116.

66. Simhan HN, Canavan TP. Preterm premature rupture of membranes: diagnosis, evaluation and management strategies. Br J Obstet Gynaecol 2005; 112(Suppl 1):32–37.

67. Bibby E, Stewart A. The epidemiology of preterm birth. Neuro Endocrinol Lett 2004; 25(Suppl 1):43–47.

68. Gomez R, Romero R, Edwin SS, David C. Pathogenesis of preterm labor and preterm premature rupture of membranes associated with intraamniotic infection. Infect Dis Clin North Am 1997; 11:135–176.

69. Dortbudak O, Eberhardt R, Ulm M, Persson GR. Periodontitis, a marker of risk in pregnancy for preterm birth. J Clin Periodontol 2005; 32:45–52.

70. Peltier MR. Immunology of term and preterm labor. Reprod Biol Endocrinol 2003; 1:122.

71. Fazeli A, Bruce C, Anumba DO. Characterization of Toll-like receptors in the female reproductivce tract in humans. Hum Reprod 2005; 20:1372–1378.

72. Holmlund U, Cebers G, Dahlfors AR et al. Expression and regulation of the pattern recognition receptors Toll-like receptor-2 and Toll-like receptor-4 in the human placenta. Immunology 2002; 107:145–151.

73. Kumazaki K, Nakayama M, Yanagihara I et al. Immunohistochemical distribution of Toll-like receptor 4 in term and preterm human placentas from normal and complicated pregnancy including chorioamnionitis. Hum Pathol 2004; 35:47–54.

74. Abrahams VM, Bole-Aldo P, Kim YM et al. Divergent trophoblast responses to bacterial products mediated by TLRs. J Immunol 2004; 173:4286–4296.

75. Hagberg H, Mallard C, Jacobsson B. Role of cytokines in preterm labour and brain injury. Br J Obstet Gynaecol 2005; 112(Suppl 1): 16–18.

76. Romero R, Espinoza J, Mazor M. Can endometrial infection/inflammation explain implantation failure, spontaneous abortion, and preterm birth after in vitro fertilization? Fertil Steril 2004; 82:805.

77. Redline RW. Placental inflammation. Semin Neonatol 2004; 9:265–274.

78. Lessin DL, Hunt JS, King CR, Wood GW. Antigen expression by cells near the maternal–fetal interface. Am J Reprod Immunol Microbiol 1988; 16:1–7.

79. Chen H-L, Yang Y, Hu X-L et al. Tumor necrosis factor-alpha mRNA and protein are present in human placental and uterine cells at early and late stages of gestation. Am J Pathol 1991; 139:327–335.

80. Kenyon S, Boulvain, M, Neilson, J. Antibiotics for preterm rupture of the membranes: a systematic review. Obstet Gynecol 2004; 104:1051–1057.

81. Fox HS, Bond BL, Parslow TG. Estrogen regulates the IFN-γ promoter. J Immunol 1991; 146:4362–4367.

82. Miller L, Hunt JS. Regulation of TNF-α production in activated mouse macrophages by progesterone. J Immunol 1998; 160: 5098–5104.

2. Free radicals, oxidative stress, and pregnancy

Lucilla Poston and Maarten Raijmakers

INTRODUCTION

Any book which focuses on inflammation in pregnancy necessarily must include discussion of oxidative stress, since inflammation and oxidative stress are inextricably linked. In common with a heightened inflammatory response, indeed in close association with it, free radicals and oxidative stress are increasingly associated with many of the common complications of pregnancy. A mild state of free radical generation has also been recognized in normal pregnancy where it may have a physiological function. This chapter introduces the reader to the theoretical and practical complexities of oxidative stress and reviews the evidence for altered redox status in normal pregnancy and the potential role of oxidative stress in abnormal pregnancy outcome.

OXIDATIVE STRESS

Oxidative stress is defined as a disturbance in the balance between pro-oxidant synthesis and antioxidant defenses, in which the balance is tipped in favor of pro-oxidants. In biological systems the most common pro-oxidants are free radicals: i.e. molecules with one or more unpaired electrons. These unpaired electrons render the molecules highly reactive and, thereby, are potentially damaging to structure and function on both the cellular and tissue level. Free radical damage is limited by a battery of antioxidant defense molecules that serve to detoxify the radicals.

BIOLOGICAL SOURCES OF FREE RADICALS

The most abundantly synthesized free radical is superoxide ($O_2^{\cdot}$), a very unstable reactive oxygen species (ROS), that is rapidly converted to the less reactive, but more stable, hydrogen peroxide (H_2O_2).

Mitochondria constantly generate ROS as a byproduct of oxidative phosphorylation, since a small percentage of respiratory oxygen (1–3%) escapes as $O_2^{\cdot}$ at complex III (ubiquinol cytochrome C reductase; EC 1.10.22).[1] Mitochondrial uncoupling of oxidative phosphorylation increases $O_2^{\cdot}$ synthesis and has been associated with apoptosis and age-related diseases.[1,2]

Recent research into biological sources of free radicals (Table 2.1) has emphasized the essential role of a family of enzymes, the NAD(P)H oxidases, that are widely expressed. These enzymes are composed of several subunits, with the major and catalytic subunit being the ubiquitously expressed gp91phox.[3,4] NAD(P)H oxidases generate $O_2^{\cdot}$ from NADPH and provide the principal source of $O_2^{\cdot}$ in neutrophils, the vascular endothelium,[5] and placental tissue, as recently shown by assessment of the activity and gene expression.[6,7] Regulation of NAD(P)H oxidase activity is under the influence of both humoral (e.g. angiotensin II, PDGF, cytokines) and hemodynamic factors (e.g. shear stress). Much of the latest research on the NAD(P)H oxidases has been focused upon their activation and potential role in vascular disease, including atherosclerosis and hypertension.[5,8]

A third potentially important source of $O_2^{\cdot}$ is xanthine oxidoreductase (EC 1.2.3.2), which exists in two interconvertible forms: xanthine dehydrogenase (EC 1.1.1.204), which predominates in vivo,

Table 2.1 Intracellular sources of free radicals

Source	Process
Mitochondria	Leakage of superoxide as byproduct of oxidative phosphorylation at complex III
Xanthine oxidase	Metabolism of xanthine to uric acid and superoxide
NAD(P)H oxidase	Conversion of oxygen and NAD(P)H to superoxide

and xanthine oxidase (EC 1.1.3.22). Xanthine oxido-reductase is expressed primarily in the liver and intestine,[9,10] but also in the placenta.[11] The enzyme is the end point of the purine metabolism pathway, converting hypoxanthine to xanthine and xanthine to urate. Normally, the enzyme exists primarily as xanthine dehydrogenase, but ischemia/reperfusion stimulates conversion of the enzyme complex to xanthine oxidase and the metabolism of purines is then coupled to the synthesis of uric acid and $O_2^{\cdot}$.[10,12] Under low oxygen tensions, xanthine oxido-reductase can also act as a source of nitric oxide by reduction of nitrate and nitrite, and can, thereby, through reaction with $O_2^{\cdot}$, form the powerful pro-oxidant peroxynitrite.[10]

ANTIOXIDANT DEFENSES

For ease of description, antioxidant defense mechanisms can be broadly divided into those that are dependent on activity of enzymes (Table 2.2) and those that are non-enzymatic (Table 2.3).

ENZYMATIC PATHWAYS

Quantitatively one of the most influential anti-oxidant pathways is the glutathione-dependent enzyme system.[13,14] Glutathione S-transferases (GSTs) provide defense against many of the breakdown products of oxidative stress (e.g. α,β-unsaturated carbonyls, epoxides, and hydroperox-

Table 2.3 Non-enzymatic antioxidants and their function

Antioxidant	Main function
Water-soluble compounds	
Glutathione	Cofactor for GSH-dependent enzymes
Vitamin C	Reduction of reactive nitrogen species and ROS
	Regeneration of vitamin E
Uric acid	Scavenging of free radicals
	Stabilization of vitamin C
Transferrin/ferritin	Binding of iron
Haptoglobin	Binding of hemoglobin
Lipid-soluble compounds	
Vitamin E	Inhibition of the propagation of lipid peroxidation
Carotenoids	Inhibition of the propagation of lipid peroxidation
	Quenching of singlet oxygen ($^1O_2$)
Ubiquinone	Membrane-associated redox reactions
Bilirubin	Inhibition of the propagation of lipid peroxidation
	Cofactor for UDP glucuronosyl transferase

ides) by the formation of a glutathione conjugate. In man, four main classes of GSTs are expressed,[13] each of which has high substrate specificity and tissue specificity, leading to varying degrees of detoxification capacity in each tissue. Glutathione peroxidases are involved in the first line of defense against ROS.[14,15] These enzymes, generally selenium-dependent, catalyze the reduction of hydrogen peroxide or organic hydrogen peroxides (e.g. lipid peroxides and DNA peroxides) into their

Table 2.2 Localization and function of enzymatic antioxidants

Enzyme system	Main localization	Function
Glutathione S-transferase	Liver (GSTα)	Reduction of organic hydroperoxides
	Placenta (GSTπ/ GSTµ)	Conjugation of oxidative breakdown products to glutathione
Glutathione peroxidase	Intracellular/cytosol (GPX-1)	Reduction of organic hydroperoxides
	Gastrointestinal (GPX-2)	Reduction of H_2O_2 to H_2O
	Extracellular/plasma (GPX-3)	
Superoxide dismutase	Cytoplasm (CuZnSOD, SOD1)	Conversion of superoxide to H_2O_2
	Mitochondria (MnSOD, SOD2)	
	Extracellular (SOD3)	
Catalase	Peroxisomal matrix	Reduction of hydrogen peroxide to H_2O and O_2
Thioredoxin/thioredoxin reductase	Intracellular	Regeneration of antioxidants

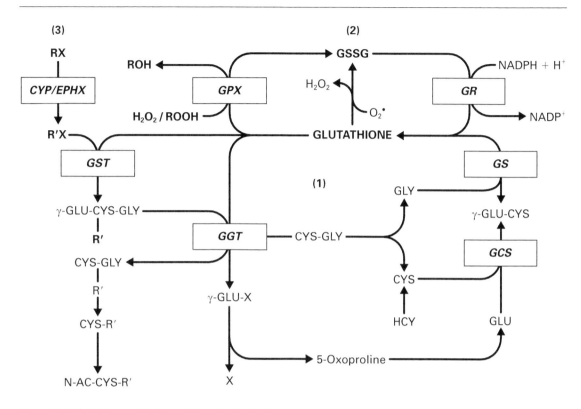

Figure 2.1 Glutathione metabolism and its antioxidant actions:
(**1**) The γ-glutamyl cycle; (**2**) the reduction of peroxides by glutatione peroxidase; and (**3**) the biotransformation pathway.

(**1**) In the γ-glutamyl cycle, glutathione is synthesized by the consecutive coupling of glutamate (GLU), cysteine (CYS), and glycine (GLY) in two steps catalyzed by γ-glutamylcysteine synthetase (GCS) and glutathione synthase (GS), respectively. Glutathione breakdown and transmembrane transfer is initiated by the cleavage of the γ-bond between cysteine and glutamate by γ-glutamyltranspeptidase (GGT). After cleavage, cysteinylglycine (CYS-GLY) is recycled. Homocysteine (HCY) is a potential source of cysteine for these reactions.

(**2**) In the defense against oxidative stress, glutathione (GSH) reduces hydrogen peroxide (H_2O_2) and organic hydroperoxides (ROOH) into H_2O or corresponding alcohols (ROH) by either direct oxidation of glutathione (GSH) or glutathione peroxidase (GPX), resulting in the formation of glutathione disulfide (GSSG). GSSG is quickly reduced to glutathione by glutathione reductase (GR), thereby consuming nicotinamide adenine dinucleotide phosphate (NADPH). The superoxide anion ($O_2^{\bullet}$) may be converted to H_2O_2 by direct oxidation of GSH.

(**3**) In phase I, the toxic compounds (RX) are activated by enzymes such as those of the cytochrome P450 mono-oxygenase (CYP) family and epoxide hydrolase (EPHX). In phase II, glutathione (γ-GLU-CYS-GLY) may be conjugated to both toxic compounds (RX/R′X) and amino acids by enzymes of the glutathione S-transferase (GST) family, thereby facilitating amino acid transport. The glutathione conjugates (GSR′) are less biologically active and more hydrophilic, thereby facilitating excretion via urine or bile, often referred to as phase III.

corresponding alcohols or to water by simultaneous oxidation of glutathione (GSH) into glutathione disulfide (GSSG; Figure 2.1). Availability of GSH is critical to the efficacy of this antioxidant pathway and glutathione reductase is therefore a crucial enzyme in this process as it catalyzes the reduction of GSSG back to GSH. Selenium, although widely but mistakenly considered to be an antioxidant, is only indirectly involved in antioxidant defense, but as a very important cofactor. Selenium deficiency, through impairment of activity of the glutathione peroxidases, can severely compromise the antioxidant defense strategy and thereby lead to oxidative stress.

Glutathione is one of a group of amino thiols that all contain the reactive –SH moiety, which is important in the above-mentioned enzyme system. The metabolism of homocysteine and cysteine are closely related to glutathione and should be included in the discussion of GSH. Cysteine is important in GSH synthesis and has a key role in redox signaling, and homocysteine plays an important role in the maintenance of cysteine in the reduced state.[16,17] The –SH group confers potent antioxidant properties on the amino thiols, making them primary regulators of the intracellular redox balance.[16–18] The reduced, oxidized, and protein-bound forms of the amino thiols exist in a dynamic equilibrium or 'redox thiol balance', which is tightly controlled and the free:oxidized ratio of thiols thus provides a sensitive estimate of cellular oxidative stress. Amino thiols may also react with nitric oxide-derived species to form S-nitrosothiols, which are potent vasodilators, acting through the guanylate cyclase pathway.[19]

In concordance with the GSH-dependent enzyme systems, other enzymes, unrelated to glutathione, provide further protection against oxidative stress: of these, superoxide dismutases, which convert $O_2^{\cdot}$ to hydrogen peroxide, are widely distributed. Three structurally different enzymes that are highly compartmentalized are described:

- CuZnSOD (SOD1) is the cytoplasmic form
- MnSOD (SOD 2) is confined to mitochondria
- extracellular SOD (SOD3) is, as the name suggests, only found in the extracellular compartment.[20]

Catalase on the other hand, which is mainly associated with the peroxisomal matrix and the inner mitochondrial membrane works cooperatively with GPX to eliminate H_2O_2,[21] Another enzyme, thioredoxin reductase (EC 1.8.1.9)[22] plays an important role in the regeneration of antioxidants such as ascorbic acid, glutathione, and ubiquinone, and in the activation of redox-sensitive transcription factors, which in turn may lead to up-regulation of antioxidant defense genes.[23]

NON-ENZYMATIC ANTIOXIDANTS

Non-enzymatic antioxidants can be broadly grouped into lipid- or water-soluble molecules. The principal lipid-soluble antioxidants are the tocopherols, more widely known as vitamin E, of which α-tocopherol predominates in man. All tocopherols inhibit the propagation step of lipid peroxidation, which is initiated by free radical attack of the cellular lipid structure. This may lead to a vicious cycle of peroxidation within the fatty acids of the cell membrane.[24,25] The carotenoids, a large family of lipid-soluble compounds that includes the precursor of vitamin A, exert antioxidant properties by two mechanisms: first, analogous to the tocopherols, they interrupt lipid peroxidation by quenching peroxyl radicals; secondly, they may also quench the reactive form of singlet oxygen.[26] Ubiquinone, a quinone derivative, also acts as an antioxidant in its reduced form, either by reducing α-tocopherol radicals (oxidized vitamin E) or directly on peroxyl radicals.[27,28] Bilirubin is also a lipid-soluble chain-breaking antioxidant scavenger of ROS. In fact, it has greater antioxidant capacity than α-tocopherol and ascorbic acid, and is the most potent chain-breaking antioxidant.[24,29]

Of the water-soluble antioxidants, ascorbic acid (vitamin C) provides an immediate defense against increased free radical synthesis. Ascorbic acid reduces ROS and reactive nitrogen species and acts synergistically with α-tocopherol by reducing the α-tocopherol radical to its antioxidant form.[23,30] In its antioxidant action, ascorbate is converted to dehydroascorbate, which is rapidly reduced to the active antioxidant form by reducing molecules such as thioredoxin and glutathione. Uric acid, the end product of oxidative purine metabolism through the action of xanthine oxidase, exhibits strong antioxidant properties against water, but not lipid-soluble free radicals, and plays an important role in the stabilization of ascorbic acid. However, it also forms potent radicals when oxidized.[31] Transferrin and ferritin, as well as heme-binding proteins (e.g. haptoglobin), indirectly act as antioxidants by chelating transition metals, particularly iron, and preventing oxidative processes initiated by these metals.[24,32]

ASSESSMENT OF OXIDATIVE STRESS

The complexities of the pro-oxidant and anti-oxidant pathways, as outlined above, illustrate the wide range of molecules that provide measurable indices of redox status (Table 2.4). The preferable approach to assess oxidative stress would be the determination of a simple and inexpensive bio-marker that combines the two arms of the oxidative stress balance, i.e. pro-oxidant and antioxidant status. Unfortunately, at the moment there is no simple 'gold standard' measure, because most biochemical assays provide an estimate of only one arm of the equation.

MARKERS OF ANTIOXIDANT DEFENSE

It would be anticipated that an increase in ROS should lead to depletion of antioxidants. Assays are available for assessment of 'total' antioxidant status; these include measurement of oxygen radical absorbance capacity (ORAC) and ferric reducing ability of plasma (FRAP),[33–35] but the latter is not all encompassing, as it does not include amino thiols.[34] Alternatively, concentrations or activity of indi-vidual antioxidants are assessed.[14,24,36,37] These can provide useful information, but may also be misleading. One antioxidant may not represent the status of all, and episodes of oxidative stress can lead to a compensatory up-regulation of enzymatic antioxidants.

ESTIMATE OF ROS SYNTHESIS

Electron spin trapping methods are available for the detection of superoxide or other free radicals. Although these are technically difficult and require specialist equipment,[38,39] they provide information on in-vivo intracellelar free radical synthesis. On the other hand, the increasingly employed assessment of superoxide generation by xanthine oxidase and NAD(P)H oxidase enzyme activity assays in blood or tissue are simpler,[5,7,40] but are not always representative of the in-vivo situation.

PRODUCTS OF OXIDATIVE MODIFICATION

Oxidative modification of lipids and proteins leads to the production of stable molecules that are amenable to measurement in plasma and tissue. As these are derived from free radical attack, they provide an alternative and generally more robust method of estimation of free radical generation. Relevant markers include products of oxidative

Table 2.4 The pros and cons of oxidative stress assessments

Assay	Pros	Cons
Redox status		
Free:oxidized ratio of thiols	Includes both arms of the oxidative stress balance	Not generally available
Free radical generation		
Spin trapping	Good representation of in-vivo situation	Technically difficult and needs specialized equipment
Xanthine oxidase activity	Simple	Only estimate of in-vitro capacity
NAD(P)H activity	Simple	Only estimate of in-vitro capacity
Oxidative damage		
Malondialdehyde (MDA)	Robust, simple method	MDA may be synthesized after sampling
F_2 isoprostanes	Very stable product	Antibodies
Antioxidants		
FRAP	Simple, inexpensive	Does not include –SH-containing moieties
Antioxidant enzymes		Up-regulated as response to increased free radical generation
Non-enzymatic enzymes	Concentrations directly influenced by free radicals	One does not reflect all

damage to lipids (e.g. conjugated dienes, malondi-aldehyde (MDA), and isoprostanes),[1,41,42] proteins (e.g. carbonyls, nitrotryosine residues),[43–46] and DNA (8-hydroxydeoxyguanosine).[47,48] However, there are methodological problems with some; e.g. MDA can also be formed by enzymatic pathways and some of the antibodies developed to members of the iso-prostane family lack specificity. In addition, most of the oxidative markers may originate from in-vitro synthesis after sampling, during storage, or in the reaction tube. Of all the assays available, MDA esti-mation is the most commonly employed, whereas the technically more demanding evaluation of isoprostanes by gas–liquid chromatography–mass spectrometry, particularly 8-iso prostaglandin $F_{2\alpha}$ ($PGF_{2\alpha}$), is likely to provide the most reliable estimate of lipid peroxidation status.

FREE RADICALS AND OXIDATIVE STRESS IN PREGNANCY

NORMAL PREGNANCY

THE PLACENTA

We have recently reported that the early human pla-centa (11–14 weeks' gestation) produces $O_2^{\cdot}$ from NAD(P)H oxidase, raising the question of a possi-ble role in normal trophoblast differentiation and proliferation.[49] Indeed Manes previously suggested that NAD(P)H oxidase could act as an 'oxygen sensor', regulating differentation from cytotro-phoblast to syncytiotrophoblast when oxygen tension increases.[6] This is a plausible, though not-proven hypothesis, as certain growth and angiogenic fac-tors are amongst those known to be redox sensi-tive.[50] Recently, gene transcription of the vascular endothelial growth factor-A, highly expressed in the placenta, was shown to be regulated by oxidative stress and the responsive site on the promoter region has been characterized.[51] Matrix metallopro-teinases (MMPs), which play an important role in cellular matrix remodeling, are also redox sensitive. Thus up-regulation of expression and/or activation of NAD(P)H oxidase could potentially play a role

in placental angiogenesis and spiral artery remodel-ing. Failure of this placentation process, or impair-ment of it, is associated with miscarriage, intrauterine growth restriction and pre-eclampsia.

Indirect evidence for this hypothesis was pro-vided by an elegant investigation in which an oxygen-sensitive probe was used to investigate the pO_2 profile throughout the placenta in the early weeks of gestation in women whose pregnancies were to be terminated.[52] This experiment showed a rapid rise in placental oxygen tension between 10 and 13 weeks' gestation, the period in which it is believed that the maternal perfusion of the placen-tal villi is slowly established when the trophoblast 'plugs' occluding the tips of the uteroplacental spiral arteries become dislodged. It would seem that the presence of highly oxygenated maternal blood represents an oxidant stress, but from the measurement of the antioxidant defense pathways it appears that the early placenta is capable of mounting a substantive defense as SOD, catalase, and GPX showed increased expression. However, it is hypothesized that a sudden or too early perfusion of the placenta in these stages of pregnancy could play a role in the above-mentioned complications of pregnancy.[52]

Alternatively, synthesis of free radicals early in pregnancy could simply represent a biological 'nuisance'. Recent studies have suggested that the early embryo is well protected against oxidative stress.[53–55] Evaluation of the concentration of antioxidants in fluid from the extraembryonic coelom (ECC) has shown high concentrations of the antioxidants taurine and vitamins A and E at 5 weeks' gestation.[55] In another study, the same group of investigators have shown a gestationally related increase in expression of catalase, CuZnSOD, and MnSOD in placental villi in early pregnancy. In addition, we and others have shown the presence of GST enzyme activity and the expression of GTSπ, GSTμ, glutathione, and cysteine in early-pregnancy placenta.[54,56] Antioxidant defenses are also active in late gestation.[57,58] Interestingly, regional antioxidant enzyme expression in term human placenta is highest around the central cavity of the cotyledon, where oxygen tension is greatest.[58]

Other clinicians have found evidence of oxidative damage, as assessed by MDA in the normal placenta, which declined with gestational age.[59] There are several reports of other markers of oxidative stress in term placentas after delivery,[57,60] but, on the other hand, also ample evidence exist for the presence of antioxidant defenses, including glutathione-related enzymes,[61,62] SOD,[59,63] catalase,[59] glutathione,[57,59,61] cysteine,[57] ascorbic acid,[59] and α-tocopherol.[59] These may play a role in protecting the fetus from toxic substances from the outside world during pregnancy and from the damaging consequences of ischemia/reperfusion, which is a likely accompaniment to uterine contractions during delivery.

THE MATERNAL CIRCULATION

It appears that normal pregnancy is a state of mild oxidative stress, although it is not known whether this has any physiological relevance. The rise in maternal free radicals in normal pregnancy is likely to be partly of placental origin (as described above), although the short half-life of ROS would necessarily implicate local effects on maternal blood lipids and proteins during placental perfusion, or indirect effects on maternal tissue through secondary mediators. Moreover, normal pregnancy is recognized to be an inflammatory state in which activation of leukocytes and associated enhanced ROS synthesis has been described.[64–66] Leukocytes are thus likely to be an important source.

Several authors have documented higher concentrations of markers of lipid peroxidation in the maternal circulation of normal pregnant women compared with the non-pregnant state,[67] suggesting an increase in free radical synthesis, although reports are not entirely consistent.[68–71] On the other hand, SOD activity[68] and concentrations of some non-enzymatic antioxidants are reported to be higher than in the non-pregnant state.[72] There are also reports of gestational profiles of lipid peroxidation products, of which one study has shown elevation of the concentrations of conjugated dienes peaking in the second trimester and falling thereafter.[73] Although there is no obvious gestational

trend for the isoprostane 8-iso-prostaglandin $F_{2\alpha}$,[74] it is, nonetheless, of a higher concentration in pregnancy than in the non-pregnant state.[75] A similar phenomenon had been found for antioxidant capacity. α-Tocopherol and the activity of GPX-3 increase throughout gestation,[73] as does SOD activity[68] and uric acid,[74] which together suggest a profile of antioxidant activity increasing in response to a free radical load. However, concentrations of ascorbic acid, generally lower than in the non-pregnant state and probably due to hemodilution or increased usage, do not rise with gestation.[74] After pregnancy, products of oxidative damage and antioxidant (e.g. α-tocopherol) levels both return to preconceptional values, showing that the move towards a state of mild oxidative stress during normal pregnancy is reversible and of a transient nature.[67]

In summary, there is evidence of enhanced free radical generation in normal pregnancy, both in the placenta and in the maternal circulation, that is obviously counterbalanced through stimulation of antioxidant pathways, resulting in an increased antioxidant capacity. Whether the generation of free radicals and products of free radical attack serve any biological role, possibly through activation of redox-sensitive genes, or whether the resultant mild oxidative stress is a byproduct of other essential pathways of metabolism and is of little physiological relevance, remains to be established.

DEVELOPMENT OF ANTIOXIDANT DEFENSES IN THE FETUS

Enzymatic mechanisms dealing with ROS, including glutathione-related enzymes, have been found in fetal tissues, including the liver, spleen, kidney, and lungs,[54,56] and, in common with placental and maternal tissues, the overall antioxidant enzymatic capacity seems to increase with gestational age. Glutathione and cysteine are also present in embryonic and early fetal tissues.[54] Umbilical cord blood contains higher enzyme activity of catalase, SOD, GPX, and GSTα[76–79] and higher concentration of urate, bilirubin, thiols, and vitamin C[80–84] compared with maternal levels, which is indicative of a highly developed antioxidant capacity. Moreover, plasma concentrations of GPX and α-tocopherol have been positively associated with birth weight.[85]

OXIDATIVE STRESS AND MISCARRIAGE

There is increasing interest in the proposal that some miscarriages may arise as a result of oxidative damage to the placenta. In an ultrasound investigation of early pregnancy in normal gestation and in women with missed miscarriage, Jauniaux and colleagues reported precocious onset of intervillous blood flow in the miscarriage group.[86] In normal pregnancy early flow was restricted to the periphery, but in missed miscarriage it was also common in the central regions of the placenta. As might be anticipated from the increased blood flow and the greater oxygen tension in the miscarriage group, samples of placenta demonstrated increased expression of two markers of oxidative stress – heat shock protein 70 and nitrotryrosine residues – as compared with placentas from normal pregnancies obtained at termination.[86] There was also evidence for oxidant stress in the peripheral tissue from normal pregnancies and the authors proposed that this may play a physiological role by inducing local tissue damage and regression of the villi, favoring formation of the chorion laeve. Although this study offers probably the most direct evidence for oxidative stress in miscarriage, other studies are also supportive. Vural et al investigated the antioxidant capacity in blood from women with recurrent early pregnancy loss and found that plasma concentrations of ascorbic acid, α-tocopherol, total thiols, and erythrocyte GSH were lower than in normal pregnancies.[87] Another report documented selenium deficiency in women with recurrent miscarriage, as assessed by determination of the selenium content of hair samples.[88] A further investigation by Sugino et al determined the MDA and $PGF_{2\alpha}$ content of decidual tissue from women who presented with a missed miscarriage and those with spontaneous vaginal abortion with bleeding, and reported high levels of both in samples from women who presented with bleeding.[89] However, decidua from those with a missed miscarriage showed no differ-

ences from normal tissue obtained from terminations. This does not entirely accord with the study of Jauniaux et al, but conditions of collection, tissue investigated, and estimation of oxidant stress were very different. Sugino et al also presented evidence for enhanced MnSOD activity and expression in the tissues from the spontaneous vaginal abortions, which may reflect a response to oxidant stress. However, activity of CuZnSOD was significantly reduced. It was concluded that oxidative stress is likely to play a role in uterine contractions associated with complete abortion, which may arise from free radical-induced stimulation of $PGF_{2\alpha}$.

OXIDATIVE STRESS AND PRE-ECLAMPSIA

A substantial weight of evidence supports a role for oxidative stress in pre-eclampsia. Oxidative damage has been implicated even at the earliest stages of pre-eclamptic pregnancies and it is now widely considered to play an important etiological role in this syndrome.

EARLY PREGNANCY

Arguably, the most important event during normal placental development is establishment of effective maternal perfusion of the placenta, achieved by the physiological conversion of the spiral arteries from highly tortuous and thick-walled vessels to flaccid sinusoidal conduits of low resistance.[90] Partial failure of the normal process of placentation, leading to only moderate remodeling of the spiral arteries and thereby to maintenance of a high resistance circulation, is a characteristic of pre-eclamptic pregnancies[91] and occurs in association with poor invasion of the vessels by the placental trophoblast.[52] As described above, in normal pregnancy, onset of placental perfusion by maternal blood occurs generally at around 10–12 weeks of gestation.[52] As proposed for miscarriage, but presumably with less immediately devastating consequences, premature perfusion of the placenta with maternal blood, or failure of the antioxidant defenses to offset the potentially damaging oxidant processes incurred at the onset of maternal blood flow, could impact upon successful trophoblast invasion. This would lead to sustained underperfusion of the placenta and so contribute to eventual development of pre-eclampsia. Indeed, a recent in-vitro study has shown that lipid peroxidation products reduce trophoblast invasion.[92] Purified extravillous cytotrophoblasts from chorionic villi of human first trimester placenta were cultured on an artificial matrix. Oxidized low-density lipoprotein (LDL) cholesterol, but not native LDL, was found to inhibit cell invasion into the gel in a concentration-dependent manner.

THE PLACENTA AS A SOURCE OF FREE RADICALS IN PRE-ECLAMPSIA

The placenta can be assumed to be an important, potentially the primary, site of free radical synthesis in pre-eclampsia, and this supposition led to a search for the biological stimulus/stimuli and pathways of synthesis. Several convincing sources of ROS are proposed. First, maintenance of the muscular coat of the maternal spiral arteries due to partial failure to remodel may lead to intermittent placental perfusion, since these vessels would inappropriately maintain the ability to constrict and relax to maternal humoral and neuronal stimuli.[93] The pre-eclamptic placenta is also prone to microthrombus formation, and frequent thrombus formation followed by clot dissolution could also lead to repeated hypoxia followed by reoxygenation. As described above, hypoxia/reoxygenation is a potent stimulus to the activation of xanthine oxidase, an enzyme abundantly expressed in cytotrophoblast, syncytiotrophoblast, and villous stromal cells.[12] Indeed placentas from women with pre-eclampsia demonstrate enhanced expression of this enzyme and it can be concluded that xanthine oxidase is an important source of placental ROS. Also an in-vitro study by Hung et al has shown without doubt that hypoxia/reperfusion enhances ROS synthesis in normal placental tissue and stimulates synthesis of biomarkers of oxidative stress.[94] The authors also showed that hypoxia/reperfusion activated pathways of apoptosis, and this is supportive of the hypothesis that apoptotic processes

lead to shedding of the placental trophoblast microparticles, which are then detectable in the maternal circulation, and which have been implicated frequently in the etiology of the maternal syndrome.[65]

The NAD(P)H oxidases must also be considered as good candidates for a source of placental ROS, particularly since known stimuli for activation of these enzymes are associated with pre-eclampsia. These include raised vascular shear stress, which is bound to occur if fetoplacental vascular resistance increases, as often happens in severe early-onset disease. The raised maternal concentrations of cytokines[65] could also influence trophoblast NAD(P)H oxidase expression and activation during the passage of maternal blood through the placental intervillous spaces. The recent demonstration by Dechend et al of enhanced NAD(P)H oxidase subunit expression in pre-eclampsia was therefore an important landmark study.[95] These authors showed a significantly enhanced expression of the p22phox, p47phox, and p67phox subunits in both trophoblast and placental vascular smooth muscle of pre-eclamptic versus control pregnancies, resulting in increased NAD(P)H oxidase activity.[95] A novel mechanism of activation has also been proposed; serum from women with pre-eclampsia has recently been shown to have a high concentration of an autoantibody to the angiotensin II receptor type 1, which upon binding to the receptor leads to activation of NAD(P)H oxidase,[96,97] thus mimicking the binding of angiotensin II. Dechend et al also reported that both angiotensin II and the autoantibody led to induction of NAD(P)H oxidase-mediated $O_2^{\cdot}$ generation, and that this activation was prevented by pre-treatment with sense but not antisense oligonucleotides against p22phox. Furthermore, both agonists led to increased expression of several NAD(P)H oxidase subunits,[95] thereby suggesting that NAD(P)H oxidases may provide a potent source of free radicals in the pre-eclamptic placenta.

Numerous authors have reported markers of oxidative stress in placentas from pre-eclamptic pregnancies. Increased concentrations in comparison to normal placentas have been reported for the F_2

isoprostanes, nitrotyrosine and 4-hydroxynonenal staining, oxidative protein damage and also in oxidizing potential.[98–101] Others have demonstrated higher than normal in-vitro production and secretion rates of F_2 isoprostanes in pre-eclamptic placentas.[102] Placental antioxidant capacity, evaluated either by measurement of vitamin E concentrations or the expression/activity of antioxidant enzymes, is also often reported to be lower than normal.[98,103] However, the higher concentrations of glutathione and glutathione peroxidase activity[61] and raised activity of catalase recorded in women with severe pre-eclampsia is likely to reflect free radical-mediated up-regulation of the relevant genes. A recent methodologically comprehensive study has convincingly shown placental oxidative stress using a wide range of assays in the same pre-eclamptic placentas.[104]

THE MATERNAL CIRCULATION

Markers of oxidant stress are also widely reported in the maternal circulation. Oxidative stress in the maternal circulation could arise indirectly from placental dysfunction and placental oxidative stress. As mentioned above, free radical-induced damage leading to apoptosis in the placenta has been proposed to cause deportation of placental microparticles, which in turn may activate maternal leukocytes.[105] Additionally, trough local cytokine synthesis maternal neutrophils may become activated by passage through the placenta. Placental release of lipid peroxides and cytokines of both placental and maternal origin may contribute to activation of maternal endothelial cells, subsequent leukocyte activation, and hence to further neutrophil activation. Isolated neutrophils from women with pre-eclampsia do indeed produce more ROS than in normal pregnancy[100] and this could originate from enhanced NAD(P)H oxidase activity.[106] The fatty acid profile in women with pre-eclampsia may also predispose to oxidative stress. Serum free fatty acids, which are prone to lipid peroxidation, are raised in pre-eclampsia.[107] The LDL particles are also smaller and more dense than those of controls and are thereby rendered more prone to oxidation.[108]

A report of raised MDA concentrations in maternal blood was one of the first observations to support a maternal state of oxidative stress,[109] and this was followed by reports of raised concentrations of thiobarbituric reactive substances, conjugate dienes, F_2 isoprostanes, antibodies to oxidized LDL, and protein carbonyls.[75,101] There is also evidence for reduced antioxidant capacity; although the widely ranging methods used have probably contributed to some ambiguity, overall, these results suggest a reduction in antioxidant capacity.[101] Women with pre-eclampsia have lower plasma GSH concentrations and lower GSH:hemoglobin concentrations when compared with control women.[110] Women with pre-eclampsia have also been shown to have lower than normal control values of selenium, when assessed by measurement in toenail clippings.[111] Interestingly, a recent study in selenium-deficient pregnant rats has shown these animals develop hypertension and proteinuria, as well as evidence of oxidative stress as assessed by a range of assays, including MDA and protein carbonyls.[112] Vitamin E concentrations, when corrected for lipid concentrations, generally have shown no consistent difference from controls.[72,74,113–117] In contrast, lower than normal plasma vitamin C concentrations, which even may occur prior to clinical onset of disease, are consistently reported.[75,99,100] A recent study, probably the most comprehensive assessment of oxidative stress yet achieved, measured a wide range of both pro- and antioxidant markers in the same women. Although the authors considered that pre-eclampsia was a mild state of oxidative stress, several of the biomarkers assayed – most notably vitamin C, which was substantially reduced – showed significant differences from normotensive controls.[118]

The maternal condition of pre-eclampsia is defined as an elevation of the blood pressure with significant proteinuria. This both belies the complexity of the syndrome and the multiorgan involvement. It has been proposed that oxidative stress could lead to many of the features of pre-eclampsia, including enhanced coagulation, vasoconstriction and hypertension, increased microvascular permeability, and proteinuria. Oxidative stress may alter vascular function by direct endothelial cell activation and by reducing synthesis and function of nitric oxide (NO), or enhancing constrictor prostaglandin and endothelin production.[119] In particular, lipid peroxides are recognized to lead to endothelial cell activation and to leukocyte adhesion and activation.[120] By reacting with NO, $O_2^{\cdot}$ leads to synthesis of peroxynitrite, which thus reduces NO availability as a relaxant, promotes necrosis and apoptosis, and causes tissue damage through its pro-oxidant activity.[119]

POTENTIAL USE OF ANTIOXIDANTS IN PREVENTION OF PRE-ECLAMPSIA

The evidence for oxidative stress, the proposed role for NAD(P)H oxidase, and the demonstration of an inflammatory state in pre-eclampsia would suggest that antioxidants could be of use in prevention of the disorder. Vitamin E has many properties that may be relevant to the pre-eclamptic state; not only does it detoxify free radicals but it also affects redox-sensitive gene expression,[25] inhibits apoptosis, and has anti-inflammatory properties.[25,121,122] Importantly, vitamin E directly inhibits monocyte NAD(P)H oxidase activity through inhibition of protein kinase C, thereby preventing phosphorylation of the p47phox subunit necessary for activation. Vitamin C would also be an obvious candidate for supplementation as plasma vitamin C levels are uniformly low – even before onset of clinical disease – in pre-eclampsia and it acts synergistically with vitamin E.[123]

In 1942, a study from the People's League of Health reported less albuminuria with hypertension in 1530 primigravidae treated daily from before 24 weeks of pregnancy onwards with a mixture of six supplements, including 100 mg vitamin C, halibut liver oil (vitamins A and D), and vitamin B_1 (200 IU), when compared with a similar number of controls taking no supplements.[124] This was a non-blinded randomized study, but as other supplements (i.e. iron, calcium, and iodine) were used, no specific benefit of antioxidants can be deduced. Two investigations undertaken in women with established severe, early-onset pre-eclampsia later

showed no benefit of vitamin E (100–300 mg/day) in a non-randomized study,[125] or of 1000 mg vitamin C, 800 IU vitamin E, and 200 mg allopurinol per day in a randomized controlled trial.[126] Our group has studied the potential benefit of antioxidants in a randomized controlled trial in women at risk of pre-eclampsia.[127] Risk was assessed on the basis of previous pre-eclampsia or by the presence of a diastolic 'notch' in the uterine artery Doppler waveform. Women were randomized to antioxidants (1000 mg vitamin C and 400 IU vitamin E daily) or placebo from 16 to 22 weeks of gestation. There was a highly significant reduction in pre-eclampsia in the supplemented group, either on the basis of the intention-to-treat cohort or the completed study cohort. The plasma concentrations of vitamin C, which were very low compared with those of normal pregnant women, were normalized in the supplemented group. Although promising, the number of women studied was too small to provide adequate power for evaluation of neonatal outcome measures. Much larger multicenter trials are now underway worldwide to investigate neonatal outcome and the potential benefit in other risk groups, including primiparous women. These clinical trials will not only determine whether antioxidants may be a beneficial prophylactic measure for pre-eclampsia prevention but also offer an excellent opportunity to investigate further the relationship between oxidative stress and the etiology of the disorder.

INTRAUTERINE GROWTH RESTRICTION

The potential role of oxidative stress in intrauterine growth restriction (IUGR) without accompanying pre-eclampsia has received little attention, although there is evidence that thioredoxin concentrations are reduced in affected placentas, which would compromise antioxidant capacity[128] and could lead to placental oxidative stress. One report suggests that women with IUGR pregnancies have lower plasma ascorbic acid concentrations and a trend towards elevation of the isoprostane 8-epi-$PGF_{2\alpha}$.[74] It has been suggested that the difference in lipid profiles between women with pre-eclampsia and those with IUGR pregnancies without pre-eclampsia could be of importance, since IUGR is not associated with a typically proatherogenic, pro-oxidative lipid profile typical of pre-eclampsia.[128] Thus, while women with IUGR pregnancies may certainly be challenged by oxidative stress in a way analogous to those who develop pre-eclampsia, they may not succumb to pre-eclampsia because of the differing lipid profiles, or perhaps because of other underlying conditions which may predispose to oxidant stress and vascular dysfunction (e.g. insulin resistance or diabetes).

PRETERM PREMATURE RUPTURE OF THE MEMBRANES

Premature rupture of the fetal chorioamnion membrane has been linked to oxidative stress.[129] The mechanism is likely to involve redox regulation of the MMPs, as fetal membrane MMP-9 is directly increased by $O_2^{\cdot-}$.[130] Women with preterm premature rupture of the membranes (pPROM) have also been shown to have lower erythrocyte selenium-dependent GPX and SOD activity, and high concentrations of MDA in maternal and umbilical venous blood compared with healthy controls.[131]

CONCLUSIONS

There is widely ranging evidence to support an association of oxidative stress with several of the common abnormalities of pregnancy outcome. There remains, however, little proof that this is causative. The ongoing clinical trials, which at present focus predominantly on pre-eclampsia, should provide evidence for or against an important role of free radicals in this disorder, while simultaneously providing insight into IUGR and pPROM. Studies of antioxidant supplementation in early pregnancy and miscarriage should heed the possibility that moderate synthesis of ROS may play a physiological role in normal early pregnancy, and at least at first, be confined to women with recurrent miscarriage.

REFERENCES

1. Lenaz G, Bovina C, D'Aurelio M et al. Role of mitochondria in oxidative stress and aging. Ann NY Acad Sci 2002; 959:199–213.
2. Chandra J, Samali A, Orrenius S. Triggering and modulation of apoptosis by oxidative stress. Free Radic Biol Med 2000; 29:323–333.
3. Bayraktutan U, Blayney L, Shah AM. Molecular characterization and localization of the NAD(P)H oxidase components gp91-phox and p22-phox in endothelial cells. Arterioscler Thromb Vasc Biol 2000; 20:1903–1911.
4. Li JM, Shah AM. Intracellular localization and preassembly of the NADPH oxidase complex in cultured endothelial cells. J Biol Chem 2002; 277:19952–19960.
5. Griendling KK, Sorescu D, Ushio-Fukai M. NAD(P)H oxidase: role in cardiovascular biology and disease. Circ Res 2000; 86:494–501.
6. Manes C. Human placental NAD(P)H oxidase: solubilization and properties. Placenta 2001; 22:58–63.
7. Raijmakers MT, Peters WH, Steegers EA, Poston L. NAD(P)H oxidase associated superoxide production in human placenta from normotensive and pre-eclamptic women. Placenta 2004; 25S:S85–S89.
8. Rajagopalan S, Kurz S, Munzel T et al. Angiotensin II-mediated hypertension in the rat increases vascular superoxide production via membrane NADH/NADPH oxidase activation. Contribution to alterations of vasomotor tone. J Clin Invest 1996; 97:1916–1923.
9. Pritsos CA. Cellular distribution, metabolism and regulation of the xanthine oxidoreductase enzyme system. Chem Biol Interact 2000; 129:195–208.
10. Harrison R. Structure and function of xanthine oxidoreductase: where are we now? Free Radic Biol Med 2002; 33:774–797.
11. Many A, Westerhausen-Larson A, Kanbour-Shakir A, Roberts JM. Xanthine oxidase/dehydrogenase is present in human placenta. Placenta 1996; 17:361–365.
12. Many A, Hubel CA, Fisher SJ, Roberts JM, Zhou Y. Invasive cytotrophoblasts manifest evidence of oxidative stress in preeclampsia. Am J Pathol 2000; 156:321–331.
13. Hayes JD, Pulford DJ. The glutathione S-transferase supergene family: regulation of GST and the contribution of the isoenzymes to cancer chemoprotection and drug resistance. Crit Rev Biochem Mol Biol 1995; 30:445–600.
14. Hayes JD, McLellan LI. Glutathione and glutathione-dependent enzymes represent a co-ordinately regulated defense against oxidative stress. Free Radic Res 1999; 31:273–300.
15. Arthur JR. The glutathione peroxidases. Cell Mol Life Sci 2000; 57:1825–1835.
16. Ueland PM, Mansoor MA, Guttormsen AB et al. Reduced, oxidized and protein-bound forms of homocysteine and other aminothiols in plasma comprise the redox thiol status – a possible element of the extracellular antioxidant defense system. J Nutr 1996; 126:1281S–1284S.
17. Hogg N. The effect of cyst(e)ine on the auto-oxidation of homocysteine. Free Radic Biol Med 1999; 27:28–33.
18. Sen CK. Redox signaling and the emerging therapeutic potential of thiol antioxidants. Biochem Pharmacol 1998; 55:1747–1758.
19. Padgett CM, Whorton AR. Regulation of cellular thiol redox status by nitric oxide. Cell Biochem Biophys 1995; 27:157–177.
20. Zelko IN, Mariani TJ, Folz RJ. Superoxide dismutase multigene family: a comparison of the CuZn-SOD (SOD1), Mn-SOD (SOD2), and EC-SOD (SOD3) gene structures, evolution, and expression. Free Radic Biol Med 2002; 33:337–349.

21. Mruk DD, Silvestrini B, Mo MY, Cheng CY. Antioxidant superoxide dismutase – a review: its function, regulation in the testis, and role in male fertility. Contraception 2002; 65:305–311.

22. Holmgren A, Bjornstedt M. Thioredoxin and thioredoxin reductase. Methods Enzymol 1995; 252:199–208.

23. Nordberg J, Arner ES. Reactive oxygen species, antioxidants, and the mammalian thioredoxin system. Free Radic Biol Med 2001; 31: 1287–1312.

24. Krinsky NI. Mechanism of action of biological antioxidants. Proc Soc Exp Biol Med 1992; 200:248–254.

25. Brigelius-Flohe R, Kelly FJ, Salonen JT et al. The European perspective on vitamin E: current knowledge and future research. Am J Clin Nutr 2002; 76:703–716.

26. Krinsky NI. The antioxidant and biological properties of the carotenoids. Ann NY Acad Sci 1998; 854:443–447.

27. Nohl H, Gille L, Staniek K. The biochemical, pathophysiological, and medical aspects of ubiquinone function. Ann NY Acad Sci 1998; 854:394–409.

28. Nohl H, Kozlov AV, Staniek K, Gille L. The multiple functions of coenzyme Q. Bioorg Chem 2001; 29:1–13.

29. Tomaro ML, Batlle AM. Bilirubin: its role in cytoprotection against oxidative stress. Int J Biochem Cell Biol 2002; 34:216–220.

30. Wilson JX. The physiological role of dehydroascorbic acid. FEBS Lett 2002; 527:5–9.

31. Sevanian A, Davies KJ, Hochstein P. Serum urate as an antioxidant for ascorbic acid. Am J Clin Nutr 1991; 54:1129S–1134S.

32. Langlois MR, Delanghe JR. Biological and clinical significance of haptoglobin polymorphism in humans. Clin Chem 1996; 42:1589–1600.

33. Benzie IF, Strain JJ. The ferric reducing ability of plasma (FRAP) as a measure of 'antioxidant power': the FRAP assay. Anal Biochem 1996; 239:70–76.

34. Cao G, Prior RL. Comparison of different analytical methods for assessing total antioxidant capacity of human serum. Clin Chem 1998; 44:1309–1315.

35. Rhemrev JP, van Overveld FW, Haenen GR et al. Quantification of the nonenzymatic fast and slow TRAP in a postaddition assay in human seminal plasma and the antioxidant contributions of various seminal compounds. J Androl 2000; 21:913–920.

36. Kamal-Eldin A, Appelqvist LA. The chemistry and antioxidant properties of tocopherols and tocotrienols. Lipids 1996; 31:671–701.

37. Mates JM, Perez-Gomez C, Nunez de Castro I. Antioxidant enzymes and human diseases. Clin Biochem 1999; 32:595–603.

38. Sikkema JM, van Rijn BB, Franx A et al. Placental superoxide is increased in pre-eclampsia. Placenta 2001; 22:304–308.

39. Valgimigli L, Pedulli GF, Paolini M. Measurement of oxidative stress by EPR radical-probe technique. Free Radic Biol Med 2001; 31:708–716.

40. Tarpey MM, White CR, Suarez E et al. Chemiluminescent detection of oxidants in vascular tissue. Lucigenin but not coelenterazine enhances superoxide formation. Circ Res 1999; 84:1203–1211.

41. Conti M, Morand PC, Levillain P, Lemonnier A. Improved fluorometric determination of malonaldehyde. Clin Chem 1991; 37:1273–1275.

42. Cracowski JL, Durand T, Bessard G. Isoprostanes as a biomarker of lipid peroxidation in humans: physiology, pharmacology and clinical implications. Trends Pharmacol Sci 2002; 23:360–366.

43. Levine RL, Williams JA, Stadtman ER, Shacter E. Carbonyl assays for determination of oxidatively modified proteins. Methods Enzymol 1994; 233:346–357.

44. Adams S, Green P, Claxton R et al. Reactive carbonyl formation by oxidative and non-oxidative pathways. Front Biosci 2001; 6:A17–A24.

45. Beal MF. Oxidatively modified proteins in aging and disease. Free Radic Biol Med 2002; 32:797–803.

46. Dalle-Donne I, Rossi R, Giustarini D, Milzani A, Colombo R. Protein carbonyl groups as biomarkers of oxidative stress. Clin Chim Acta 2003; 329:23–38.

47. Takimoto E, Ishida J, Sugiyama F et al. Hypertension induced in pregnant mice by placental renin and maternal angiotensinogen [see comments]. Science 1996; 274:995–998.

48. Hong YC, Lee KH, Yi CH, Ha EH, Christiani DC. Genetic susceptibility of term pregnant women to oxidative damage. Toxicol Lett 2002; 129:255–262.

49. Raijmakers MT, Burton GJ, Jauniaux E et al. Placental NAD(P)H oxidase mediated superoxide generation in early pregnancy. Placenta 2005; 27:158–163.

50. Irani K. Oxidant signaling in vascular cell growth, death, and survival: a review of the roles of reactive oxygen species in smooth muscle and endothelial cell mitogenic and apoptotic signaling. Circ Res 2000; 87:179–183.

51. Schafer G, Cramer T, Suske G et al. Oxidative stress regulates vascular endothelial growth factor-A gene transcription through Sp1- and Sp3-dependent activation of two proximal GC-rich promoter elements. J Biol Chem 2003; 278:8190–8198.

52. Jauniaux E, Watson AL, Hempstock J et al. Onset of maternal arterial blood flow and placental oxidative stress. A possible factor in human early pregnancy failure. Am J Pathol 2000; 157:2111–2122.

53. Van Lieshout EM, Knapen MF, Lange WP, Steegers EA, Peters WH. Localization of glutathione S-transferases alpha and pi in human embryonic tissues at 8 weeks gestational age. Hum Reprod 1998; 13:1380–1386.

54. Raijmakers MT, Steegers EA, Peters WH. Glutathione S-transferases and thiol concentrations in embryonic and early fetal tissues. Hum Reprod 2001; 16:2445–2450.

55. Jauniaux E, Cindrova-Davies T, Johns J et al. Distribution and transfer pathways of antioxidant molecules inside the first trimester human gestational sac. J Clin Endocrinol Metab 2004; 89:1452–1458.

56. Pacifici GM, Franchi M, Colizzi C, Giuliani L, Rane A. Glutathione S-transferase in humans: development and tissue distribution. Arch Toxicol 1988; 61:265–269.

57. Raijmakers MT, Bruggeman SW, Steegers EA, Peters WH. Distribution of components of the glutathione detoxification system across the human placenta after uncomplicated vaginal deliveries. Placenta 2002; 23:490–496.

58. Hempstock J, Bao YP, Bar-Issac M et al. Intralobular differences in antioxidant enzyme expression and activity reflect the pattern of maternal arterial bloodflow within the human placenta. Placenta 2003; 24:517–523.

59. Qanungo S, Sen A, Mukherjea M. Antioxidant status and lipid peroxidation in human feto-placental unit. Clin Chim Acta 1999; 285:1–12.

60. Zusterzeel PL, Rutten H, Roelofs HM, Peters WH, Steegers EA. Protein carbonyls in decidua and placenta of pre-eclamptic women as markers for oxidative stress. Placenta 2001; 22:213–219.

61. Knapen MF, Peters WH, Mulder TP et al. Glutathione and glutathione-related enzymes in decidua and placenta of controls and women with pre-eclampsia. Placenta 1999; 20:541–546.

62. Zusterzeel PL, Peters WH, De Bruyn MA et al. Glutathione S-transferase isoenzymes in decidua and placenta of preeclamptic pregnancies. Obstet Gynecol 1999; 94:1033–1038.

63. Telfer JF, Thomson AJ, Cameron IT, Greer IA, Norman JE. Expression of superoxide dismutase and xanthine oxidase in myometrium, fetal membranes and placenta during normal human pregnancy and parturition. Hum Reprod 1997; 12:2306–2312.

64. Sacks GP, Studena K, Sargent K, Redman CW. Normal pregnancy and preeclampsia both produce inflammatory changes in peripheral blood leukocytes akin to those of sepsis. Am J Obstet Gynecol 1998; 179:80–86.

65. Redman CW, Sacks GP, Sargent IL. Preeclampsia: an excessive maternal inflammatory response to pregnancy. Am J Obstet Gynecol 1999; 180:499–506.

66. Luppi P, Haluszczak C, Trucco M, DeLoia JA. Normal pregnancy is associated with peripheral leukocyte activation. Am J Reprod Immunol 2002; 47:72–81.

67. Little RE, Gladen BC. Levels of lipid peroxides in uncomplicated pregnancy: a review of the literature. Reprod Toxicol 1999; 13: 347–352.

68. Loverro G, Greco P, Capuano F et al. Lipoperoxidation and antioxidant enzymes activity in pregnancy complicated with hypertension. Eur J Obstet Gynecol Reprod Biol 1996; 70:123–127.

69. Gladen BC, Tabacova S, Baird DD, Little RE, Balabaeva L. Variability of lipid hydroperoxides in pregnant and nonpregnant women. Reprod Toxicol 1999; 13:41–44.

70. Kharb S. Total free radical trapping antioxidant potential in preeclampsia. Int J Gynaecol Obstet 2000; 69:23–26.

71. Ilhan N, Ilhan N, Simsek M. The changes of trace elements, malondialdehyde levels and superoxide dismutase activities in pregnancy with or without preeclampsia. Clin Biochem 2002; 35: 393–397.

72. Uotila JT, Kirkkola AL, Rorarius M, Tuimala RJ, Metsa-Ketela T. The total peroxyl radical-trapping ability of plasma and cerebrospinal fluid in normal and preeclamptic parturients. Free Radic Biol Med 1994; 16:581–590.

73. Uotila J, Tuimala R, Aarnio T, Pyykko K, Ahotupa M. Lipid peroxidation products, selenium-dependent glutathione peroxidase and vitamin E in normal pregnancy. Eur J Obstet Gynecol Reprod Biol 1991; 42:95–100.

74. Chappell LC, Seed PT, Briley A et al. A longitudinal study of biochemical variables in women at risk of preeclampsia. Am J Obstet Gynecol 2002; 187:127–136.

75. Hubel CA. Oxidative stress in the pathogenesis of preeclampsia. Proc Soc Exp Biol Med 1999; 222:222–235.

76. Novak Z, Kovacs L, Pal A et al. Comparative study of antioxidant enzymes and lipid peroxidation in cord and maternal red blood cells. Acta Paediatr Hung 1990; 30:391–397.

77. Karsdorp VH, Dekker GA, Bast A et al. Maternal and fetal plasma concentrations of endothelin, lipid hydroperoxides, glutathione peroxidase and fibronectin in relation to abnormal umbilical artery velocimetry. Eur J Obstet Gynecol Reprod Biol 1998; 80:39–44.

78. Knapen MF, van der Wildt B, Sijtsma EG et al. Glutathione S-transferase Alpha 1-1 and aminotransferases in umbilical cord blood. Early Hum Dev 1999; 54:129–135.

79. Mihailovic M, Cvetkovic M, Ljubic A et al. Selenium and malondialdehyde content and glutathione peroxidase activity in maternal and umbilical cord blood and amniotic fluid. Biol Trace Elem Res 2000; 73:47–54.

80. Kiely M, Morrissey PA, Cogan PF, Kearney PJ. Low molecular weight plasma antioxidants and lipid peroxidation in maternal and cord blood. Eur J Clin Nutr 1999; 53:861–864.

81. Kiely M, Cogan PF, Kearney PJ, Morrissey PA. Concentrations of tocopherols and carotenoids in maternal and cord blood plasma. Eur J Clin Nutr 1999; 53:711–715.

82. Raijmakers MT, Roes EM, Steegers EA, van der Wildt B, Peters WH. Thiols in umbilical cord and maternal plasma in normal pregnancy. Clin Chem 2001; 47:749–751.

83. Baydas G, Karatas F, Gursu MF et al. Antioxidant vitamin levels in term and preterm infants and their relation to maternal vitamin status. Arch Med Res 2002; 33:276–280.

84. Raijmakers MT, Roes EM, Steegers EA, van der WB, Peters WH. Umbilical glutathione levels are higher after vaginal birth than after cesarean section. J Perinat Med 2003; 31:520–522.

85. Ripalda MJ, Rudolph N, Wong SL. Developmental patterns of antioxidant defense mechanisms in human erythrocytes. Pediatr Res 1989; 26:366–369.

86. Jauniaux E, Hempstock J, Greenwold N, Burton GJ. Trophoblastic oxidative stress in relation to temporal and regional differences in maternal placental blood flow in normal and abnormal early pregnancies. Am J Pathol 2003; 162:115–125.

87. Vural P, Akgul C, Yildirim A, Canbaz M. Antioxidant defense in recurrent abortion. Clin Chim Acta 2000; 295:169–177.

88. Al Kunani AS, Knight R, Haswell SJ, Thompson JW, Lindow SW. The selenium status of women with a history of recurrent miscarriage. BJOG 2001; 108:1094–1097.

89. Sugino N, Nakata M, Kashida S et al. Decreased superoxide dismutase expression and increased concentrations of lipid peroxide and prostaglandin F(2alpha) in the decidua of failed pregnancy. Mol Hum Reprod 2000; 6:642–647.

90. Pijnenborg R, Anthony J, Davey DA et al. Placental bed spiral arteries in the hypertensive disorders of pregnancy. Br J Obstet Gynaecol 1991; 98:648–655.

91. Brosens IA, Robertson WB, Dixon HG. The role of the spiral arteries in the pathogenesis of preeclampsia. Obstet Gynecol Annu 1972; 1:177–191.

92. Pavan L, Tsatsaris V, Hermouet A et al. Oxidized low-density lipoproteins inhibit trophoblastic cell invasion. J Clin Endocrinol Metab 2004; 89:1969–1972.

93. Burton GJ, Hung TH. Hypoxia-reoxygenation; a potential source of placental oxidatives stress in normal pregnancy and preeclampsia. Fetal Matern Med Rev 2003; 14:97–117.

94. Hung TH, Skepper JN, Charnock-Jones DS, Burton GJ. Hypoxia-reoxygenation: a potent inducer of apoptotic changes in the human placenta and possible etiological factor in preeclampsia. Circ Res 2002; 90:1274–1281.

95. Dechend R, Viedt C, Muller DN et al. AT1 receptor agonistic antibodies from preeclamptic patients stimulate NADPH oxidase. Circulation 2003; 107:1632–1639.

96. Wallukat G, Homuth V, Fischer T et al. Patients with preeclampsia develop agonistic autoantibodies against the angiotensin AT1 receptor. J Clin Invest 1999; 103:945–952.

97. Xia Y, Wen H, Bobst S, Day MC, Kellems RE. Maternal autoantibodies from preeclamptic patients activate angiotensin receptors on human trophoblast cells. J Soc Gynecol Investig 2003; 10:82–93.

98. Walsh SW. Maternal–placental interactions of oxidative stress and antioxidants in preeclampsia. Semin Reprod Endocrinol 1998; 16:93–104.

99. Poston L, Raijmakers MT. Trophoblast oxidative stress, antioxidants and pregnancy outcome. Placenta 2004; S25:S72–S78.

100. Raijmakers MT, Dechend R, Poston L. Oxidative stress and preeclampsia; the rationale for antioxidant clinical trials. Hypertension 2004; 44:1–7.

101. Raijmakers MT, Peters WH, Steegers EA, Poston L. Amino thiols, detoxification and oxidative stress in pre-eclampsia and other disorders of pregnancy. Curr Pharm Des 2005; 11(6):711–734.

102. Walsh SW, Vaughan JE, Wang Y, Roberts LJ. Placental isoprostane is significantly increased in preeclampsia. FASEB J 2000; 14: 1289–1296.

103. Wang Y, Walsh SW. Antioxidant activities and mRNA expression of superoxide dismutase, catalase, and glutathione peroxidase in normal and preeclamptic placentas. J Soc Gynecol Investig 1996; 3: 179–184.

104. Vanderlelie J, Venardos K, Clifton VL et al. Increased biological oxidation and reduced anti-oxidant enzyme activity in pre-eclamptic placentae. Placenta 2005; 26:53–58.

105. Redman CW, Sargent IL. Pre-eclampsia, the placenta and the maternal systemic inflammatory response – a review. Placenta 2003; 24 (Suppl A):S21–S27.

106. Lee VM, Quinn PA, Jennings SC, Ng LL. Neutrophil activation and production of reactive oxygen species in pre-eclampsia. J Hypertens 2003; 21:395–402.

107. Hubel CA, Mclaughlin MK, Evans RW et al. Fasting serum triglycerides, free fatty acids, and malondialdehyde are increased in preeclampsia, are positively correlated, and decrease within 48 hours post partum. Am J Obstet Gynecol 1996; 174:975–982.

108. Hubel CA, Shakir Y, Gallaher MJ, Mclaughlin MK, Roberts JM. Low-density lipoprotein particle size decreases during normal pregnancy in association with triglyceride increases. J Soc Gynecol Investig 1998; 5:244–250.

109. Hubel CA, Roberts JM, Taylor RN et al. Lipid peroxidation in pregnancy: new perspectives on preeclampsia. Am J Obstet Gynecol 1989; 161:1025–1034.

110. Knapen MF, Mulder TP, Van Rooij IA, Peters WH, Steegers EA. Low whole blood glutathione levels in pregnancies complicated by preeclampsia or the hemolysis, elevated liver enzymes, low platelets syndrome. Obstet Gynecol 1998; 92:1012–1015.

111. Rayman MP, Abou-Shakra FR, Ward NI, Redman CW. Comparison of selenium levels in pre-eclamptic and normal pregancies. Biol Trace Elem Res 1996; 55:9–20.

112. Vanderlelie J, Venardos K, Perkins AV. Selenium deficiency as a model of experimental pre-eclampsia in rats. Reproduction 2004; 128:635–641.

113. Schiff E, Friedman SA, Stampfer M et al. Dietary consumption and plasma concentrations of vitamin E in pregnancies complicated by preeclampsia. Am J Obstet Gynecol 1996; 175:1024–1028.

114. Hubel CA, Kagan VE, Kisin ER, Mclaughlin MK, Roberts JM. Increased ascorbate radical formation and ascorbate depletion in plasma from women with preeclampsia: implications for oxidative stress. Free Radic Biol Med 1997; 23:597–609.

115. Valsecchi L, Cairone R, Castiglioni MT, Almirante GM, Ferrari A. Serum levels of alpha-tocopherol in hypertensive pregnancies. Hypertens Pregnancy 1999; 18:189–195.

116. Zhang C, Williams MA, Sanchez SE et al. Plasma concentrations of carotenoids, retinol, and tocopherols in preeclamptic and normotensive pregnant women. Am J Epidemiol 2001; 153:572–580.

117. Zusterzeel PL, Steegers-Theunissen RP, Harren FJ et al. Ethene and other biomarkers of oxidative stress in hypertensive disorders of pregnancy. Hypertens Pregnancy 2002; 21:39–49.

118. Llurba E, Gratacos E, Martin-Gallan P, Cabero L, Dominguez C. A comprehensive study of oxidative stress and antioxidant status in preeclampsia and normal pregnancy. Free Radic Biol Med 2004; 37:557–570.

119. Davidge ST. Oxidative stress and altered endothelial cell function in preeclampsia. Semin Reprod Endocrinol 1998; 16:65–73.

120. Taylor RN, de Groot CJ, Cho YK, Lim K-H. Circulating factors as markers and mediators of endothelial cell dysfunction in preeclampsia. Semin Reprod Endocrinol 1998; 16:17–31.

121. Rossig L, Hoffmann J, Hugel B et al. Vitamin C inhibits endothelial cell apoptosis in congestive heart failure. Circulation 2001; 104: 2182–2187.

122. Takacs P, Green KL, Nikaeo A, Kauma SW. Increased vascular endothelial cell production of interleukin-6 in severe preeclampsia. Am J Obstet Gynecol 2003; 188:740–744.

123. Chan AC. Partners in defense, vitamin E and vitamin C. Can J Physiol Pharmacol 1993; 71:725–731.

124. Nutrition of expectant and nursing mothers. Interim report of the People's League of Health. Lancet 1942; 4:10–12.

125. Stratta P, Canavese C, Porcu M et al. Vitamin E supplementation in preeclampsia. Gynecol Obstet Invest 1994; 37:246–249.

126. Gülmezoglu AM, Hofmeyr GJ, Oosthuizen MM. Antioxidants in the treatment of severe pre-eclampsia: an explanatory randomised controlled trial. Br J Obstet Gynaecol 1997; 104:689–696.

127. Chappell LC, Seed PT, Briley AL et al. Effect of antioxidants on the occurrence of pre-eclampsia in women at increased risk: a randomised trial. Lancet 1999; 345:810–816.

128. Sahlin L, Ostlund E, Wang H, Holmgren A, Fried G. Decreased expression of thioredoxin and glutaredoxin in placentae from pregnancies with pre-eclampsia and intrauterine growth restriction. Placenta 2000; 21:603–609.

129. Buhimschi IA, Weiner CP. Oxygen free radicals and disorders of pregnancy. Fetal Mat Med Rev 2002; 12:273–298.

130. Buhimschi IA, Kramer WB, Buhimschi CS, Thompson LP, Weiner CP. Reduction–oxidation (redox) state regulation of matrix metalloproteinase activity in human fetal membranes. Am J Obstet Gynecol 2000; 182:458–464.

131. Woods JR Jr. Reactive oxygen species and preterm premature rupture of membranes – a review. Placenta 2001; 22 (Suppl A):S38–S44.

3. Pregnancy-related changes to maternal host immune defenses

Denise G Hemmings and Larry J Guilbert

INTRODUCTION

The potential immunologic conflict between the mother and her antigenically different fetus suggests that modulation of the maternal host immune responses is essential for survival of the conceptus.[1] A unique homeostasis between different systems of the body exists in pregnancy, the end result of which favors the development of the fetus while preserving maternal health. Indeed, although there are numerous (and often conflicting) reports of alterations in numbers, distribution and function of maternal host defense components in normal pregnancy, there does not appear to be an overall compromise of acquired maternal immune defenses against the usual assaults. However, research in the past two decades suggests that pregnancy entails a shift in the balance between the different arms of the maternal immune response leading to less aggressive, but nonetheless competent, forms of immunity. It is also becoming increasingly clear that innate defenses play a critical role in maternal host defenses during pregnancy. We shall review the effect of pregnancy on maternal host immune defenses with illustrative examples of specific autoimmune disorders and infectious diseases which will then be related to both local and systemic mechanisms of pregnancy maintenance. Finally, we shall discuss how the maternal host immune response affects pregnancy outcome.

PREGNANCY AND THE MATERNAL IMMUNE SYSTEM

After a simplified overview of host immune defenses including innate, humoral and cell-mediated immunity, the effects of pregnancy on each of these components will be described followed by a discussion of the pregnancy-related changes in maternal immune responses in autoimmunity and to specific pathogens.

HOST IMMUNE DEFENSE SYSTEMS

We shall simplify host immune defense into three systems.

INNATE DEFENSES

Innate defense mechanisms do not depend on classical immunological memory and are the first line of defense against microbial invasion. They are mediated by cells of the myeloid lineage: neutrophils, eosinophils, and mononuclear phagocytes, as well as by natural killer (NK) cells. Circulating NK cells form a small proportion of peripheral blood lymphocytes and are involved in the lysis and elimination of virus-infected and neoplastic cells. They lack the classical cell surface antigen receptors of T and B lymphocytes and are not antigen-specific. NK cells are regulated by activating/inhibitory receptors such as Ly49, CD94/NKG2, p58, p49, and KIR, that interact with cell surface MHC molecules on potential target cells.[2] Toll-like receptors (TLRs), which are expressed by myeloid and lymphoid cells, recognize conserved molecular structures found only on microbial pathogens and play a key role in the innate antimicrobial host defense.[3] Additional innate defenses include proteins such as cationic antimicrobial proteins[4] and complement components.[5]

ACQUIRED HUMORAL IMMUNITY

Acquired humoral immunity involves recognition of specific extracellular antigens by antibodies. Antibody production proceeds via clonal, antigen-specific B-lymphocyte expansion that, for protein antigens, requires help from a subset of antigen-specific, CD4+ T lymphocytes (T helper type 2 [Th2] cells). Antibody can disrupt cellular or microbial function and enhance microbial or macromolecule uptake by phagocytic cells.

ACQUIRED CELL-MEDIATED IMMUNITY

Acquired cell-mediated immunity (CMI) is mediated by immune cells, often involving inflammatory activation, and leads to death of intracellular infectious pathogens and infected or altered cells. There are three general categories:

- Antigen-specific cytotoxic T lymphocytes (CTL) recognize peptides presented by class I major histocompatibility complex antigens (MHC class I) on the surface of target cells. CD8+ CTL (more common than CD4+ CTL) responses proceed via clonal, antigen-specific CD8+ T-cell expansion that requires help from another subset of antigen-specific CD4+ T helper cells (Th1 cells).
- Macrophages, NK cells, eosinophils, and neutrophils (active in innate defenses) exhibit acquired CMI via antibody-dependent cellular cytotoxicity (ADCC).
- Th1 cells also release inflammatory mediators such as interferon-γ (IFN-γ) that activate killing by macrophages (delayed-type hypersensitivity, DTH).

INTERACTIONS AMONG IMMUNE DEFENSE SYSTEMS

The three systems that make up the host immune defense are strongly interactive (Figure 3.1). Signals derived from the innate system determine the direction of acquired immune responses by driving the development of appropriate antigen-specific Th1 or Th2 cells,[5–9] including those with suppressor or tolerance-inducing function.[10] For example, macrophage infection by intracellular parasites such as *Toxoplasma gondii* initiates a feed-forward inflammatory loop as follows: infected macrophages release interleukin-12 (IL-12), which stimulates NK cell release of IFN-γ, which in turn enhances macrophage release of IL-12.[7,11] This local accumulation of IFN-γ and IL-12 constitutes an effective innate defense and also leads to antigen-specific Th1 cell development and the cell-mediated acquired responses most effective against intracellular parasites.[12] Other elements of the innate system that regulate acquired responses include complement components such as C3d[5] and TLR activation on antigen-presenting cells (APCs) such as dendritic cells, B cells, and macrophages. Signals through the TLRs modulate immune cell activities, including release of products that impact acquired immune function such as prostaglandin E$_2$ (PGE$_2$), tumor necrosis factor-α (TNF-α) and interleukins IL-10, IL-12, and IL-6.[8,9] In addition, effector elements of innate responses are enhanced by specific antibody during an acquired humoral response (ADCC) or by inflammatory mediators (TNF-α, IFN-γ) released by T lymphocytes during acquired CMI. In addition, humoral and CMI responses to a given antigen polarize by cross-inhibiting each other: Th1 cell release of IFN-γ during CMI inhibits Th2 cell replication, and Th2 cell release of TGF-β and IL-10 during a humoral response inhibits Th1 cell cytokine release.[6,13]

THE EFFECT OF PREGNANCY ON HOST IMMUNE DEFENSE SYSTEMS

PREGNANCY AND INNATE DEFENSE

The number of circulating polymorphonuclear leukocytes (PMN) increases slightly in pregnant women and, depending on the measure of activity, PMN activity is either increased (CD11b, CD14, CD64)[14] or reduced (adherence, chemotactic response, oxidative metabolism, bacterial killing)[15] during pregnancy (Table 3.1).

Peripheral blood monocytes are also elevated in pregnancy, probably as a result of constitutive uterine production of the hematopoietic growth factor,

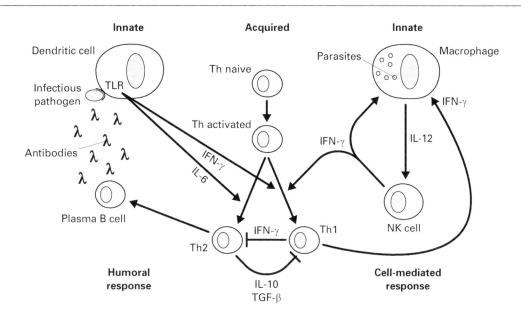

Figure 3.1 Interaction of innate and acquired immune responses. Stimulation of cells involved in the innate immune response such as macrophages and dendritic cells by different types of pathogens leads to activation of the most appropriate acquired immune response to remove that pathogen. For example, macrophages infected with a parasite produce IL-12, which then stimulates natural killer (NK) cells to produce IFN-γ. This feedforward loop not only further activates the macrophages to destroy the parasites but also the cytokines produced stimulate activation of the Th1 or cell-mediated arm of the acquired immune response, which is essential for clearance of this type of infection. On the other hand, when dendritic cells expressing toll-like receptors (TLRs) come into contact with molecules expressed on infectious pathogens such as bacteria, they begin to produce a number of cytokines, including IL-6, which then stimulates the Th2 or humoral arm of the acquired immune response, resulting in production of bacteria-specific antibodies. In addition, cross-inhibition occurs between Th1 and Th2 cells, where production of IFN-γ by Th1 cells inhibits proliferation of Th2 cells, and production of IL-10 and TGF-β by Th2 cells inhibits cytokine production by Th1 cells.

macrophage colony-stimulating factor (CSF-1),[16] and the estrogen-induced sensitivity of bone marrow monocyte precursors to this growth factor.[17] Monocyte activation markers/indicators CD11b, CD14, CD64, basal levels of reactive oxygen intermediates, phagocytosis, and oxidative burst capacity have all been shown to be elevated during pregnancy.[18] However, pregnancy-associated hormones (e.g. progesterone) inactivate mononuclear phagocyte functions such as cytokine production and inducible nitric oxide synthase (iNOS) expression.[19]

During gestation, total numbers of circulating cytotoxic NK cells (CD56, CD16+ cells) remain fairly constant and within the range observed in normal non-pregnant controls. However, the activity of peripheral blood NK cells isolated from pregnant women is decreased when tested in vitro.[20] Indeed, activation of NK cells in mice is detrimental to pregnancy outcome, leading to increased fetal resorptions.[21] In contrast to circulating NK cells, a distinct NK cell type appears uniquely in the uterus during the luteal phase of ovulation and in the early (implantation/placentation) stages of pregnancy.[22] These cells have a much higher expression of CD56 and a much lower expression of CD16 than do circulating NK cells and are suggested to be important in the processes of implantation, placentation, and pregnancy maintenance.[23]

In normal pregnancy, the gradual increase in plasma levels of complement components such as C3, C4, and CH50 parallels that of other

Table 3.1 Impact of pregnancy on innate, humoral, and cell-mediated immune defenses

Cells/functions	Effect of pregnancy	Comments
Innate defense		
Neutrophil (PMN) levels	↑	
Neutrophil (PMN) activity	↑↓	Depends on marker
Monocyte number	↑	
Monocyte activity	↑↓	Depends on marker
Peripheral NK cell number	=	
Peripheral NK cell activity	↓	
Acute-phase proteins	↑	
Toll-like receptors	?	
Complement components	↑	
Humoral responses		
B-lymphocyte number	=	
IgM	=	
IgA	=	
IgG	=	
Humoral immune response	↓=	Equal when corrected for volume
Cell-mediated responses		
CD4 lymphocyte number	↓	
CD8 lymphocyte number	=	
Mixed lymphocyte response	↓	
Paternal antigen-specific CTL	↓	Third-party CTL not changed
Third-party antigen-specific DTH	↓	

acute-phase reactants, including ceruloplasmin, α_1-antitrypsin, and haptoglobin.[24] It has been suggested that increases in such innate effectors compensates for decreases in the cell-mediated arm of immunity during pregnancy.[18] However, recent studies have also demonstrated the adverse effects of complement activation in combination with antiphospholipid antibodies[25,26] and in maternal diseases such as pre-eclampsia and systemic lupus erythematosus.[24,27]

PREGNANCY AND ACQUIRED HUMORAL IMMUNITY

Pregnancy-related changes in humoral or antibody-mediated immunity can be assessed by examining the number of circulating B cells, levels of immunoglobulin (Ig), and antigen-specific responses. The percentage of circulating B lymphocytes in gravid women is not altered.[28] However, the percentage of CD5+ B cells, which predominate

early in B-cell ontogeny and are implicated in the production of polyreactive autoantibodies, is greatly reduced.[29] A similar inhibition of bone marrow B lymphopoiesis occurs in pregnant mice.[30]

Serum IgA and IgM levels do not change significantly during gestation,[28] although there is a reduction in IgG levels that can be attributed to increased blood volume. Of note, autoantibodies are found in abnormal pregnancies, especially in those associated with hypertension and intrauterine growth restriction (IUGR), and elevated levels are associated with pregnancy loss.[31]

Human pregnancy does not significantly alter the humoral response to vaccines[32] and antibody responses in pregnant mice are not reduced (in contrast to cell-mediated responses, see below).[33] Specific maternal antibody responses to paternal antigens are common but appear not to predict pregnancy failure.[34] In fact, in a mouse model of rapid tumor rejection, probably mediated by antibodies, pregnancy did not affect the rejection of tumors bearing paternal MHC.[35] This is in sharp contrast to the effect of pregnancy on cell-mediated rejection of tumors bearing paternal MHC (see below).

PREGNANCY AND ACQUIRED CELL-MEDIATED IMMUNITY

Pregnancy induces a transient acute involution of the thymus, indicating a profound effect on T-cell lymphopoiesis.[36] This manifests as a gradual decrease in the percentage of CD4+ T cells, with little or no increase in the CD8+ population in the peripheral blood of women during normal pregnancy,[37] resulting in a decreased CD4/CD8 ratio most evident in the third trimester.[38] It is important to note that many of these changes in T-cell populations are subtle, and that alterations in antigen-specific Th1, Th2, CTL, or suppresser T-cell subpopulations have not yet been systematically examined during pregnancy.

Physiological depression of maternal CMI has been proposed to play a fundamental role in the prevention of fetal rejection.[39] There is some controversy whether and to what extent pregnancy increases the susceptibility and/or worsens the natural course of diseases in which CMI plays an important role. However, pregnancy does appear to mute antigen-specific CMI against several intracellular infections (see below) and reduces symptoms of the cell-mediated autoimmune disease rheumatoid arthritis.[40] Further evidence of suppressed CMI during pregnancy include the prolongation of skin grafts[41] and the reversible suppression of cell-mediated rejection of tumors bearing paternal MHC.[42] Proliferative or cytokine responses against several recall antigens are also reduced during pregnancy, including responses against cytomegalovirus (CMV),[38,43,44] herpes simplex virus-1 (HSV-1),[44] tuberculin,[43] tetanus,[45] influenza,[45] and other antigens and mitogens.[46]

PREGNANCY AND THE Th1/Th2 BALANCE

It has been reported that pregnancy both does[47] and does not[48,49] induce a shift towards Th2 cells/cytokines (thus away from a CMI response) in the peripheral circulation of humans and mice (Table 3.2). In women having repeated spontaneous abortions, trophoblast antigen-induced Th2 cytokine production is decreased (and that of Th1 cytokines increased) in peripheral lymphocytes.[50] T cells found in the decidua also produce reduced Th2 cytokines, IL-4 and LIF (leukocyte inhibitory factor).[51] These latter observations suggest that both local and systemic Th2 responses to paternal antigens are important to a successful human pregnancy. In addition, the observations that the pregnancy products progesterone,[52] estrogen,[53] and glucocorticoids[54] strongly bias T-helper development towards Th2 while decreasing Th1-type responses suggests a mechanism for the Th2 shift during pregnancy. On the other hand, there is evidence to support the importance of some Th1-type responses for reproductive success, including functional uterine NK cells and local levels of newly defined Th1-type cytokines, although this has recently been challenged.[55] These results suggest that the immune changes in pregnancy are considerably more complicated than a simple systemic shift towards a Th2-type profile and away from a Th1-type response.[56,57]

THE EFFECT OF PREGNANCY ON AUTOIMMUNITY

Mitigation of inflammatory diseases by pregnancy is most strikingly exemplified by the clinical improvement during pregnancy (Table 3.3) observed in about 75% of women suffering from rheumatoid arthritis.[40] Improvement in both synovitis and extra-articular features manifests in the first trimester, but increases until term. Involvement of specific immunity is indicated by the observation that the degree of improvement corresponds to the magnitude of MHC incompatibility between mother and fetus.[58] It is likely that anti-inflammatory cytokine production during pregnancy may be involved in the improvement of this inflammatory

Table 3.2 Effect of pregnancy on cytokine expression

Mediator	Main source	Action	Pregnancy levels
Th1 cytokines:	T cells, macrophages, decidua, placenta	Regulation of cell-mediated and acute inflammatory responses; macrophage activation	?↓[a]
IL-2 IFN-γ TNF-α			
Th2 cytokines:	T cells, macrophages, decidua, placenta	Inhibition of Th1 responses; B-cell proliferation; antibody formation; induction of tolerance	?↑[a]
IL-4 TGF-β IL-10			

[a] ? Systemic levels (circulating or tissue associated) not determined for all cytokines of the type during human pregnancy. Arrows indicate reported local and/or systemic levels in experimental animals.

Table 3.3 Impact of pregnancy on autoimmune diseases

Disease	Immune involvement	Effect of pregnancy on symptoms
Rheumatic arthritis	CMI	↓
Multiple sclerosis	CMI	↓
Systemic lupus erythematosus	CMI/antibody	=↑
Myasthenia gravis	Antibody	↑

disease.[59] Amelioration of symptoms during gestation is frequently followed by postpartum flares, which are also seen in other types of autoimmune arthritis.[59] Likewise, disease activity in multiple sclerosis, a chronic inflammatory disease of the central nervous system, shows a decrease in the second half of pregnancy and a return to prepregnancy levels in the first months postpartum. A shift towards a Th2 response during pregnancy, which then shifts back towards a Th1 profile postpartum, may explain these results.[60] In rabbits, pregnancy suppresses the development of the inflammatory disease autoimmune allergic encephalomyelitis, an animal model of multiple sclerosis.[61]

In contrast, about 40% of women suffering from myasthenia gravis may experience exacerbations during gestation,[62] particularly in the first trimester. Pathogenesis in this autoimmune condition appears to be mediated mainly by anti-acetylcholine receptor autoantibodies. In about 15% of pregnancies, transplacentally transferred IgG induces a transient form of myasthenia gravis in the newborn.[63] Whether pregnancy alters the course of systemic lupus erythematosus, another complex antibody-associated autoimmune disorder that frequently affects women in their childbearing years, remains controversial.[27,58]

Taken together, these observations indicate that pregnancy-induced immunological profiles are closely related to the mechanisms that control autoimmune disease activity: autoimmune inflammatory diseases tend to regress and antibody-mediated diseases tend to worsen during gestation (Figure 3.2).

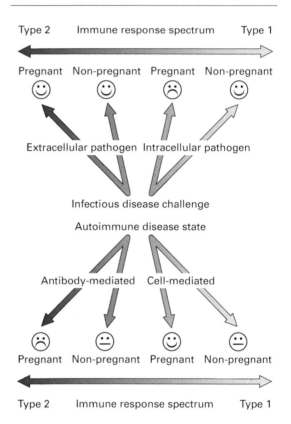

Figure 3.2 Pregnancy-induced shifts in maternal immunity and their influence on the course of maternal diseases. During pregnancy, the shift away from Th1-type immunity (depicted on the right side of the graph with lighter arrows) may be beneficial for those women suffering from autoimmune disorders with a predominant Th1-linked pathogenesis (lower quadrant), but impairs their resistance against microbial pathogens whose containment depend on Th1 responses (upper quadrant). The physiological tilt towards Th2-type immunity (left side of the graph, darker arrows) does not affect or may even facilitate the elimination of pathogens combated by antibody-mediated mechanisms (upper quadrant), but could exacerbate the Th2-associated pathological features of certain autoimmune disorders (lower quadrant).

MATERNAL IMMUNE DEFENSES AGAINST SPECIFIC PATHOGENS

Infectious pathogens have evolved host defense avoidance mechanisms that can affect both humoral and cell-mediated arms of acquired immunity; thus, defense against them is rarely confined to a single arm of the host defense system. Given the multitude of potential microbial pathogens and the complexity of the immune responses they elicit, it is therefore not surprising that reports of the impact of pregnancy on maternal infections are multiple and conflicting (summarized in Table 3.4). In general, despite well-documented exceptions such as primiparous malaria,[64] most infections do not pose a significant threat for the pregnant woman (see Figure 3.2). Indeed, even in cases in which an infection is very advanced and normal defense mechanisms have been overwhelmed, there appear to be physiological mechanisms that primarily induce fetal demise in order to spare the mother.[65]

PREGNANCY AND BACTERIAL INFECTION

Common extracellular bacterial infections, combated by antibody-mediated immunity, do not appear more frequent or take an abnormal course in pregnant women.[66] Likewise, the paucity of comment on the effect of pregnancy on the course of common pyogenic infections, also combated by antibody-mediated immunity, argues that the humoral arm of immunity remains intact during pregnancy.

Whether gestation increases the susceptibility to, or severity of, listerial, syphilitic, or gonorrheal infections, host defenses against which are partly or completely cell-mediated, is controversial.[66–68] Although listerial infections may occur more frequently but not more severely during gestation,[68] there is agreement that the consequences of maternal listeriosis are ominous for the conceptus.[69] Pregnancy also appears to be a risk factor for infections by *Coxiella burnetii*, an intracellular bacteria causing Q fever.[70] Cell-mediated immunity is also important for resistance to intracellular mycobacterial infections, including both tuberculosis (TB)[71] and leprosy.[72] Although early studies suggested pregnancy to be a risk factor for TB reactivation,[39] more recent evidence indicates that TB is neither more frequent nor more severe in pregnant compared with non-pregnant women.[73] However, leprosy may reactivate or relapse in about 40% of gravid women, especially during the third trimester.[74]

Table 3.4 Effect of pregnancy on maternal defense against infectious agents

Infection	Defenses	Effect of pregnancy on defense mechanism	Comments
Human			
Pyogenic bacteria	Antibody	=	
Tuberculosis	CMI	=	
Leprosy	CMI	↓	Recurrence
Listeriosis	CMI	↓	Severity, recurrence
Q fever	CMI	↓	Incidence
Hepatitis E	CMI	↓	Incidence, severity
Cytomegalovirus	CMI/antibody	=	Recurrence
Variola virus	CMI/antibody	↓	Mortality
Other viruses	CMI/antibody	=	
Gut parasites	Antibody	=	
Trypanosoma cruzi	CMI	↓	Parasite density
Plasmodium falciparum	CMI	↓	Incidence, recurrence, placental disease
Toxoplasma gondii	CMI/antibody	=	
Leishmaniasis	CMI/antibody	=	
Mouse model			
Listeriosis	CMI	↓	Placental disease
Toxoplasma gondii	CMI	↓	
Leishmania major	CMI	↓	

PREGNANCY AND VIRAL INFECTIONS

The effect of pregnancy on defenses against viral infections is variable, probably because of the requirement for both humoral and cell-mediated immune responses. Although primary infections by the common Betaherpesvirinae CMV (cytomegalovirus) do not appear more often during pregnancy, it is well established that reactivation occurs more frequently.[66] Mouse CMV reactivation requires the combined deletion of T-helper cells, CTL, and NK cells,[75] suggesting that cell-mediated immunity is crucial to maintenance of latency and that latency is overcome in pregnancy. Under all circumstances, maternal CMV infections are more serious for the fetus than the mother.[39] Pregnant women are particularly susceptible to fulminant hepatitis E infections, but not to other hepatitis viruses.[76] It is a consistent observation that human immunodeficiency virus (HIV)-infected pregnant women appear no more likely to progress in their acquired immunodeficiency syndrome (AIDS) status (CDC class III/IV) than non-pregnant women.[77] Pregnancy also does not appear to increase maternal susceptibility to the coronavirus causing severe acute respiratory syndrome (SARS), but there are deleterious effects on fetal well-being.[78] Pregnant women who contract variola virus (agent causing smallpox) have higher mortality rates possibly because of the reduced Th1 and increased Th2 responses associated with pregnancy.[79]

PREGNANCY AND PARASITIC INFECTIONS

Defense against intestinal worms, which are mainly combated by antibody-mediated immunity,[13] does not appear to be altered during pregnancy nor is pregnancy outcome affected by a worm infestation.[66] In contrast, infections with intracellular parasites such as plasmodia and trypanosomes, against which cell-mediated immune defenses are essential,[80,81] represent a health risk for both mother and fetus. The incidence and the severity of malaria are well known to be greater in pregnant women, particularly primigravidae.[64] In many cases, persistent parasitemia can be demonstrated even after chloroquine treatment.[82] A greater degree of parasitemia has also been observed in pregnant women chronically infected with *Trypanosoma cruzi*.[83]

Pregnant mice are more susceptible to infections by the intracellular parasites *Leishmania major* and *Toxoplasma gondii*,[67,84] the clearance of which requires a strong cell-mediated response.[84,85] However, even the muted immune response against *L. major* compromises pregnancy at both pre- and postimplantation stages,[65] indicating the sensitivity of pregnancy outcome to cell-mediated immune defenses. Although pregnant mice are more susceptible to *T. gondii*, the incidence of leishmaniasis or the relapse of pre-existing toxoplasmosis in humans during pregnancy is considered rare,[66,86,87] with the outcome again more serious for the fetus than the mother.[39,86]

WHY AND HOW DOES PREGNANCY AFFECT MATERNAL IMMUNITY?

Maternal host defense must accommodate antigenically foreign paternal antigens, both locally at the maternal–fetal interface and systemically after antigen leakage from the conceptus.[88] Whereas the former would lead to fetal rejection, the latter would subject the mother to an intolerable level of inflammation. Neither of these scenarios occurs,[35,42] which argues for multiple and flexible mechanisms of immune suppression to allow for adequate maternal defense against a myriad of possible infections and yet still accommodate antigenically foreign paternal antigens. How does this occur? One possible explanation is derived from the danger/non-danger hypothesis[57,89] where fetal paternal antigens would be declared non-dangerous and thus ignored, whereas antigens from maternal infections would be considered dangerous with an ensuing protective immune response. But how are paternal antigens declared non-dangerous operationally? The answer is: through parallel and overlapping mechanisms (see below),[57,90] the number of which grows as we understand the immune system better.

The literature cited above argues that pregnancy does not greatly alter antibody-mediated responses to infectious diseases. In pregnant women – with notable exceptions such as listeriosis, hepatitis E infections, malaria, Q fever, and toxoplasmosis – cell-mediated immune responses also do not appear to be greatly suppressed nor is there increased susceptibility to intracellular infections in general. In the exceptions listed above, it is difficult to precisely identify alterations in the maternal host immune response that result in increased susceptibility; however, infections are rarely combated by a single arm of immunity and the relative contributions of antibody-mediated and cell-mediated immune responses to infections during pregnancy require carefully constructed animal models. The best documented examples are leishmania,[84] toxoplasmosis,[67] and listeriosis[67,91] mouse models. In each of these models, there is strong and well-documented support for pregnancy decreasing host resistance against intracellular infections. However, there is also evidence that the placenta/decidua is a favorable growth environment for the replication of *Plasmodium falciparum*,[64] *Coxiella burnetii*,[70] and *Listeria monocytogenes*.[92] Thus, the increased susceptibility of pregnant women to the above infections could arise from one or both of the following: the absence of an effective local host immune defense within the pregnant uterus (which then acts as a disease reservoir) and/or an overall systemically reduced cell-mediated immunity during pregnancy. These two situations have been documented in two different mouse models of infections. The parasite *Leishmania major* never reaches the placenta of pregnant mice, but systemic antigen-specific cell-mediated immunity is suppressed.[65,84] On the other hand, although maternal cell-mediated resistance remains very strong during an infection of pregnant mice with *Listeria monocytogenes*, the bacteria thrives in the placental environment.[92] Thus, an understanding of how and why pregnancy induces susceptibility to particular infections must accommodate both possibilities, and each of these must also relate to the host requirements for maintaining pregnancies.

We shall therefore review recently proposed immune mechanisms localized within the utero-placental environment that prevent/lead to unexplained pregnancy loss (spontaneous abortion with no identified chromosomal abnormalities), then extend these understandings to systemic down-regulation of maternal cell-mediated immune responses (Figure 3.3).

LOCAL UTEROPLACENTAL INTERACTIONS IMPLICATED IN PREGNANCY MAINTENANCE

CYTOKINES

The events leading to pregnancy loss are thought to originate within the decidua, a maternal cellular response to the implanted conceptus. The observation that the largest concentration of perforin (a granule component in mature CTL and NK cells crucial to their killing functions) in the body is present in the decidua during pregnancy[93] suggests that strong mechanisms for termination are already present in normal pregnancy. Active inhibition of termination must therefore also involve regulation of NK and lymphocyte responses. Since cytokines are central regulators of immune cell proliferation, differentiation, and function, their roles in reproductive success have been closely examined. Expression of type 1 cytokines (those associated with Th1 cells and thus cell-mediated immunity) is associated with spontaneous abortion and type 2 (associated with Th2 cells) with pregnancy maintenance.[94] The possible cytotoxic effects of the Th1 inflammatory cytokines IFN-γ and TNF-α on the placenta and the regulation of these effects by the Th2/Th3 cytokines IL-10 and TGF-β have been recently reviewed[11,95] and are summarized below (Figure 3.4A).

Both IFN-γ and TNF-α strongly stimulate cell-mediated immune functions and both induce mouse pregnancy loss.[94] IFN-γ, in combination with TNF-α, has direct cytotoxic effects on villous trophoblasts.[96] IFN-γ is suggested to indirectly compromise the placental blood supply and thereby trigger spontaneous abortion through stimulation of the prothrombinase fg12 in vascular endothelium or trophoblasts, with subsequent chemotaxis and activation of neutrophils.[11,97] Paradoxically,

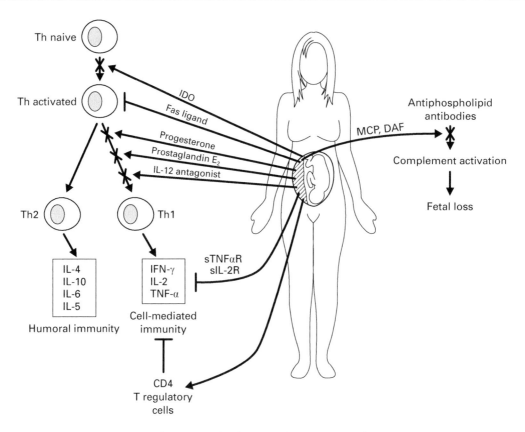

Figure 3.3 Effect of pregnancy on maternal immunity. The placenta produces a number of factors that act directly at the maternal–fetal interface (Fas ligand, complement inhibitory factors) and factors that may act both locally and systemically (cytokines, hormones, soluble receptors, IDO) to reduce a potentially damaging Th1-type immune response. IDO, indoleamine 2,3-dioxygenase; sTNFαR, soluble TNF-α receptor; sIL-2R, soluble IL-2 receptor; MCP, membrane cofactor protein; DAF, decay-accelerating factor.

IFN-γ is expressed in the mouse decidua/placenta throughout mouse pregnancy[49] and appears to have an important trophic effect, but only in the first pregnancy.[98] This effect may be related to its ability to stimulate secretion of the macrophage/trophoblast product indoleamine 2,3-dioxygenase (IDO; see below).[99]

The presence of both TGF-β and IL-10 in decidua[100,101] helps to maintain pregnancy by reducing the effects of inflammatory cytokines such as TNF-α and IFN-γ. TGF-β is potently immunosuppressive and is suggested to be the major product of another subset of T-helper lym-phocytes, Th3 cells.[13] The TGF-β2-like molecule released by decidual cells is a potent immune suppressor.[101] IL-10, in addition to inhibiting Th1 cell cytokine release through potential immune cross-regulation (Figures 3.1, 3.4A)[13] has also been reported to induce protective (against NK cells) expression of the non-classical MHC molecule HLA-G on extravillous cytotrophoblast.[102] It is unlikely that extravillous cytotrophoblasts themselves express IL-10;[103] however, they do express IL-10 receptors, and the functional predominance of TGF-β and IL-10 in the decidua is suggested to maintain pregnancy.[11,104]

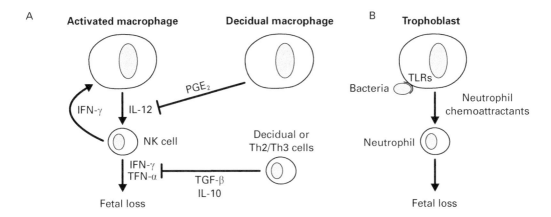

Figure 3.4 Mechanisms of fetal loss. (A) Activated macrophages produce IL-12, which then activates natural killer (NK) cells to produce IFN-γ and TNF-α. These cytokines are known to induce fetal loss. However, macrophages resident in the decidua produce prostaglandin E$_2$ (PGE$_2$), which prevents production of IL-12 by activated macrophages. Local uterine production of TGF-β and IL-10 counteract these detrimental effects. (B) Trophoblasts express toll-like receptors (TLRs) and are able to recognize and respond to a bacterial infection by producing neutrophil attractants. Accumulation of neutrophils at the maternal–fetal interface not only removes the bacterial threat but may also compromise pregnancy.

INDOLEAMINE 2,3-DIOXYGENASE

IDO degrades the essential amino acid tryptophan and in doing so acts both as a potent innate defense mechanism against intracellular pathogens and prevents rejection of allogeneic conceptuses in animal models possibly by inhibition of T-lymphocyte activation.[99] If IDO activity is inhibited, abortion of allogenic, but not syngeneic, pregnancies occurs, suggesting its importance in local uterine immune responses to foreign tissue (rejection). The importance of IDO in human pregnancies has been exemplified by a recent study demonstrating strong expression of IDO on invading first trimester extravillous trophoblasts.[105]

Another example in which allogenic, but not syngeneic, fetuses are rejected involves the elimination of CD25+, CD4+ T cells (T-regulatory cells) and impaired IDO production.[106] The authors of this study showed a pregnancy-dependent increase in levels of T-regulatory cells both peripherally in lymph nodes and blood and specifically in the uterus of pregnant mice. They suggest that the importance of these cells to allogenic pregnancies is through their ability to bind to decidual APC via CD80–CD86, which induces the APC-dependent production of IDO.[107] It is highly likely that these interactions also occur in human pregnancies, since these CD25+, CD4+ T-regulatory cells,[108] along with potently active antigen-presenting dendritic cells,[109] are also found in human decidua.

UTERINE NK CELLS

Uterine NK cells are thought to be central producers/mediators of cytokines affecting pregnancy.[23] This unique population of NK cells in the pregnant uterus appears to retain cytolytic activity but also strongly produce cytokines, especially IFN-γ. The interaction of NK cell receptors with HLA-C, HLA-E, and HLA-G on extravillous cytotrophoblasts is suggested to inhibit the cytotoxic activity of these cells.[90,95] However, it is clear that complete elimination of decidual NK cells in the tgε26 mouse model compromises pregnancy, an effect reversed by re-addition of functional NK cells.[110] Moreover, uterine NK interactions with extravillous trophoblasts are clearly important in the precise control of decidual trophoblast invasion, which, when impaired, may lead to shallow invasion and pre-eclampsia.[23] Thus,

NK cells, just like IFN-γ, have multiple and opposing effects on pregnancy.

Interactions of uterine NK cells with activated macrophages may induce NK cell cytokine production (IFN-γ and TNF-α) that leads to fetal loss.[11] Interactions between these two cell types have previously been suggested to lead to spontaneous abortions mediated by nitric oxide release.[111] However, resident decidual macrophages in a normal pregnancy situation tend to produce prostaglandin E$_2$ (PGE$_2$), which acts to suppress cell-mediated immune responses by inhibiting APC production of IL-12[95] (see Figure 3.4A).

The concept of uteroplacental NK cell and macrophage interactions leading to abortions has been challenged by the demonstration that there are no F4/80+ (a specific marker of macrophages) cells in the mouse decidua. However, under inflammatory conditions, the presence of Mac-1+ neutrophils may lead to abortion.[92] These authors suggest the existence of an alternative interaction in the decidua, with macrophages being replaced by trophoblasts (as previously suggested).[112] In this model, trophoblasts, activated by infection potentially through TLRs,[113,114] release neutrophil chemoattractants, leading to a localized accumulation of neutrophils, which then act as antimicrobial effectors and probably also abortion effectors, as previously described.[97] Thus, trophoblasts are postulated to be part of a pregnancy-specific innate immune defence system[92,112] (see Figure 3.4B).

TROPHOBLAST DEFENSE MECHANISMS

In normal pregnancy, trophoblasts also function to inhibit potentially cytotoxic T-cell activity against the allogeneic fetus (Table 3.5). Peripheral and local γ/δ T cells are increased in normal human pregnancy. However, peripheral γ/δ T cells express Vγ9/Vδ2 TCR (Th1 phenotype), whereas γ/δ T cells located in the decidua primarily express Vδ1 (Th2 phenotype). Trophoblasts express HLA-E, which, when recognized by Vδ2-expressing cells, provides an inhibitory signal to these γ/δ T cells, preventing a Th1 type of response.[115]

Trophoblasts also express Fas ligand (CD95L),[90] which is involved in immune protection of privileged sites such as the eye and the testes. Activated T cells which express Fas (CD95) undergo apoptosis when in contact with cells expressing Fas ligand. Cultured human trophoblasts induce apoptosis in activated T cells through Fas/Fas ligand interactions,[116] providing a mechanism to eliminate potentially damaging T cells. Interestingly, although trophoblasts also express Fas,[117] the apoptotic pathway appears to be inactive. Fas ligand-deficient mice show massive leukocyte accumulation at the decidua–placenta interface, suggesting the importance of this mechanism in the control of lymphocyte trafficking during pregnancy.[118]

Trophoblasts are also refractory to the effects of complement through production of inhibitory molecules such as membrane cofactor protein (CD46), which is a cofactor of C3b-inactivator,

---

Table 3.5 Trophoblast function and maternal immune responses

Trophoblast function	Effect on maternal immune responses
Anatomical barrier	Blocks access of fetal cells to maternal immune system
Negative for HLA class I classic antigens	No cytotoxic killing by CTLs
Positive for HLA class I non-classic antigens	No cytotoxic killing by NK cells; inhibits peripheral γδ T-cell activity
Complement inhibitor expression	Refractory to complement-mediated killing
Fas ligand expression	Induces apoptosis in Fas-expressing T-cells
Inactive Fas	No Fas-induced apoptosis
Production of IDO	Degrades tryptophan and inhibits T-cell activity
Production of progesterone, estrogen, glucocorticoids	Increases Th2- and reduces Th1-type responses
Production of prostaglandin E$_2$	Prevents Th1 cell development
Production of soluble TNF-α, IL-6, and IL-2 receptors	Blocks activity of these cytokines, reducing Th1-type immune responses
Production of IL-12 homologue, EBI3	Potential IL-12 antagonist, preventing macrophage and NK cell activation

and decay-accelerating factor (CD55), which increases the destruction rate of complement.[95] The importance of complement inhibition at the maternal–fetal interface has been shown recently in a mouse model in which a complement regulator has been knocked out (Crry), resulting in lethality in utero.[119] In addition, the important role of complement activation in the antiphospholipid syndrome of pregnancy in which autoantibodies lead to severe pregnancy complications emphasizes the importance of complement inhibition at the decidua–trophoblast interface.[26]

It is clear that the human decidua–placenta region is strongly anti-inflammatory. In addition to the presence of anti-inflammatory cytokines IL-10[100] and TGF-β[101] in the decidua, the villous placenta releases an arsenal of anti-inflammatory agents into the intervillous space/maternal circulation (Figure 3.3). These include progesterone, which specifically inhibits Th1 cell development[52] and inhibits macrophage effector function;[19] PGE$_2$, which also inhibits Th1 cell development;[95] IDO;[99] the IL-12 homologue EBI3,[120] which may be an IL-12 antagonist; and soluble TNF-α, IL-6, and IL-2 receptors,[121] which reduce active levels of these cytokines by complex formation. Release of these anti-inflammatory agents from the villous placenta into maternal circulation not only suppresses inflammation within the placental intervillous space but also provides a likely mechanism of systemic suppression of CMI in pregnant women.

HOW THE REQUIREMENTS OF PREGNANCY MAY AFFECT SYSTEMIC MATERNAL IMMUNITY

The underlying biological rationale for generalized systemic CMI suppression during pregnancy is not as clear as for suppression of local decidual–placental immune responses. It is, however, possible that cytokines and activated leukocytes generated during a strong CMI could 'spill over' into the decidual compartment and there engage abortion-promoting interactions between leukocytes and trophoblasts (a bystander effect). This possibility is supported by observations that systemic injections of IL-2, TNF-α, or IFN-γ, along with bacterial lipopolysaccharide, induce mouse pregnancy loss.[122] In addition, these same cytokines and activated leukocytes may cause excessive damage to the villous placenta, a possibility supported by observations of villous placental inflammation (villitis) coincident with recurrent pregnancy loss and IUGR.[123] Thus, general suppression of Th1 responses could limit both 'bystander effect' abortions and placental damage and thereby confer evolutionary advantages.

Teleologically, this generalized suppression of maternal cell-mediated immunity should prevent maternal inflammatory responses to specific paternal antigens. However, priming (development) of Th1 cells or CTL specific to paternal alloantigens could still lead to damaging responses after migration of these cells to the maternal–fetal interface or into the fetus. Transgenic mouse models have been used to determine if specific immune suppression to paternal antigens occurs during pregnancy. Generation of CTL responses against paternal MHC, but not third-party MHC, are in fact transiently suppressed during mouse pregnancy in transgenic models;[42] thus, the mother is immunologically aware of foreign allogeneic fetal cells and responds in a paternal antigen-specific manner to suppress CMI. This awareness could arise either from maternal T cell or APC surveillance of the fetus or from interactions at the maternal–fetal interface. Although maternal cells are found in fetuses after blastocyst transplantation in mice,[124] there is as yet little evidence for sustained immunosurveillance. There is, however, good evidence for release of fetal cells into the mother,[88] presumably through ruptures in the villous placenta. Notwithstanding the results in transgenic mice, in normal mice, CTL responses[35] and CD4+ and CD8+ T-cell IFN-γ responses (K Trejo-Oliver, LJ Guilbert, and TR Mosmann, unpublished work) can be induced against paternal antigens during pregnancy. This raises the possibility that there are multiple layers for prevention of alloreactive attack: first, sequestration of fetal cells at the maternal–fetal interface, leading to maternal ignorance of paternal antigens; and secondly, under more stressful conditions, induction of tolerance.

Transgenic mice may be an example of stressful conditions, in that they have high alloreactive T-cell frequencies and lack normal immune reactivity to infections.

THE EFFECT OF MATERNAL IMMUNE DEFENSES ON PREGNANCY OUTCOME

There are several pregnancy disorders in which an adverse maternal host immune defense appears to be part of the presentation. These include abortion, miscarriages, IUGR, preterm birth, and pre-eclampsia. Infectious origins for each of these disorders have been postulated, and maternal host immune defenses are clearly implicated.

Maternal infections that lead to increased fetal wastage or IUGR are candidates for maternal immune dysfunction during pregnancy: toxoplasmosis,[86] plasmodium (malaria),[64] parvovirus,[125] mumps,[126] rubella,[127] measles,[128] CMV,[129] listeriosis,[68] SARS,[78] subclinical maternal bacteremia, possibly originating in the urinary tract,[69] brucellosis,[130] enterovirus,[125] and syphilis.[131] In addition, most cases of recurring miscarriage (>3 consecutive losses, ~1% of all pregnancies in the United States) are ascribed to maternal–fetal immune incompatibility.[132] It is, however, not known whether previous or simultaneous infections are part of the cause. IUGR or low birth weight is a complication in most of the diseases or disorders leading to fetal demise listed above and, as previously discussed, may result from excessive damage of the villous placenta through placental inflammation or villitis.[123]

Preterm labor and birth are associated with amniotic or uterine inflammation, infections, or maternal host defenses.[133] SARS[78] and maternal *Ureaplasma urealyticum*[134] are also associated with preterm birth. Mouse models of intrauterine inflammation show that activation of TLR-4 (receptors involved in innate antimicrobial host defense), located on trophoblasts, may induce preterm labor.[113] Activation of TLR-2 on first-trimester human trophoblasts leads to increased trophoblast apoptosis, suggesting a mechanism by which localized uterine infections could affect pregnancy outcome.[114]

Pre-eclampsia is a hypertensive disorder of pregnancy that has been described as a state of elevated inflammation;[14] it is also a risk factor for IUGR and demonstrates placental pathology consistent with an inflammatory disorder.[135] Although it is generally thought that both pre-eclampsia and IUGR may stem from shallow implantation and the resulting restricted arterial blood flow,[136] evidence of inflammation, including excessive Th1 cytokine production, link the disorder to maternal host immune defenses[14,137,138] and possibly to infection.[139,140] However, systemic Th1 and Th2 immune responses to both paternal and vaccination antigens did not differ in women with or without pre-eclampsia,[141] suggesting a localized rather than systemic immunopathological effect may occur in pre-eclampsia.

SUMMARY

Maternal and fetal well-being are in a remarkable immunological balance that sometimes, but not always, puts the mother at risk for infections normally defended by inflammatory responses or diseases exacerbated by antibody responses. Although there does not appear to be a general compromise of maternal immunity to infectious diseases, there is an increased susceptibility to some, but not all, intracellular infections. This increased susceptibility appears to be related to a favorable (anti-inflammatory) growth environment in the pregnant uterus for some pathogens and to a systemic muting of cell-mediated immunity in others. We argue that the observed local uterine and systemic suppression of cell-mediated immunity is required to limit both pregnancy loss and placental damage.

Given that many inflammatory immune responses are detrimental to pregnancy, the question arises as to why pregnancy has not evolved resistance to such an important arm of immunity. The answer may lie in the consistent observation that when a pregnant woman is immunologically stressed beyond compromise or if the fetus is malformed or itself diseased, the fetus is removed or rejected to the benefit of the mother, who can conceive again. Thus, mammalian evolution retains the option to abort a fetus under a variety of situations, and the mechanism of such an action appears essentially immunological (cell-mediated) in nature. In this regard, it is useful to recall that pregnancy and the mammalian immune system have coevolved, and that each has shaped the other.

REFERENCES

1. Medawar PB. Some immunological and endocrinological problems raised by the evolution of viviparity in vertebrates. Symp Soc Exp Biol 1953; 7:320–338.
2. Moretta L, Bottino C, Pende D et al. Different checkpoints in human NK-cell activation. Trends Immunol 2004; 25:670–676.
3. Abreu MT, Arditi M. Innate immunity and toll-like receptors: clinical implications of basic science research. J Pediatr 2004; 144:421–429.
4. Levy O. Antimicrobial proteins and peptides: anti-infective molecules of mammalian leukocytes. J Leukoc Biol 2004; 76:909–925.
5. Carroll MC. The complement system in regulation of adaptive immunity. Nat Immunol 2004; 5:981–986.
6. Kidd P. Th1/Th2 balance: the hypothesis, its limitations, and implications for health and disease. Altern Med Rev 2003; 8:223–246.
7. Raulet DH. Interplay of natural killer cells and their receptors with the adaptive immune response. Nat Immunol 2004; 5:996–1002.
8. Hoebe K, Janssen E, Beutler B. The interface between innate and adaptive immunity. Nat Immunol 2004; 5:971–974.
9. Iwasaki A, Medzhitov R. Toll-like receptor control of the adaptive immune responses. Nat Immunol 2004; 5:987–995.
10. Jiang H, Chess L. An integrated view of suppressor T cell subsets in immunoregulation. J Clin Invest 2004; 114:1198–1208.
11. Arck P, Dietl J, Clark D. From the decidual cell internet: trophoblast-recognizing T cells. Biol Reprod 1999; 60:227–233.
12. Seder RA, Gazzinelli RT. Cytokines are critical in linking the innate and adaptive immune responses to bacterial, fungal, and parasitic infection. Adv Intern Med 1999; 44:353–388.
13. Mosmann TR, Sad S. The expanding universe of T-cell subsets: Th1, Th2 and more. Immunol Today 1996; 17:138–146.
14. Sacks GP, Studena K, Sargent K, Redman CW. Normal pregnancy and preeclampsia both produce inflammatory changes in peripheral blood leukocytes akin to those of sepsis. Am J Obstet Gynecol 1998; 179:80–86.
15. Krause PJ, Ingardia CJ, Pontius LT et al. Host defense during pregnancy: neutrophil chemotaxis and adherence. Am J Obstet Gynecol 1987; 157:274–280.
16. Bartocci A, Pollard JW, Stanley ER. Regulation of colony-stimulating factor 1 during pregnancy. J Exp Med 1986; 164:956–961.
17. Maoz H, Kaiser N, Halimi M et al. The effect of estradiol on human myelomonocytic cells. 1. Enhancement of colony formation. J Reprod Immunol 1985; 7:325–335.
18. Sacks G, Sargent I, Redman C. An innate view of human pregnancy. Immunol Today 1999; 20:114–118.
19. Hunt JS, Miller L, Platt JS. Hormonal regulation of uterine macrophages. Dev Immunol 1998; 6:105–110.
20. Baley JE, Schacter BZ. Mechanisms of diminished natural killer cell activity in pregnant women and neonates. J Immunol 1985; 134:3042–3048.
21. Kinsky R, Delage G, Rosin N et al. A murine model of NK cell mediated resorption. Am J Reprod Immunol 1990; 23:73–77.
22. King A, Loke YW, Chaouat G. NK cells and reproduction. Immunol Today 1997; 18:64–66.
23. Parham P. NK cells and trophoblasts: partners in pregnancy. J Exp Med 2004; 200:951–955.
24. Abramson SB, Buyon JP. Activation of the complement pathway: comparison of normal pregnancy, preeclampsia, and systemic lupus erythematosus during pregnancy. Am J Reprod Immunol 1992; 28:183–187.
25. Caucheteux SM, Kanellopoulos-Langevin C, Ojcius DM. At the innate frontiers between mother and fetus: linking abortion with complement activation. Immunity 2003; 18:169–172.
26. Salmon JE, Girardi G. The role of complement in the antiphospho-lipid syndrome. Curr Dir Autoimmun 2004; 7:133–148.
27. Warren JB, Silver RM. Autoimmune disease in pregnancy: systemic lupus erythematosus and antiphospholipid syndrome. Obstet Gynecol Clin North Am 2004; 31:345–372, vi–vii.
28. Falkoff R. Maternal immunologic changes during pregnancy: a critical appraisal. Clin Rev Allerg 1987; 5:287–300.
29. Bhat NM, Mithal A, Bieber MM, Herzenberg LA, Teng NN. Human CD5+ B lymphocytes (B-1 cells) decrease in peripheral blood during pregnancy. J Reprod Immunol 1995; 28:53–60.
30. Medina KL, Kincade PW. Pregnancy-related steroids are potential negative regulators of B lymphopoiesis. Proc Natl Acad Sci USA 1994; 91:5382–5386.
31. Shoenfeld Y, Blank M. Autoantibodies associated with reproductive failure. Lupus 2004; 13:643–648.
32. Gill TJ 3rd, Repetti CF, Metlay LA et al. Transplacental immunization of the human fetus to tetanus by immunization of the mother. J Clin Invest 1983; 72:987–996.
33. Dresser DW. The potentiating effect of pregnancy on humoral immune responses of mice. J Reprod Immunol 1991; 20:253–266.
34. Cowchock FS, Smith JB. Predictors for live birth after unexplained spontaneous abortions: correlations between immunologic test results, obstetric histories, and outcome of next pregnancy without treatment. Am J Obstet Gynecol 1992; 167:1208–1212.
35. Wegmann TG, Waters CA, Drell DW, Carlson GA. Pregnant mice are not primed but can be primed to fetal alloantigens. Proc Natl Acad Sci USA 1979; 76:2410–2414.
36. Clarke AG, Kendall MD. Histological changes in the thymus during mouse pregnancy. Thymus 1989; 14:65–78.
37. Castilla JA, Rueda R, Vargas ML et al. Decreased levels of circulating CD4+ T lymphocytes during normal human pregnancy. J Reprod Immunol 1989; 15:103–111.
38. Sabahi F, Rola-Plesczcynski M, O'Connell S, Frenkel LD. Qualitative and quantitative analysis of T lymphocytes during normal human pregnancy. Am J Reprod Immunol 1995; 33:381–393.
39. Weinberg ED. Pregnancy-associated depression of cell-mediated immunity. Rev Infect Dis 1984; 6:814–831.
40. Russell AS, Johnston C, Chew C, Maksymowych WP. Evidence for reduced Th1 function in normal pregnancy: a hypothesis for the remission of rheumatoid arthritis. J Rheumatol 1997; 24:1045–1050.
41. Andresen RH, Monroe CW, Swartzbaugh S, Madden DA. Influence of the pregnant uterus upon the rejection of adult homografts; a preliminary study. Am J Obstet Gynecol 1965; 93:693–701.

42. Tafuri A, Alferink J, Moller P, Hammerling GJ, Arnold B. T cell awareness of paternal alloantigens during pregnancy. Science 1995; 270:630–633.

43. Tanaka A, Hirota K, Takahashi K, Numazaki Y. Suppression of cell mediated immunity to cytomegalovirus and tuberculin in pregnancy employing the leukocyte migration inhibition test. Microbiol Immunol 1983; 27:937–943.

44. Kumar A, Madden DL, Nankervis GA. Humoral and cell-mediated immune responses to herpesvirus antigens during pregnancy – a longitudinal study. J Clin Immunol 1984; 4:12–17.

45. Bermas BL, Hill JA. Proliferative responses to recall antigens are associated with pregnancy outcome in women with a history of recurrent spontaneous abortion. J Clin Invest 1997; 100:1330–1334.

46. Gehrz RC, Christianson WR, Linner KM et al. A longitudinal analysis of lymphocyte proliferative responses to mitogens and antigens during human pregnancy. Am J Obstet Gynecol 1981; 140:665–670.

47. Marzi M, Vigano A, Trabattoni D et al. Characterization of type 1 and type 2 cytokine production profile in physiologic and pathologic human pregnancy. Clin Exp Immunol 1996; 106:127–133.

48. Matthiesen L, Ekerfelt C, Berg G, Ernerudh J. Increased numbers of circulating interferon-gamma- and interleukin-4-secreting cells during normal pregnancy. Am J Reprod Immunol 1998; 39:362–367.

49. Platt JS, Hunt JS. Interferon-gamma gene expression in cycling and pregnant mouse uterus: temporal aspects and cellular localization. J Leukoc Biol 1998; 64:393–400.

50. Hill JA, Polgar K, Anderson DJ. T-helper 1-type immunity to trophoblast in women with recurrent spontaneous abortion. JAMA 1995; 273:1933–1936.

51. Piccinni MP, Beloni L, Livi C et al. Defective production of both leukemia inhibitory factor and type 2 T-helper cytokines by decidual T cells in unexplained recurrent abortions. Nat Med 1998; 4: 1020–1024.

52. Piccinni MP, Romagnani S. Regulation of fetal allograft survival by hormone-controlled Th1- and Th2-type cytokines. Immunol Res 1996; 15:141–150.

53. Salem ML. Estrogen, a double-edged sword: modulation of Th1- and Th2-mediated inflammations by differential regulation of Th1/Th2 cytokine production. Curr Drug Targets Inflamm Allergy 2004; 3:97–104.

54. Elenkov IJ. Glucocorticoids and the Th1/Th2 balance. Ann NY Acad Sci 2004; 1024:138–146.

55. Barber EM, Pollard JW. The uterine NK cell population requires IL-15 but these cells are not required for pregnancy nor the resolution of a *Listeria monocytogenes* infection. J Immunol 2003; 171:37–46.

56. Chaouat G, Ledee-Bataille N, Dubanchet S et al. Th1/Th2 paradigm in pregnancy: paradigm lost? Cytokines in pregnancy/early abortion: reexamining the Th1/Th2 paradigm. Int Arch Allergy Immunol 2004; 134:93–119.

57. Moffett A, Loke YW. The immunological paradox of pregnancy: a reappraisal. Placenta 2004; 25:1–8.

58. Varner MW. Autoimmune disorders and pregnancy. Semin Perinatol 1991; 15:238–250.

59. Oestensen M, Forger F, Nelson JL et al. Pregnancy in patients with rheumatic disease: anti-inflammatory cytokines increase in pregnancy and decrease post partum. Ann Rheum Dis 2004; 64:839–844.

60. Al-Shammri S, Rawoot P, Azizieh F et al. Th1/Th2 cytokine patterns and clinical profiles during and after pregnancy in women with multiple sclerosis. J Neurol Sci 2004; 222:21–27.

61. Evron S, Brenner T, Abramsky O. Suppressive effect of pregnancy on the development of experimental allergic encephalomyelitis in rabbits. Am J Reprod Immunol 1984; 5:109–113.

62. Plauche WC. Myasthenia gravis in mothers and their newborns. Clin Obstet Gynecol 1991; 34:82–99.

63. Giacoia GP, Azubuike K. Autoimmune diseases in pregnancy: their effect on the fetus and newborn. Obstet Gynecol Surv 1991; 46:723–732.

64. Brabin BJ, Romagosa C, Abdelgalil S et al. The sick placenta – the role of malaria. Placenta 2004; 25:359–378.

65. Krishnan L, Guilbert LJ, Wegmann TG, Belosevic M, Mosmann TR. T helper 1 response against Leishmania major in pregnant C57BL/6 mice increases implantation failure and fetal resorptions. Correlation with increased IFN-gamma and TNF and reduced IL-10 production by placental cells. J Immunol 1996; 156:653–662.

66. Brabin BJ. Epidemiology of infection in pregnancy. Rev Infect Dis 1985; 7:579–603.

67. Luft BJ, Remington JS. Effect of pregnancy on resistance to *Listeria monocytogenes* and *Toxoplasma gondii* infections in mice. Infect Immun 1982; 38:1164–1171.

68. Southwick FS, Purich DL. Intracellular pathogenesis of listeriosis. N Engl J Med 1996; 334:770–776.

69. Lessing JB, Amster R, Berger SA, Peyser MR. Bacterial infection and human fetal wastage. J Reprod Med 1989; 34:975–976.

70. Maurin M, Raoult D. Q fever. Clin Microbiol Rev 1999; 12:518–553.

71. Barnes PF, Lu S, Abrams JS et al. Cytokine production at the site of disease in human tuberculosis. Infect Immun 1993; 61:3482–3489.

72. Modlin RL. Th1-Th2 paradigm: insights from leprosy. J Invest Dermatol 1994; 102:828–832.

73. Ormerod P. Tuberculosis in pregnancy and the puerperium. Thorax 2001; 56:494–499.

74. Duncan ME. An historical and clinical review of the interaction of leprosy and pregnancy: a cycle to be broken. Soc Sci Med 1993; 37:457–472.

75. Polic B, Hengel H, Krmpotic A et al. Hierarchical and redundant lymphocyte subset control precludes cytomegalovirus replication during latent infection. J Exp Med 1998; 188:1047–1054.

76. Kane MA. Hepatitis viruses and the neonate. Clin Perinatol 1997; 24:181–191.

77. Coyne BA, Landers DV. The immunology of HIV disease and pregnancy and possible interactions. Obstet Gynecol Clin North Am 1990; 17:595–606.

78. Wong SF, Chow KM, Leung TN et al. Pregnancy and perinatal outcomes of women with severe acute respiratory syndrome. Am J Obstet Gynecol 2004; 191:292–297.

79. Hassett DE. Smallpox infections during pregnancy, lessons on pathogenesis from nonpregnant animal models of infection. J Reprod Immunol 2003; 60:13–24.

80. Silva JS, Morrissey PJ, Grabstein KH et al. Interleukin 10 and interferon gamma regulation of experimental *Trypanosoma cruzi* infection. J Exp Med 1992; 175:169–174.

81. von der Weid T, Langhorne J. The roles of cytokines produced in the immune response to the erythrocytic stages of mouse malarias. Immunobiology 1993; 189:397–418.

82. Mvondo JL, James MA, Campbell CC. Malaria and pregnancy in Cameroonian women. Effect of pregnancy on *Plasmodium falciparum* parasitemia and the response to chloroquine. Trop Med Parasitol 1992; 43:1–5.

83. Menezes CA, Bittencourt AL, Mota E, Sherlock I, Ferreira J. [The assessment of parasitemia in women who are carriers of *Trypanosoma cruzi* infection during and after pregnancy]. Rev Soc Bras Med Trop 1992; 25:109–113.

84. Krishnan L, Guilbert LJ, Russell AS et al. Pregnancy impairs resistance of C57BL/6 mice to Leishmania major infection and causes decreased

antigen-specific IFN-gamma response and increased production of T helper 2 cytokines. J Immunol 1996; 156:644–652.

85. Scott P, Pearce E, Cheever AW, Coffman RL, Sher A. Role of cytokines and CD4+ T-cell subsets in the regulation of parasite immunity and disease. Immunol Rev 1989; 112:161–182.

86. Montoya JG, Liesenfeld O. Toxoplasmosis. Lancet 2004; 363: 1965–1976.

87. Figueiro-Filho EA, Duarte G, El-Beitune P, Quintana SM, Maia TL. Visceral leishmaniasis (kala-azar) and pregnancy. Infect Dis Obstet Gynecol 2004; 12:31–40.

88. Johnson KL, Bianchi DW. Fetal cells in maternal tissue following pregnancy: what are the consequences? Hum Reprod Update 2004; 10:497–502.

89. Anderson CC, Matzinger P. Danger: the view from the bottom of the cliff. Semin Immunol 2000; 12:231–238; discussion 257–344.

90. Thellin O, Coumans B, Zorzi W, Igout A, Heinen E. Tolerance to the foeto–placental 'graft': ten ways to support a child for nine months. Curr Opin Immunol 2000; 12:731–737.

91. Abram M, Schluter D, Vuckovic D et al. Murine model of pregnancy-associated *Listeria monocytogenes* infection. FEMS Immunol Med Microbiol 2003; 35:177–182.

92. Guleria I, Pollard JW. The trophoblast is a component of the innate immune system during pregnancy. Nat Med 2000; 6:589–593.

93. Zheng LM, Ojcius DM, Young JD. Distribution of perforin-containing cells in normal and pregnant mice. Eur J Immunol 1993; 23:2085–2091.

94. Wegmann TG, Lin H, Guilbert L, Mosmann TR. Bidirectional cytokine interactions in the maternal–fetal relationship: is successful pregnancy a Th2 phenomenon? Immunol Today 1993; 14:353–356.

95. Bulla R, Fischetti F, Bossi F, Tedesco F. Feto–maternal immune interaction at the placental level. Lupus 2004; 13:625–629.

96. Yui J, Garcia-Lloret M, Wegmann TG, Guilbert LJ. Cytotoxicity of tumour necrosis factor-alpha and gamma-interferon against primary human placental trophoblasts. Placenta 1994; 15: 819–835.

97. Clark DA, Chaouat G, Arck PC, Mittruecker HW, Levy GA. Cytokine-dependent abortion in CBA × DBA/2 mice is mediated by the procoagulant fgl2 prothrombinase [correction of prothrombinase]. J Immunol 1998; 160:545–549.

98. Ashkar AA, Croy BA. Interferon-gamma contributes to the normalcy of murine pregnancy. Biol Reprod 1999; 61:493–502.

99. Mackler AM, Barber EM, Takikawa O, Pollard JW. Indoleamine 2,3-dioxygenase is regulated by IFN-gamma in the mouse placenta during *Listeria monocytogenes* infection. J Immunol 2003; 170: 823–830.

100. Lin H, Mosmann TR, Guilbert L, Tuntipopipat S, Wegmann TG. Synthesis of T helper 2-type cytokines at the maternal–fetal interface. J Immunol 1993; 151:4562–4573.

101. Lea RG, Flanders KC, Harley CB et al. Release of a transforming growth factor (TGF)-beta 2-related suppressor factor from post-implantation murine decidual tissue can be correlated with the detection of a subpopulation of cells containing RNA for TGF-beta 2. J Immunol 1992; 148:778–787.

102. Moreau P, Adrian-Cabestre F, Menier C et al. IL-10 selectively induces HLA-G expression in human trophoblasts and monocytes. Int Immunol 1999; 11:803–811.

103. Sacks GP, Clover LM, Bainbridge DR, Redman CW, Sargent IL. Flow cytometric measurement of intracellular Th1 and Th2 cytokine production by human villous and extravillous cytotrophoblast. Placenta 2001; 22:550–559.

104. Guilbert LJ. There is a bias against type 1 (inflammatory) cytokine expression and function in pregnancy. J Reprod Immunol 1996; 32:105–110.

105. Honig A, Rieger L, Kapp M et al. Indoleamine 2,3-dioxygenase (IDO) expression in invasive extravillous trophoblast supports role of the enzyme for materno–fetal tolerance. J Reprod Immunol 2004; 61:79–86.

106. Aluvihare VR, Kallikourdis M, Betz AG. Regulatory T cells mediate maternal tolerance to the fetus. Nat Immunol 2004; 5:266–271.

107. Fallarino F, Grohmann U, Hwang KW et al. Modulation of tryptophan catabolism by regulatory T cells. Nat Immunol 2003; 4: 1206–1212.

108. Annunziato F, Cosmi L, Liotta F et al. Phenotype, localization, and mechanism of suppression of CD4(+)CD25(+) human thymocytes. J Exp Med 2002; 196:379–387.

109. Kammerer U, Schoppet M, McLellan AD et al. Human decidua contains potent immunostimulatory CD83(+) dendritic cells. Am J Pathol 2000; 157:159–169.

110. Guimond M, Wang B, Croy BA. Immune competence involving the natural killer cell lineage promotes placental growth. Placenta 1999; 20:441–450.

111. Haddad EK, Duclos AJ, Baines MG. Early embryo loss is associated with local production of nitric oxide by decidual mononuclear cells. J Exp Med. 1995; 182:1143–1151.

112. Guilbert L, Robertson SA, Wegmann TG. The trophoblast as an integral component of a macrophage-cytokine network. Immunol Cell Biol 1993; 71 (Pt 1):49–57.

113. Elovitz MA, Wang Z, Chien EK, Rychlik DF, Phillippe M. A new model for inflammation-induced preterm birth: the role of platelet-activating factor and Toll-like receptor-4. Am J Pathol 2003; 163:2103–2111.

114. Abrahams VM, Bole-Aldo P, Kim YM et al. Divergent trophoblast responses to bacterial products mediated by TLRs. J Immunol 2004; 173:4286–4296.

115. Szekeres-Bartho J, Barakonyi A, Miko E, Polgar B, Palkovics T. The role of gamma/delta T cells in the feto–maternal relationship. Semin Immunol 2001; 13:229–233.

116. Coumans B, Thellin O, Zorzi W et al. Lymphoid cell apoptosis induced by trophoblastic cells: a model of active foeto–placental tolerance. J Immunol Methods 1999; 224:185–196.

117. Payne SG, Smith SC, Davidge ST, Baker PN, Guilbert LJ. Death receptor Fas/Apo-1/CD95 expressed by human placental cyto-trophoblasts does not mediate apoptosis. Biol Reprod 1999; 60:1144–1150.

118. Hunt JS, Vassmer D, Ferguson TA, Miller L. Fas ligand is positioned in mouse uterus and placenta to prevent trafficking of activated leukocytes between the mother and the conceptus. J Immunol 1997; 158:4122–4128.

119. Xu C, Mao D, Holers VM et al. A critical role for murine complement regulator crry in fetomaternal tolerance. Science 2000; 287:498–501.

120. Devergne O, Coulomb-L'Hermine A, Capel F, Moussa M, Capron F. Expression of Epstein–Barr virus-induced gene 3, an interleukin-12 p40-related molecule, throughout human pregnancy: involvement of syncytiotrophoblasts and extravillous trophoblasts. Am J Pathol 2001; 159:1763–1776.

121. Lien E, Liabakk NB, Austgulen R. Detection of soluble receptors for tumor necrosis factor, interleukin-2 and interleukin-6 in retroplacental serum from normal pregnant women. Gynecol Obstet Invest 1996; 41:1–4.

122. Chaouat G. Synergy of lipopolysaccharide and inflammatory cytokines in murine pregnancy: alloimmunization prevents

abortion but does not affect the induction of preterm delivery. Cell Immunol 1994; 157:328–340.

123. Labarrere CA, Faulk WP. Immunopathology of human extraembryonic tissues. In: Coulam CB, Faulk WP, McIntyre JA, eds. Immunological Obstetrics. New York: WW Norton & Co; 1992: 439–463.

124. Piotrowski P, Croy BA. Maternal cells are widely distributed in murine fetuses in utero. Biol Reprod 1996; 54:1103–1110.

125. Petersson K, Norbeck O, Westgren M, Broliden K. Detection of parvovirus B19, cytomegalovirus and enterovirus infections in cases of intrauterine fetal death. J Perinat Med 2004; 32:516–521.

126. Garcia AG, Pereira JM, Vidigal N et al. Intrauterine infection with mumps virus. Obstet Gynecol 1980; 56:756–759.

127. Zheng F, Du J, Hu Y. A study of rubella virus infection during pregnancy. Zhonghua Fu Chan Ke Za Zhi 2002; 37:391–394.

128. Chiba ME, Saito M, Suzuki N, Honda Y, Yaegashi N. Measles infection in pregnancy. J Infect 2003; 47:40–44.

129. Griffiths PD, Baboonian C. A prospective study of primary cytomegalovirus infection during pregnancy: final report. Br J Obstet Gynaecol 1984; 91:307–315.

130. Makhseed M, Harouny A, Araj G, Moussa MA, Sharma P. Obstetric and gynecologic implication of brucellosis in Kuwait. J Perinatol 1998; 18:196–199.

131. Labbe AC, Mendonca AP, Alves AC et al. The impact of syphilis, HIV-1, and HIV-2 on pregnancy outcome in Bissau, Guinea-Bissau. Sex Transm Dis 2002; 29:157–167.

132. Stirrat GM. Recurrent spontaneous abortion. In: Coulam CB, Faulk WP, McIntyre JA, eds. Immunological Obstetrics. New York: WW Norton & Co; 1992: 357–379.

133. Gomez R, Romero R, Edwin SS, David C. Pathogenesis of preterm labor and preterm premature rupture of membranes associated with intraamniotic infection. Infect Dis Clin North Am 1997; 11:135–176.

134. Kundsin RB, Leviton A, Allred EN, Poulin SA. Ureaplasma urealyticum infection of the placenta in pregnancies that ended prematurely. Obstet Gynecol 1996; 87:122–127.

135. Salafia CM, Minior VK, Pezzullo JC et al. Intrauterine growth restriction in infants of less than thirty-two weeks' gestation: associated placental pathologic features. Am J Obstet Gynecol 1995; 173:1049–1057.

136. Kaufmann P, Black S, Huppertz B. Endovascular trophoblast invasion: implications for the pathogenesis of intrauterine growth retardation and preeclampsia. Biol Reprod 2003; 69:1–7.

137. Dekker GA, Robillard PY, Hulsey TC. Immune maladaptation in the etiology of preeclampsia: a review of corroborative epidemiologic studies. Obstet Gynecol Surv 1998; 53:377–382.

138. Saito S, Sakai M. Th1/Th2 balance in preeclampsia. J Reprod Immunol 2003; 59:161–173.

139. Herrera JA, Chaudhuri G, Lopez-Jaramillo P. Is infection a major risk factor for preeclampsia? Med Hypotheses 2001; 57:393–397.

140. von Dadelszen P, Magee LA. Could an infectious trigger explain the differential maternal response to the shared placental pathology of preeclampsia and normotensive intrauterine growth restriction? Acta Obstet Gynecol Scand 2002; 81:642–648.

141. Jonsson Y, Ekerfelt C, Berg G et al. Systemic Th1/Th2 cytokine responses to paternal and vaccination antigens in preeclampsia: no differences compared with normal pregnancy. Am J Reprod Immunol 2004; 51:302–310.

4. Implantation, trophoblast/decidual interactions, and local inflammatory changes

Siobhan Quenby, Gill Vince, and Mark A Turner

INTRODUCTION

Successful pregnancy is dependent on the embryo attaching to the uterine endometrium and on invading the uterine wall. Trophoblast invasion must ensure that the supply of oxygen and nutrients to the fetus is appropriate, without compromising the health of the mother. Recently, research on early pregnancy has led to a much improved understanding of which processes are involved in this delicate balance. The aim of this chapter is to introduce the interested clinician to this area of research. This summary will have three themes:

- many molecules and molecular interactions are involved in embryo implantation and trophoblast invasion
- the causal pathways or regulatory networks linking these molecules together are not understood at present
- approaches that integrate laboratory and clinical work are required for further progress.

IMPLANTATION

Implantation is the process by which the blastocyst comes into contact with, adheres to and starts to penetrate the uterine endometrium.[1] Implantation depends on the blastocyst emerging from the zona pellucida (hatching) and on the endometrium becoming receptive to the blastocyst (decidualization). A large number of molecules appear to be relevant to these processes,[1] including ovarian hormones acting on the uterus (estrogen, progesterone); vasoactive factors (uterine histamine acting on the blastocyst); and growth factors (such as members of the epidermal growth factor (EGF) family), cytokines, and endocannabinoids (secreted by, and acting on, both uterus and blastocyst). A range of intracellular regulatory processes appear to be relevant in both blastocyst and uterus. These regulatory processes include homeobox genes, nuclear receptors, cell cycle regulators, and developmental genes. Ovarian hormones (estrogen and progesterone) coordinate the initial uterine response, whereas the blastocyst looks after itself until it has hatched, at which point a complex bidirectional system evolves.[2] It has been suggested that the blastocyst secretes a 'preimplantation factor' which modulates the maternal immune system.[3] One interesting hypothesis is that the blastocyst adhesion depends on the same mechanisms as neutrophil adhesion during inflammation.[4] Multiple extracellular molecules involved in the physical attachment of the blastocyst to endometrium have been described, including connexins, cadherins, MUC1, heparin sulfate, integrin $\alpha_v\beta_3$ and integrin subunit β_1[5] – see Figure 4.1. The importance of each of these molecules is currently unknown. Each molecule could contribute to hierarchical mechanisms or could be a necessary but not sufficient part of a causal network.

INVASION

Invasion refers to the processes by which extra-embryonic tissues differentiate and enter maternal tissues. The principal cell type in these processes is extravillous trophoblast (EVT). Trophoblast invasion lays the foundations for placentation, as the extent of invasion determines the quality of anchorage and depth of the placenta, ensuring that it will not detach. Trophoblast invasion of the maternal spiral arteries is important in ensuring appropriate fetal oxygen and nutrient supply. The timing of fetal oxygen delivery is crucial: too much oxygen too

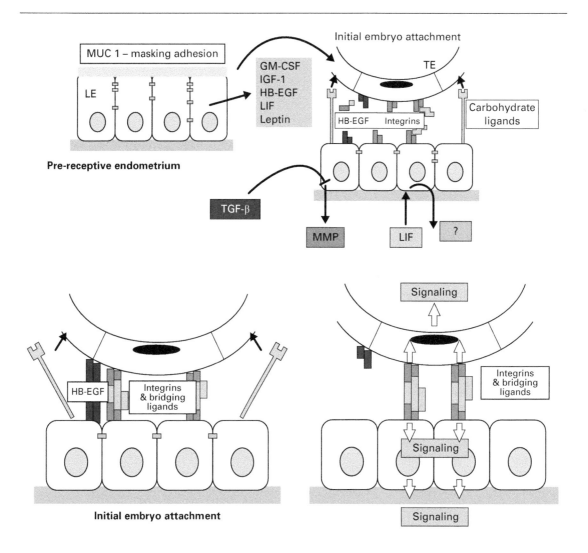

Figure 4.1 Stages in the attachment of the embryo and relevant molecular interactions. Adapted from Aplin and Kimber.[5]

soon is associated with evidence of oxidative stress and poor pregnancy outcome.[6] Poor invasion can cause obstetric complications, including miscarriage, pre-eclampsia, intrauterine growth restriction, placental abruption, and intrauterine death. Excessive invasion leads to placenta acreta, persistent trophoblastic disease, or invasive cancer (choriocarcinoma) with its attendant severe risk to the mother's life. Thus, trophoblast invasion can be considered as a balance between the demands of the fetus to invade the mother and those of the mother to survive this invasion. This balance is even more remarkable when it is considered that the majority (90%) of karyotypically abnormal pregnancies miscarry in the first trimester and the majority (93%) of karyotypically normal pregnancies continue.[7]

Hence, miscarriage, considered to be failed trophoblast invasion, can be viewed as 'nature's quality control'.[8] Factors that affect invasion, positively or negatively, will duly determine the success or failure of pregnancy. Normal pregnancy is a model of successfully controlled tissue invasion, in which trophoblasts penetrate the maternal decidua without destruction of tissue or rejection.[9]

INITIAL DEVELOPMENT OF THE TROPHOBLAST

On the 5th day after conception, an additional round of division causes the 32-celled morula to reach the blastocyst stage. This hollow ball is composed of an inner cell mass, eventually giving rise to the fetal and embryonic tissues,[10] and an attached outer shell of cells known as the trophoblast, which will ultimately give rise to the chorion. By the 10th day, the invading trophoblast has formed two distinct layers, known as the cytotrophoblast and the syncytiotrophoblast. The cytotrophoblast (the inner layer) is composed of individual, well-defined, and rapidly proliferating cells. In their undifferentiated form these cells are small, cuboid in shape, lacking distinct cell borders, and mononuclear, with the round vesicular nucleus containing evenly dispersed chromatin.[11] The outer and thicker layer, the syncytiotrophoblast, comprises multinucleated cells with indistinct cell borders. The trophoblast differentiates along two main pathways:

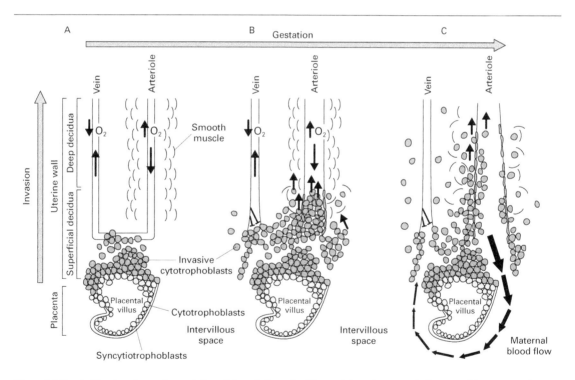

Figure 4.2 Trophoblast invasion and remodeling of the spiral arteries. Placental tissue is seen at the bottom of the image, with invasion occurring upwards. At stage A, extravillous trophoblast (EVT) has adopted an invasive phenotype. At stage B, EVT has continued to invade. Some EVT has adopted an endovascular phenotype and is plugging a partially remodeled arteriole. At stage C, a fully remodeled arteriole has been unplugged and blood flow has commenced in the intervillous space. Miscarriage is thought to reflect poor EVT invasion at stage A and before. Poor progress between stages B and C is thought to contribute to the etiology of pre-eclampsia. (Adapted from Red Horse et al.[16])

- villous – from the placental villous tree the site of maternal–fetal gas and nutrient exchange
- extravillous – that invade the maternal decidua beyond the endometrial–myometrial border until the inner third of the myometrium.[12,13]

Work using gene deletion techniques (knockout experiments) in the mouse has shown that multiple genes are involved in trophoblast differentiation.[14] Mouse studies can be particularly powerful because of the ability to examine what happens when a knockout fetus has a wild-type placenta[14] or when a gene deletion is only expressed in the placenta.[15] The relevance of these genes to human development is unclear. Furthermore, the regulatory network controlling gene expression has not been elucidated.

In order to maintain itself throughout pregnancy, the trophoblast must maintain a population of stem cells. In the mouse, trophoblast stem cells are maintained by fibroblast growth factor (FGF) family members, although FGF does not sustain a trophoblast stem cell population in humans.[16]

EXTRAVILLOUS TROPHOBLAST

EVTs invade the uterine tissue initially through the proliferating stem cells at the basement membrane of anchoring villi – see Figure 4.2. Stem villous cytotrophoblast undergoes a proliferative burst and differentiates into cells of the cytotrophoblast column, anchoring peripheral villi to the uterus.[17] Transition to the postproliferative invasive phenotype takes place several cell layers distant.[18] This transition from the cytotrophoblast into the migratory EVT is mediated by contact of the tip of the first-trimester mesenchymal villous with decidual extracellular matrix (ECM). Adhesion to a permissive ECM stimulates cytotrophoblast proliferation and differentiation along the extravillous lineage.[17] Subsequently, cells detach in large numbers from the periphery of the column and become migratory infiltrative cells. This step is dependent on paracrine signaling from the mesenchymal cells that lie directly beneath the villous basement membrane.[17]

Integrin–fibronectin interactions also contribute significantly to anchorage of the placenta to uterine extracellular matrix in vivo.[19] Integrin expression by invasive trophoblast is spatially and temporally regulated.[20]

EVTs differentiate into two populations of cells:

- Interstitial EVTs, which invade as far as the inner third of the myometrium, move towards the spiral arteries of the decidua, and differentiate into giant multinuclear cells.[21–23]
- endovascular EVTs, which form loose plugs in the apical portion of the spiral arteries.[24]

EVT FUNCTIONS

For successful invasion to occur, EVT has to perform a range of functions: transform the maternal spiral arteries, tolerate hypoxia, proliferate and die by apoptosis (programmed cell death), differentiate, adhere to and digest the extracellular matrix, and move and interact with the maternal immune system. EVT also contributes to the production of hormones required for pregnancy maintenance, e.g. hPL (human placental lactogen). Each of these functions has multiple overlapping control systems, so that trophoblast invasion is a finely controlled balance of competing mechanisms.

SPIRAL ARTERIES

Placental bed spiral arteries are muscular arteries, the terminations of uterine radial arteries.[25] A huge increase in blood flow (3.5-fold) through these arteries is required during pregnancy so that the blood supply into the placental intervillous space is adequate to support fetal growth. This is accomplished by the complete remodeling of the spiral artery wall entering the distal segments of these vessels,[21] a process completed at about 20–22 weeks' gestation.[22,26] The local maternal microvascular system vanishes and the remaining upstream arteries, up to the aorta, undergo physiological changes[27] such as an increase in length and circumference in a process known as remodeling. The remodeling leads to the disappearance of the muscle layer of the spiral arteries and the replacement of endothelial cells by endovascular trophoblasts. There is also endothelial swelling causing compensatory hypertrophy of individual smooth muscle cells of the tunica media, and edema and disruption of the vessel architecture.[23] Despite the disruptive nature of this arterial remodeling, which includes the degradation and resynthesis of ECM, there is minimal evidence of cell death or arterial damage.[28] Arterial remodeling is dependent on pregnancy, but not on contact with trophoblast, and has started by 8 weeks of pregnancy at the latest.[29] In vitro, remodeling is more effective if the targets are uterine arteries from pregnant women rather than omental arteries or uterine arteries from non-pregnant women: this suggests a maternofetal dialogue.[26]

Changes in the uterine vasculature are reflected in changes in the blood flow through the uterine arteries. Changes in the blood flow through the uterine arteries can be detected using Doppler ultrasound. Doppler ultrasound can detect different patterns of change during the first trimester of pregnancy. The clinical significance of these changes is discussed elsewhere (see Chapter 00).

HYPOXIA

The placental circulation is not established until 8–12 weeks of pregnancy.[24] This implies that initial trophoblast invasion takes place in an environment with relatively low oxygen tension.[29] There is considerable controversy over whether trophoblast invasiveness is increased or decreased under low oxygen concentrations.[30–33] However, the relatively low levels of oxygen appear to be important. There is evidence that excessive oxygen delivery to the embryo before 12 weeks has an adverse impact.[34]

Uterine artery remodeling is well advanced before blood flow to the placental intervillous space is established. Blood flow to the intervillous space could occur earlier than it does. Between 8 and 12 weeks, uterine arteries could deliver more oxygen than the embryo and placenta could tolerate. The paradox between the timing of arterial remodeling and the apparent lack of damage from excessive exposure to oxygen is resolved by the endovascular EVT. Endovascular EVT forms plugs in the remodeling arteries. These plugs are thought to prevent blood flow in the remodeled arteries until the placenta and fetus are ready to deal with relatively high levels of oxygen.[16] Under this model, successful execution of the pathway that specifies expression of the endovascular trophoblast phenotype at the right time in the right place is essential for successful pregnancy – see Figure 4.2.

The reader should note that the understanding of 'hypoxia' in the literature has changed. Many older papers use the term 'normoxia' to indicate that experiments were performed in room air. 'Hypoxia' was used to indicate that experiments were performed in conditions that involved less ambient oxygen than room air. Work in the late 1990s showed that the normal level of oxygen at the maternofetal interface in early pregnancy is 5–10%.[29] This work led to the appreciation that hypoxia is a relative state: relative to the conditions that would pertain under in-vivo conditions in normal pregnancy. Thus, the focus now is on expressing the actual conditions under which experiments were performed and relating those conditions to estimates of the corresponding in-vivo conditions.[35] However, there are significant technical problems with measuring oxygen tension.[36]

FACTORS DETERMINING CELL FATE IN EVT

As noted above, EVT is a dynamic cell lineage that expresses multiple phenotypes. Coordinated expression of these phenotypes is essential for successful pregnancy and we will now consider factors that regulate the expression of EVT phenotypes.

PROLIFERATION/APOPTOSIS

The proliferative burst occurs early in the EVT lineage. An important feature of the proliferative burst is endoreduplication.[37] Endoreduplication is continued rounds of DNA synthesis without intervening mitoses. The process of trophoblast proliferation is comparable to that of neoplastic tissues, but is one in which the stages are far more stringently regulated.[38]

The control of trophoblast population expansion as trophoblast invasion occurs is likely to involve tumour suppressor genes. We have previously shown that first-trimester EVTs express tumor suppressor genes in a well-defined sequence as they invade the maternal decidua.[39] The most differentiated and furthest invading trophoblast cell type, the multinucleated trophoblast, expresses a combination of genes that may indicate a high apoptotic rate. The co-occurrence of proto-oncogenes and the products of tumor suppressor genes in EVT suggests an important role not only in the negative regulation of cellular invasion but also in population expansion through the presence of oncogenes and antiapoptotic proteins.[39]

Further evidence suggesting a role for apotosis in limiting trophoblast invasion comes from the study of Fas. The Fas ligand (FasL) is a membrane-bound protein that induces apoptosis following interaction with Fas.[40] FasL has been found in trophoblasts in humans[40] and differentiating human cytotrophoblasts in cell culture.[41] Furthermore, apoptosis has been detected in EVT in first-trimester decidual tissue.[42]

DIFFERENTIATION

Proliferation gives way to differentiation and invasion. Differentiation and invasion occur in parallel. Initial invasion of the maternal uterine stroma is controlled by the transcription factor Gcm1.[43] Differentiation is associated with expression of factors such as human leukocyte antigen-G (HLA-G) and hPL and by several other phenotypic changes.

As trophoblast differentiates to the invasive phenotype, its adhesion molecule phenotype changes from epithelial to endothelial.[20] This involves a series of 'integrin switches'. These are regulated by a range of factors, including vascular endothelial growth factor-C (VEGF-C) and placenta growth factor (PlGF), which are secreted by invading trophoblast,[44] by the transforming growth factor-β (TGF-β) family, including endoglin, a component of the TGF-β receptor, and by tumor necrosis factor-α (TNF-α).[45] Acquisition of this endothelial phenotype allows cytotrophoblast to exist in the maternal

uterine vasculature under the guise of normal endothelium or smooth muscle, and is part of the process of arterial remodeling.[46] These integrin switches are modified in cases of pre-eclampsia.[47] This suggests that well-controlled differentiation of EVT is a key feature of normal pregnancy. The integrin switches are less prominent in ectopic pregnancy.[18] This suggests that the local environment contributes to the regulation of EVT differentiation.

MIGRATION

EVTs have been shown, in vitro and in vivo, to be highly migratory,[48] reflected in their decreasing glycogen and lipid (energy) stores as migration continues. Growth factors – e.g. hepatocyte growth factor (HGF), VEGF, and PIGF – have been shown to stimulate EVT motility.[49,50]

ADHERENCE TO AND DIGESTION OF THE EXTRACELLUAR MATRIX

In order to migrate through the ECM, trophoblast cells produce matrix metalloproteinases (MMPs). This family of gelatinase enzymes has the capacity to digest ECMs of host tissues.[51] Specifically, in pregnancy, these enzymes are there to degrade the endometrial basement membranes and the ECM.[52] MMPs are stimulated by interleukin (IL)-1, IL-6, leptin, and TNF-α, all of endometrial origin. Indeed, IL-6 has been shown to be an endometrial regulator of cytotrophoblastic gelatinases.[53] The promoter region of the *MMP-9* gene has two AP-1 binding sites, AP-1 being a transcription factor made up of the *c-fos* and *c-jun* oncogenes. It has therefore been suggested that transactivation of these two oncogenes, and activation of AP-1, promotes the invasive cytotrophoblastic phenotype, inducing the production of MMP-9.[54,55] Another means of control appears to be the presence of GCMa, a transcription factor specific for the placenta and one that is required for placental development.[56]

Stromelysin-3, another MMP, is expressed by differentiated and non-proliferative villous trophoblast and EVT cells in early and late placental beds and villi. Its pattern of expression evolves during pregnancy and there is strong evidence that it could play a role in placentation.[52]

Another regulator of trophoblastic invasion is TGF-β_1,[57] which inhibits the proteolytic activity of cytotrophoblast.[58] It most probably works by inducing multiple independent signals to check the proliferative potential of human trophoblastic cells, facilitating their functional differentiation, although as yet there is no definitive proof that this is the case.

DEFECTIVE EVT INVASION IN ANTIPHOSPHOLIPID SYNDROME

First- and second-trimester miscarriages,[59] pre-eclampsia, and intrauterine growth restriction[60] are more likely in women with antiphospholipid antibodies. In other conditions, antiphospholipid antibodies are associated with a tendency to form blood clots, thrombi, that could compromise pregnancy outcome by occluding placental blood supply. However, examination of placentas and first-trimester decidua from pregnancies in women with antiphospholipid syndrome (APS) has found little evidence of specific thrombotic placental pathology.[61–64] On the other hand, there is evidence that defective trophoblast invasion is an underlying feature of obstetric pathology associated with APS. Defective decidual endovascular trophoblast invasion was the most frequent histological abnormality in APS-associated early pregnancy loss.[63] We have developed a model of EVT function that measures movement and differentiation of freshly isolated EVTs into giant multinuclear cells.[65] We found that antiphospholipid antibodies inhibited EVT function in this model.[65] This was in agreement with other workers who have found a direct effect of antiphospholipid antibodies on in-vitro tropho-blast cell function when using choriocarcinoma cell lines or primary villous trophoblast.[66–70] These findings indicate that a consideration of maternal factors such as APS and smoking,[71] and maternal medication such as heparin[72] or anticonvulsants[73] will be necessary to complement our understanding of the how interactions between mother and off-spring contribute to the events of early pregnancy.

MATERNOFETAL INTERACTION IN THE DECIDUA

The uterine decidua is not necessary to trigger EVT invasion, but is likely to limit its extent and to accelerate the onset of EVT migration.[74] The mechanisms of the interaction between embryo and decidua have been outlined in the preceding paragraphs. Here we focus on cellular aspects of the interface. In the maternal decidua, immunocompetent maternal cells and allogenically different EVTs coexist. The most abundant immunocompetent cells in the maternal decidua are the uterine natural killer (uNK) cells, also known as large granular lymphocytes (LGLs) or CD56+ cells. The origin and function of these cells is unclear.[75]

Increased numbers of uNK cells were found in the preimplantation endometrium of recurrent miscarriage (RM) patients compared with controls.[76,77] Furthermore, uNK cells are more numerous in the decidua from chromosomally abnormal miscarriages than in chromosomally normal miscarriages.[78] There were more activated leukocytes in the decidua taken from the miscarriages of women with unexplained RM and a normal fetal karyotype compared with that taken from women with RM and abnormal fetal karyotype.[79] This, again, suggests different cellular immunity associated with the miscarriage of karyotypically normal and abnormal pregnancies; i.e. uNK cells may have a role in the control of trophoblast invasion and the recognition of normal and abnormal pregnancies.

EVT and uNK cells can directly interact. EVTs do not express standard class I and class II HLA molecules, so that maternal immune cells cannot stage a rejection response as they would to an organ transplant. EVTs do express the class I HLA molecules (HLA-C, HLA-G, and HLA-E), which can be specifically recognized by different receptors on LGLs.[80] The following EVT–uNK, ligand–receptor interactions have been described:

- uNKs express killer immunoglobulin-like receptors (KIR), some of which are inhibitory and some activatory. These KIR recognize HLA-C on fetal EVT, and the repertoire of KIR expressed by decidual uNK is heterogeneous.[81] Therefore, a different KIR repertoire on maternal LGLs may occur in RM. EVTs express both the maternal and paternal allele of HLA-C, and HLA-C expression is up-regulated by interferon-γ (IFN-γ).[80] Thus, HLA-C may vary in normal and pathological pregnancies.
- HLA-G is only expressed by EVT and is thought to have a major role in maternofetal tolerance. HLA-G expression has been reported to be different in normal and pathological pregnancies. HLA-G can be recognized by receptors on uNKs, from the immunoglobulin-like-transcript (ILT) family. ILT2 and 4 are associated with the binding of HLA-G.[80]
- HLA-E expressed by EVT binds to CD94/NKG2 receptors, which are highly expressed on decidual uNKS and mediate inhibition of killing.[80]

Other systems that control the fetal–maternal cellular interaction in the decidua include:

Siglecs

Siglecs are members of the Ig superfamily that bind to sialic acid (Sia) and are mainly expressed by cellular members of the hematopoietic system.[82] Recognition of Sia by Siglecs plays a role in the regulation of the innate immune system.[82] Siglec-6 is expressed predominantly by trophoblast and Siglec-7 has been identified as an inhibitory NK-cell receptor using a redirected killing assay.[82]

Tryptophan metabolism

It has been proposed that, in mice, placental indolamine 2,3-dioxygenase (IDO) metabolizes tryptophan to cause a localized depletion of tryptophan at the site of placentation. This tryptophan depletion is then thought to inhibit T cells and thus prevent them from attacking the invading placenta.[83] In human pregnancy, placental IDO activity can be activated by IFN-γ and inhibited by IL-4.[84]

Corticotropin-releasing hormone

Corticotropin-releasing hormone (CRH) secreted by the trophoblast and decidua in rats promotes blastocyst implantation by killing activated T cells.[85] Furthermore, inhibition of the CRH receptor in pregnant rats reduced the number of implantation sites. CRH is secreted by the human EVT and maternal decidua but its role in human miscarriage has yet to be tested.[85]

Growth factors

Some evidence exists of positive regulatory control by cytokines and growth factors derived from the endometrium;[58] one of these is insulin-like growth factor binding protein-1 (IGFBP-1), the principal secretory product of the decidua. Also involved in positive regulation are insulin-like growth factor II (IGF-II) and uPA.[86]

Some evidence exists to suggest that activation of the thrombin receptor PAR1 (protease activated receptor-1), expressed by invasive EVTs, influences placentation;[87] proteolysis of this receptor enhances normal and pathological cellular invasion.

LOCAL INFLAMMATORY CHANGES

In general terms, inflammation involves three main elements: soluble mediators, cells, and effector mechanisms. Each of these is present at the maternofetal interface in early pregnancy.

SOLUBLE MEDIATORS

A very large number of mediators of inflammation are expressed at the materno–fetal interface.[88] In mice, the maternofetal interface can be neatly summarized by a comparison with cytokine secretion by T-cell subsets, namely Th1 vs Th2. However, in humans this comparison is not complete.[89]

There is some direct evidence that certain cytokines are required for reproductive success, at least in the mouse. One example is leukemia inhibitory factor (LIF), which plays a pivotal role mediating the effects of ovarian hormones on uterus and blastocyst in the mouse: understanding how relevant this is to the human is difficult and requires investigation with multiple techniques.[90] Knockout of the gene for IL-11 receptor-α leads to poor decidualization and reduced implantation.[91] Deleting cytokine genes from mice can have quantitative effects on pregnancy. IL-10 knockout mice show more implantation sites and deliver pups who are heavier at birth,[92] whereas granulocyte–macrophage colony-stimulating factor (GM-CSF) knockout mice deliver pups who are lighter at birth.[93] Other cytokines have not been amenable to study using mouse models. For example, blockade of the IL-1 receptor with a specific antagonist is associated with reduced success of implantation.[94] However, repeated attempts to examine which cytokines are active using gene knockouts in mice have not found a member of the IL-1 family that is essential to implantation, or other aspects of reproductive success.[2] Signaling pathways that are required for implantation include wnt/b-catenin[95] and signal transducer and activation of transcription 3 (Stat 3).[96]

CELLS

The materno–fetal interface expresses a specific array of immune cells. Whereas the predominant decidual leukocyte is the uNK cell (see above), macrophages and T cells are also present, although B cells and granulocytes are normally absent.[97] Cells derived from other lineages (e.g. trophoblast) can express mediators of inflammation so that telling the story of inflammation is likely to be complicated given that multiple regulatory networks are active.

EFFECTOR MECHANISMS

Inflammation involves tissue remodeling and defense against an aggressor. Tissue remodeling is performed by enzymes that act on the ECM. The ECM, in turn, modifies the behavior of the cells embedded in it. The materno–fetal interface expresses a rich array of these enzymes. Mechanisms that are clearly relevant to outcome have been delineated, although it is unclear how important each mechanism is. Defense against aggressors include chemical attack (e.g. complement system) and cellular attack. Trophoblast is resistant to lysis by T cells (antibody and cell-activated), macrophages, and conventional NK cells.[98] However, trophoblast can sustain injury from NK cells stimulated with IL-2.[98] Monocytes stimulated with lipopolysaccharide can induce apoptosis in syncytiotrophoblast, if the syncytiotrophoblast has been primed with IFN-γ.[99]

Complement

Complement is an effector component of the innate immune system. Its regulation is needed to protect tissues from inflammation. Mouse embryos deficient in the complement regulator Crry all died in pregnancy as a result of placental complement activation and inflammation.[100] In humans, complement regulatory proteins CD46, CD55, and CD59 are expressed on trophoblast in the first trimester from both normal and miscarried pregnancies.[101,102]

Implantation is often described as a proinflammatory reaction similar to labor, and in contrast to the maintenance of pregnancy, which is often described as anti-inflammatory. However, the incomplete mapping between events during reproduction and classic inflammation mean that these descriptions are probably more useful in planning research than as analogies to explain what is happening. For example, the concept of the 'fetal allograft' has yielded a fruitful line of research but does not accurately represent events because it does not direct attention to the right cells.[103]

Intrauterine infection may be present during implantation. Evidence of intrauterine infection is associated with reduced rates of implantation during in vitro fertilization (IVF).[104] Thus, as well as negotiating between the maternal and fetal needs, the materno–fetal interface may also be simultaneously fending off exogenous attack.

REVIEW OF METHODS

A review of methods in this area is pertinent for two reasons:

1. In order to make sense of experimental results, it is necessary to have a basic understanding of the experimental methods.
2. Some models are better at identifying hierarchies of molecules (e.g. signaling cascades), whereas other models are better at establishing which molecules are important when there is significant redundancy.[105]

This section will summarize the most popular experimental techniques.

TISSUE CULTURE TECHNIQUES

Culture of first-trimester placental explants has been reviewed recently:[35] production of explants involves dissecting tissue and mounting it in a culture system; characterization involves assessing the viability and determining the nature of the culture material. Seemingly homogeneous placental tissue can yield several different types of explant, e.g. arising from different types of villi. Explants provide the opportunity to explore how phenotypes develop and to investigate the relevance of mechanisms through experimental manipulation. Central to the interpretation of results from explants is an explicit understanding of how experimental conditions relate to the corresponding in-vivo conditions. The conditions of explant culture can yield insights into the biology, e.g. the effect of the matrix for invasion. Explants retain tissue architecture: this is a strength in that cells are likely to retain the influences that act on them in vivo; this is a weakness in that the actions of individual cell types are difficult to isolate. For this reason, tissue culture techniques have traditionally been more useful when identifying the members of molecular ensembles and examining the time-course of coordinated processes.

CELL CULTURE

Cell culture allows reproducible experiments on a single cell line.[106] There is a trade-off between the clarity arising from well-controlled conditions and the ability to generalize. Primary culture is closer to the in-vivo situation and may facilitate generalization but at the price of greater variability between individual preparation. Primary culture of first-trimester EVT is difficult. Models of EVT from third-trimester tissue have been described and have the advantages of availability and the quantity of cells obtained from each individual.[65] Established cell lines offer greater control, but the process of cell immortalization may hinder generalization to the in-vivo situation. Several EVT cell lines have been used, including SGHPL4.[50]

The utility of culture techniques can be enhanced by manipulating the expression of specific genes using transfection (overexpression or antisense) or siRNA. Gene array studies can report the simultaneous expression of many thousands of transcripts. These results will clearly identify members of the molecular ensemble. Moving from catalogues of active genes to mechanistic hierarchies or causal combinations depends upon careful experimental design concerning specific questions about well-defined end points, such as clear-cut clinical events.

Animal models, especially gene knockouts in mice, allow specific genes to be targeted. Results cannot always be generalized, because they vary with the genetic background of the mouse and because of differences between species. Nevertheless, mouse studies can provide important 'proof of concept' concerning specific molecules and can implicate molecules in placental development that would not otherwise be suspected. The effects of gene disruption can be targeted to the embryo only (using tetraploid rescue strategies) and to the placenta (using tissue-specific expression strategies).

RESEARCH DIRECTIONS

In general, our current understanding of implantation and subsequent events provides a descriptive catalogue rather than an explanation of poor outcome or a sound basis to suggest novel interventions. Improved understanding of specific issues can develop from the application of multiple techniques, e.g. LIF.[90]

Each finding discussed in this chapter can be interpreted in multiple ways and could, or could not, relate to clinically important events. This implies that hypothesis-driven work is required to identify how key players fit together and explain differences in outcomes. Sources of mechanistic hypotheses include:

- analogies concerning processes (inflammation/ tumors/transplants/neutrophils)
- analogies involving whole animals (mice, primates, and comparative genomics)
- clinical phenotypes.

Analogies about processes have limitations, e.g. the limitations of transplant rejection as an analogy were noted above. The value of such analogies will lie in their ability to suggest interactions, but the weakness of analogies is that hidden assumptions may facilitate unjustified generalization. It has been suggested that one way to determine whether a process found in well-controlled laboratory conditions can be generalized to other conditions is to examine how common the process is in other species.[107] This approach is in its infancy in reproductive medicine, although a comparative genomic approach has been used to narrow down the possibilities in other disease states that show complex regulatory networks.[108] Clinical phenotypes can yield useful insight, e.g. integrin expression in ectopic pregnancy.[109]

Continuities through pregnancy can offer opportunities and present challenges. Events early in pregnancy appear to be reflected in the histology of term placenta (aberrant trophoblast differentiation, aberrant remodeling of maternal blood vessels). These findings may allow improved understanding of the consequences of events during the first trimester. However, as with all placental studies, difficulties can arise from inconsistent sampling.[110] Some processes are consistently found in complicated pregnancies, no matter what gestational age is sampled. Processes that are found in complicated pregnancies at all gestational ages include infection[111] and aberrant cell kinetics.[112] Processes that extend between pregnancies may yield insights into the events of early pregnancy.[76]

Our current understanding of early pregnancy does not provide reasons why some adverse events occur in some women some of the time. In order to bridge this gap, studies will need to identify sources of variation during early pregnancy (such as gene polymorphisms) and relate these to clear descriptions of clinical events. This implies that the interested clinician can expect a period of observational consolidation before novel interventions can be proposed from a rational basis.

CONCLUSION

Trophoblast invasion is an important determinant of pregnancy outcome and is tightly controlled. Trophoblastic diseases, pre-clampsia, and some unexplained miscarriages could be attributed to the dysfunction of these control processes, the manifestations of which are excessive or insufficient invasion and 'shallow' placenta formation. A more comprehensive understanding of all aspects of trophoblast invasion, particularly at the levels of regulation, would enable the development of interventional methods of treatment. This understanding requires the integration of laboratory results with clinical phenotyping.

REFERENCES

1. Dey SK, Lim H, Das SK et al. Molecular cues to implantation. Endocr Rev 2004; 25:341–373.

2. Stewart CL, Cullinan EB. Preimplantation development of the mammalian embryo and its regulation by growth factors. Dev Genet 1997; 21:91–101.

3. Barnea ER. Insight into early pregnancy events: the emerging role of the embryo. Am J Reprod Immunol 2004; 51:319–322.

4. Genbacev OD, Prakobphol A, Foulk RA et al. Trophoblast L-selectin-mediated adhesion at the maternal–fetal interface. Science 2003; 299:405–408.

5. Aplin JD, Kimber SJ. Trophoblast–uterine interactions at implantation. Reprod Biol Endocrinol 2004; 2:48.

6. Jauniaux E, Hempstock J, Greenwold N, Burton GJ. Trophoblastic oxidative stress in relation to temporal and regional differences in maternal placental blood flow in normal and abnormal early pregnancies. Am J Pathol 2003; 162:115–125.

7. McFadyen IR. Early fetal loss. In: Rodeck, C, ed. Fetal Medicine Oxford: Blackwell Scientific, 1989.

8. Quenby S, Vince G, Farquharson R, Aplin J. Recurrent miscarriage: a defect in nature's quality control? Hum Reprod 2002; 17:1959–1963.

9. Knoeller S, Lim E, Aleta L et al. Distribution of immunocompetent cells in decidua of controlled and uncontrolled (choriocarcinoma/hydatidiform mole) trophoblast invasion. Am J Reprod Immunol 2003; 50:41–47.

10. Aplin JD. The cell biological basis of human implantation. Baillière's Best Pract Res Clin Obstet Gynaecol 2000; 14:757–764.

11. Jones CJ, Fox H. Ultrastructure of the normal human placenta. Electron Microsc Rev 1991; 4:129–178.

12. Meekins JW, Pijnenborg R, Hanssens M, McFadyen IR, Van Asshe A. A study of placental bed spiral arteries and trophoblast invasion in normal and severe pre-eclamptic pregnancies. Br J Obstet Gynaecol 1994; 101:669–674.

13. Benirscke K, Kaufmann P. Pathology of the Human Placenta, 4th edn. Berlin: Springer; 2000.

14. Cross JC. How to make a placenta: mechanisms of trophoblast cell differentiation in mice – a review. Placenta 2005; 26 (Suppl A):S3–9.

15. Constancia M, Hemberger M, Hughes J et al. Placental-specific IGF-II is a major modulator of placental and fetal growth. Nature 2002; 417(6892):945–948.

16. Red-Horse K, Zhou Y, Genbacev O et al. Trophoblast differentiation during embryo implantation and formation of the maternal–fetal interface. J Clin Invest 2004; 114(6):744–754.

17. Aplin JD, Haigh T, Lacey H, Chen CP, Jones CJ. Tissue interactions in the control of trophoblast invasion. J Reprod Fertil Suppl 2000; 55:57–64.

18. Kemp B, Kertschanska S, Kadyrov M et al. Invasive depth of extravillous trophoblast correlates with cellular phenotype: a comparison of intra- and extrauterine implantation sites. Histochem Cell Biol 2002; 117:401–414.

19. Aplin JD, Haigh T, Jones CJ, Church HJ, Vicovac L. Development of cytotrophoblast columns from explanted first-trimester human placental villi: role of fibronectin and integrin alpha5beta1. Biol Reprod 1999; 60:828–838.

20. Damsky CH, Fisher SJ. Trophoblast pseudo-vasculogenesis: faking it with endothelial adhesion receptors. Curr Opin Cell Biol 1998; 10:660–666.

21. Pijnenborg R, Dixon G, Robertson WB, Brosens I. Trophoblastic invasion of human decidua from 8 to 18 weeks of pregnancy. Placenta 1980; 1:3–19.

22. Pijnenborg R, Robertson WB, Brosens I, Dixon G. Review article: trophoblast invasion and the establishment of haemochorial placentation in man and laboratory animals. Placenta 1981; 2:71–91.

23. Pijnenborg R, Bland JM, Robertson WB, Brosens I. Uteroplacental arterial changes related to interstitial trophoblast migration in early human pregnancy. Placenta 1983; 4:397–413.

24. Burton GJ, Jauniaux E, Watson AL. Maternal arterial connections to the placental intervillous space during the first trimester of human pregnancy: the Boyd collection revisited. Am J Obstet Gynecol 1999; 181:718–724.

25. Lyall F. The human placental bed revisited. Placenta 2002; 23: 555–562.

26. Crocker IP, Wareing M, Ferris GR et al. The effect of vascular origin, oxygen, and tumour necrosis factor alpha on trophoblast invasion of maternal arteries in vitro. J Pathol 2005; 206(4):476–485.

27. Moll W. Structure adaptation and blood flow control in the uterine arterial system after hemochorial placentation. Eur J Obstet Gynecol Reprod Biol 2003; 110(Suppl):S19–27.

28. Blankenship TN, Enders AC. Trophoblast cell-mediated modifications to uterine spiral arteries during early gestation in the macaque. Acta Anat (Basel) 1997; 158:227–236.

29. Jauniaux E, Watson A, Burton G. Evaluation of respiratory gases and acid–base gradients in human fetal fluids and uteroplacental tissue between 7 and 16 weeks' gestation. Am J Obstet Gynecol 2001; 184:998–1003.

30. Genbacev O, Zhou Y, Ludlow JW, Fisher SJ. Regulation of human placental development by oxygen tension. Science 1997; 277:1669–1672.

31. Zhou Y, Genbacev O, Damsky CH, Fisher SJ. Oxygen regulates human cytotrophoblast differentiation and invasion: implications for endovascular invasion in normal pregnancy and in pre-eclampsia. J Reprod Immunol 1998; 39:197–213.

32. Perkins J, St John J, Ahmed A. Modulation of trophoblast cell death by oxygen and EGF. Mol Med 2002; 8:847–856.

33. Kilani RT, Mackova M, Davidge ST, Guilbert LJ. Effect of oxygen levels in villous trophoblast apoptosis. Placenta 2003; 24:826–834.

34. Hempstock J, Jauniaux E, Greenwold N, Burton GJ. The contribution of placental oxidative stress to early pregnancy failure. Hum Pathol 2003; 34:1265–1275.

35. Miller RK, Genbacev O, Turner MA et al. Human placental explants in culture: approaches and assessments. Placenta 2005; 26:439–448.

36. Newby D, Marks L, Lyall F. Dissolved oxygen concentration in culture medium: assumptions and pitfalls. Placenta 2005; 26:353–357.

37. Zybina TG, Kaufmann P, Frank HG et al. Genome multiplication of extravillous trophoblast cells in human placenta in the course of differentiation and invasion into endometrium and myometrium. I. Dynamics of polyploidization. Tsitologiia 2002; 44:1058–1067.

38. Bamberger AM, Makrigiannakis A, Roser K et al. Expression of the high-mobility group protein HMGI(Y) in human trophoblast: potential role in trophoblast invasion of maternal tissue. Virchows Arch 2003; 443:649–654.

39. Quenby S, Brazeau C, Drakeley A, Lewis-Jones DI, Vince G. Oncogene and tumour suppressor gene products during trophoblast differentiation in the first trimester. Mol Hum Reprod 1998; 4:477–481.

40. Uckan D, Steele A, Cherry Wang BY et al. Trophoblasts express Fas ligand: a proposed mechanism for immune privilege in placenta and maternal invasion. Mol Hum Reprod 1997; 3:655–662.

41. Runic, R, Lockwood CJ, Ma Y, Dipasquale B, Guller S. Expression of Fas ligand by human cytotrophoblasts: implications in placentation and fetal survival. J Clin Endocrinol Metab 1996; 81:3119–3122.

42. von Rango U, Krusche CA, Kertschanska S et al. Apoptosis of extravillous trophoblast cells limits the trophoblast invasion in uterine but

not in tubal pregnancy during first trimester. Placenta 2003; 24:929–940.

43. Baczyk D, Satkunaratnam A, Nait-Oumesmar B et al. Complex patterns of GCM1 mRNA and protein in villous and extravillous trophoblast cells of the human placenta. Placenta 2004; 25: 553–559.

44. Zhou Y, Bellingard V, Feng KT, McMaster M, Fisher SJ. Human cytotrophoblasts promote endothelial survival and vascular remodeling through secretion of Ang2, PlGF, and VEGF-C. Dev Biol 2003; 263:114–125.

45. Fukushima K, Miyamoto S, Komatsu H et al. TNFalpha-induced apoptosis and integrin switching in human extravillous trophoblast cell line. Biol Reprod 2003; 68:1771–1778.

46. Zhou Y, Damsky CH, Fisher SJ. Preeclampsia is associated with failure of human cytotrophoblasts to mimic a vascular adhesion phenotype. One cause of defective endovascular invasion in this syndrome? J Clin Invest 1997; 99:2152–2164.

47. Zhou Y, Fisher SJ, Janatpour M et al. Human cytotrophoblasts adopt a vascular phenotype as they differentiate. A strategy for successful endovascular invasion? J Clin Invest 1997; 99:2139–2151.

48. Genbacev O, Jensen KD, Powlin SS, Miller RK. In vitro differentiation and ultrastructure of human extravillous trophoblast (EVT) cells. Placenta 1993; 14:463–475.

49. Lash GE, Cartwright JE, Whitley GS, Trew AJ, Baker PN. The effects of angiogenic growth factors on extravillous trophoblast invasion and motility. Placenta 1999; 20:661–667.

50. Cartwright JE, Tse WK, Whitley GS. Hepatocyte growth factor induced human trophoblast motility involves phosphatidylinositol-3-kinase, mitogen-activated protein kinase, and inducible nitric oxide synthase. Exp Cell Res 2002; 279:219–226.

51. Bischof P, Campana A. Molecular mediators of implantation. Baillières Best Pract Res Clin Obstet Gynaecol 2000; 14:801–814.

52. Maqoui E, Polette M, Nawrocki B et al. Expression of stromelysin-3 in the human placenta and placental bed. Placenta 1997; 18:277–285.

53. Meisser A, Cameo P, Islami D, Campana A, Bischof P. Effects of interleukin-6 (IL-6) on cytotrophoblastic cells. Mol Hum Reprod 1999; 5:1055–1058.

54. Bischof P, Truong K, Campana A. Regulation of trophoblastic gelatinases by proto-oncogenes. Placenta 2003; 24:155–163.

55. Peters TJ, Albieri A, Bevilacqua E et al. Differentiation-dependent expression of gelatinase B/matrix metalloproteinase-9 in trophoblast cells. Cell Tissue Res 1999; 295:287–296.

56. Yu C, Shen K, Lin M et al. GCMa regulates the syncytin-mediated trophoblastic fusion. J Biol Chem 2002; 277:50062–50068.

57. Rama, S, Suresh Y, Rao AJ. TGF beta1 induces multiple independent signals to regulate human trophoblastic differentiation: mechanistic insights. Mol Cell Endocrinol 2003; 206:123–136.

58. Bischof P, Meisser A, Campana A. Mechanisms of endometrial control of trophoblast invasion. J Reprod Fertil Suppl 2000; 55:65–71.

59. Lockshin MD, Qamar T, Druzin ML, Goei S. Antibody to cardiolipin, lupus anticoagulant, and fetal death. J Rheumatol 1987; 14:259–262.

60. Backos M, Rai R, Baxter N et al. Pregnancy complications in women with recurrent miscarriage associated with antiphospholipid antibodies treated with low dose aspirin and heparin. Br J Obstet Gynaecol 1999; 106:102–107.

61. Salafia CM, Cowcock FS. Placental pathology and antiphospholipid syndrome: a descriptive study. Am J Perinatol 1997; 14:435–441.

62. Salafia CM, Parke AL. Placental pathology in systemic lupus erythematosus and phospholipid antibody-syndrome. Clin Rheum Dis 1997; 23:85–97.

63. Sebire NJ, Fox H, Backos M et al. Defective endovascular trophoblast invasion in primary antiphospholipid antibody syndrome-associated early pregnancy failure. Hum Reprod 2002; 17:1067–1071.

64. Sebire NJ, Backos M, El Gaddal S, Goldin RD, Regan L. Placental pathology antiphospholipid antibodies and pregnancy outcome in recurrent miscarriage patients. Obstet Gynecol 2003; 101:258–263.

65. Quenby S, Mountfield S, Cartwright JE et al. Antiphospholipid antibodies prevent extravillous trophoblast differentiation. Fertil Steril 2005; 83:691–698.

66. Rote NS, Chang J, Katsuragawa H et al. Expression of phosphatidylserine-dependent antigens on the surface of differentiating BeWo human choriocarcinoma cells. Am J Reprod Immunol 1995; 33:14–21.

67. Katsuragawa H, Kanzaki H, Inoue T et al. Monoclonal antibody against phosphatidylserine inhibits in vitro human trophoblastic hormone production and invasion. Biol Reprod 1997; 56:50–58.

68. Chamley LW, Duncalf AM, Mitchell MD, Johnson PM. Action of anti-cardiolipin and antibodies to beta2-glycoprotein-I on trophoblast proliferation as a mechanism for fetal death. Lancet 1998; 352:1037–1038.

69. Di Simone N, Ferrazzani S, Castellani R et al. Heparin and low-dose aspirin restore placental human chorionic gonadotrophin secretion abolished by antiphospholipid antibody-containing sera. Hum Reprod 1997; 12:2061–2065.

70. Di Simone N, Caliandro D, Castellani R et al. Low-molecular weight heparin restore in-vitro trophoblast invasiveness and differentiation in presence of immunoglobulin G fractions obtained from patients with antiphospholipid syndrome. Hum Reprod 1999; 14:489–495.

71. Genbacev O, McMaster MT, Lazic J et al. Concordant in situ and in vitro data show that maternal cigarette smoking negatively regulates placental cytotrophoblast passage through the cell cycle. Reprod Toxicol 2000; 14:495–506.

72. Quenby S, Mountfield S, Cartwright JE, Whitley GS, Vince G. Effects of low-molecular-weight and unfractionated heparin on trophoblast function. Obstet Gynecol 2004; 104:354–361.

73. Quenby S, Amin S, Bates M, Neilson J, Vince G. The effect of anti-epileptic drugs on trophoblast function. Placenta 2005; 26:A65.

74. Goffin F, Munaut C, Malassine A et al. Evidence of a limited contribution of maternofetal interactions to trophoblast differentiation along the invasive pathway. Tissue Antigens 2003; 62:104–116.

75. Trundley A, Moffett A. Human uterine leukocytes and pregnancy. Tissue Antigens 2004; 63:1–12.

76. Quenby S, Bates M, Doig T et al. Pre-implantation endometrial leukocytes in women with recurrent miscarriage. Hum Reprod 1999; 14:2386–2391.

77. Clifford K, Flanagan AM, Regan L. Endometrial CD56+ natural killer cells in women with recurrent miscarriage: a histomorphometric study. Hum Reprod 1999; 14:2727–2730.

78. Yamamoto T, Takahashi Y, Kase N, Mori H. Role of decidual natural killer (NK) cells in patients with missed abortion: differences between cases with normal and abnormal chromosome. Clin Exp Immunol 1999; 116:449–452.

79. Quack KC, Vassiliadou N, Pudney J, Anderson DJ, Hill JA. Leukocyte activation in the decidua of chromosomally normal and abnormal fetuses from women with recurrent abortion. Hum Reprod 2001; 16:949–955.

80. King A, Burrows TD, Hiby SE et al. Surface expression of HLA-C antigen by human extravillous trophoblast. Placenta 2000; 21:376–387.

81. Loke YW, King A. Decidual natural-killer-cell interaction with trophoblast: cytolysis or cytokine production? Biochem Soc Trans 2000; 28:196–198.

82. Crocker PR, Varki A. Siglecs, sialic acids and innate immunity. Trends Immunol 2001; 22:337–342.

83. Munn DH, Zhou M, Attwood JT et al. Prevention of allogeneic fetal rejection by tryptophan catabolism. Science 1998; 281:1191–1193.

84. Kudo Y, Boyd CA, Sargent IL, Redman CW. Tryptophan degradation by human placental indoleamine 2,3-dioxygenase regulates lymphocyte proliferation. J Physiol 2001; 535:207–215.

85. Makrigiannakis A, Zoumakis E, Kalantaridou S et al. Corticotropin-releasing hormone promotes blastocyst implantation and early maternal tolerance. Nat Immunol 2001; 2:1018–1024.

86. Lala PK, Chakraborty C. Factors regulating trophoblast migration and invasiveness: possible derangements contributing to pre-eclampsia and fetal injury. Placenta 2003; 24:575–587.

87. O'Brien PJ, Koi H, Parry S et al. Thrombin receptors and protease-activated receptor-2 in human placentation: receptor activation mediates extravillous trophoblast invasion in vitro. Am J Pathol 2003; 163:1245–1254.

88. Saito S. Cytokine network at the feto–maternal interface. J Reprod Immunol 2000; 47:87–103.

89. Sacks GP, Redman CW, Sargent IL. Monocytes are primed to produce the Th1 type cytokine IL-12 in normal human pregnancy: an intracellular flow cytometric analysis of peripheral blood mononuclear cells. Clin Exp Immunol 2003; 131:490–497.

90. Kimber SJ. Leukaemia inhibitory factor in implantation and uterine biology. Reproduction 2005; 130:131–145.

91. Robb L, Dimitriadis E, Li R, Salamonsen LA. Leukemia inhibitory factor and interleukin-11: cytokines with key roles in implantation. J Reprod Immunol 2002; 57(1–2):129–141.

92. White CA, Johansson M, Roberts CT, Ramsay AJ, Robertson SA. Effect of interleukin-10 null mutation on maternal immune response and reproductive outcome in mice. Biol Reprod 2004; 70:123–131.

93. Robertson SA, O'Connell A, Pensa K, Ramsay A. Impaired implantation, fetal development and parturition in interleukin-6 deficient mice. Am J Reprod Immunol 2001; 46:69.

94. Simon C, Frances A, Piquette GN et al. Embryonic implantation in mice is blocked by interleukin-1 receptor antagonist. Endocrinology 1994; 134(2):521–528.

95. Mohamed OA, Jonnaert M, Labelle-Dumais C et al. Uterine Wnt/beta-catenin signaling is required for implantation. Proc Natl Acad Sci USA 2005; 102(24):8397–8398.

96. Catalano RD, Johnson MH, Campbell EA et al. Inhibition of Stat3 activation in the endometrium prevents implantation: a nonsteroidal approach to contraception. Proc Natl Acad Sci USA 2005; 102(24):8585–8590.

97. Vince G, Johnson P. Leucocyte populations and cytokine regulation in human uteroplacental tissues. Biochem Soc Trans 2000; 28:191–195.

98. Arck P, Dietl J, Clark D. From the decidual cell internet: trophoblast-recognizing T cells. Biol Reprod 1999; 60(2):227–233.

99. Garcia-Lloret MI, Winkler-Lowen B, Guilbert LJ. Monocytes adhering by LFA-1 to placental syncytiotrophoblasts induce local apoptosis via release of TNF-alpha. A model for hematogenous initiation of placental inflammations. J Leukoc Biol 2000; 68(6):903–908.

100. Xu C, Mao D, Holers VM et al. A critical role for murine complement regulator crry in fetomaternal tolerance. Science 2000; 287:498–501.

101. Hill JA, Melling GC, Johnson PM. Immunohistochemical studies of human uteroplacental tissues from first-trimester spontaneous abortion. Am J Obstet Gynecol 1995; 173:90–96.

102. Nishikori K, Noma J, Hirakawa S, Amano T, Kudo T. The change of membrane complement regulatory protein in chorion of early pregnancy. Clin Immunol Immunopathol 1993; 69:167–174.

103. Moffett A, Loke YW. The immunological paradox of pregnancy: a reappraisal. Placenta 2004; 25(1):1–8.

104. Kamiyama S, Teruya Y, Nohara M, Kanazawa K. Impact of detection of bacterial endotoxin in menstrual effluent on the pregnancy rate in in vitro fertilization and embryo transfer. Fertil Steril 2004; 82:788–792.

105. Paria BC, Reese J, Das SK, Dey SK. Deciphering the cross-talk of implantation: advances and challenges. Science 2002; 296(5576):2185–2188.

106. Sullivan MH. Endocrine cell lines from the placenta. Mol Cell Endocrinol 2004; 228:103–119.

107. Paulesu L, Romagnoli R, Bigliardi E. Materno–fetal immunotolerance: is interleukin-1 a fundamental mediator in placental viviparity? Dev Comp Immunol 2005; 29:409–415.

108. Emison ES, McCallion AS, Kashuk CS et al. A common sex-dependent mutation in a RET enhancer underlies Hirschsprung disease risk. Nature 2005; 434(7035):857–863.

109. Kemp B, Kertschanska S, Kadyrov M et al. Invasive depth of extravillous trophoblast correlates with cellular phenotype: a comparison of intra- and extrauterine implantation sites. Histochem Cell Biol 2002; 117(5):401–414.

110. Redline RW, Boyd T, Campbell V et al. Maternal vascular underperfusion: nosology and reproducibility of placental reaction patterns. Pediatr Dev Pathol 2004; 7(3):237–249.

111. Romero R, Espinoza J, Mazor M. Can endometrial infection/inflammation explain implantation failure, spontaneous abortion, and preterm birth after in vitro fertilization? Fertil Steril 2004; 82(4):799–804.

112. Crocker IP, Tansinda DM, Baker PN. Altered cell kinetics in cultured placental villous explants in pregnancies complicated by pre-eclampsia and intrauterine growth restriction. J Pathol 2004; 204(1):11–18.

5. Inflammation and recurrent pregnancy loss

Susan Laird and Tin-Chiu Li

INTRODUCTION

Recurrent miscarriage (RM) is defined as the loss of three or more consecutive pregnancies in the first trimester of pregnancy. It occurs in approximately 0.5–3% of women. The etiology of repeated pregnancy loss is multifactorial and includes coagulation defects, autoimmune disorders, endocrine disorders, uterine structure anomalies, endometrial defects, and parental and fetal chromosomal abnormalities.[1] The etiology in approximately 50% of cases is unknown, but it has been postulated that a proportion of these repeated pregnancy losses may be due to immune causes.

In general, inflammation may be a consequence of either infection or an autoimmune process. During pregnancy the implanting embryo may evoke an inflammatory response in the endometrium. Miscarriage may occur as a consequence of an abnormal inflammatory response secondary to infection, autoimmune disease, or an abnormal response to implantation. During the first trimester of pregnancy, ascending infection is a rare cause of miscarriage. Severe systemic infection, including several viral infections such as rubella, toxoplasmosis, and cytomegalovirus infection in the first trimester, may also result in miscarriage, although the likelihood of miscarriage following these viral infections is not high. Whereas infection may occasionally cause miscarriage, it is most unusual for it to be a cause of recurrent miscarriage. On the other hand, abnormal inflammation resulting in RM is far more likely to be a consequence of autoimmune disease or an abnormal implantation response.

During pregnancy the female reproductive tract is exposed to paternal antigens expressed in tissue of the developing fetus. This would normally result in a maternal immune response and destruction of the 'foreign' tissue. In successful pregnancies this obviously does not occur. Although the mechanisms which prevent this are not clearly understood, it is postulated that one reason for recurrent pregnancy loss may be the breakdown in these protective mechanisms.

MODELS USED TO STUDY RECURRENT MISCARRIAGE

In women with RM, pregnancy loss usually occurs during the first trimester. Obtaining placental tissue, prior to the recognition of the pregnancy loss, at this time in human pregnancy is obviously not possible and therefore the mechanisms of abnormal development postulated to occur in pregnancies destined to miscarry are difficult to study. Various alternative approaches have been adopted to study the role of factors in the etiology of recurrent miscarriage. These include the analysis of immune cell populations and cytokines in:

- the peripheral blood of women who suffer RM and normal fertile women either before pregnancy or at the time of miscarriage[2,3]
- endometrial tissue obtained from women with RM and normal fertile women in the peri-implantation period in the non-pregnant state[4,5]
- placental tissue obtained at the time of miscarriage from women with a history of RM, from women with a spontaneous, non-recurrent miscarriage, and from women requesting terminations of normal pregnancy.[6,7]

Whereas the study of placental tissue might appear to be the best approach, there are difficulties, particularly with respect to factors involved in inflammatory processes, in determining whether observed differences are due to proinflammatory events as a consequence of the miscarriage. More recently, comparisons have been made between placental tissue from women with unexplained RM with chromosomally normal and abnormal fetuses;[8,9] as both these groups of women have undergone similar miscarriage events, differences observed in the women with normal fetuses may be of more use in gaining an understanding of the mechanism of repeated miscarriage. However, even in this case, the differences seen may result from different mechanisms of miscarriage resulting from embryonically driven and maternally driven causes and a molecule or cell that is important in both causes would be missed.

RECURRENT MISCARRIAGE AND ABNORMAL EMBRYO IMPLANTATION

Embryo implantation is a highly invasive process. It involves attachment of the embryo to the luminal surface of the endometrial epithelium via its trophectoderm. The embryo then passes through this epithelial layer and embeds itself in the underlying stroma. The trophoblast cells differentiate into a number of different cell types. Villous cytotrophoblast cells invade the maternal blood supply and fuse to form syncytiotrophoblast. Extravillous trophoblast cells are present in the maternal decidua and form two types: non-invasive anchoring cell columns and invasive villous cytotrophoblast cells which migrate out from these columns through the maternal decidua. During early pregnancy, interactions between maternal and fetal cells will occur in two compartments:

- between the fetal cytotrophoblast cells and maternal decidual cells
- between the fetal syncytiotrophoblast cells and the maternal blood supply.

Interactions between the fetal cytotrophoblast cells and the maternal decidual cells are thought to be important in controlling the invasiveness of the cytotrophoblast cells. Abnormal control of embryo implantation can lead to a number of disorders. Increased invasiveness results in placenta acreta (invasion through to the myometrium) and preeclampsia. Recurrent pregnancy loss may be due to abnormal fetoplacental development, a consequence of decreased invasiveness or detrimental interactions between the maternal decidua and fetal trophoblast cells.

CYTOKINES AND RECURRENT MISCARRIAGE

Cytokines have traditionally been divided into families dependent upon the immune cell of origin and the immunological effects that they bring about. CD4+ T helper (Th) cells are the major immune cells involved in cytokine production and these can be divided into three functional subsets based on their cytokine production. Th1 cells produce interferon-γ (IFN-γ), interleukin-2 (IL-2), and tumor necrosis factor-β (TNF-α/β), and these are the main effectors of cell-mediated immune responses. Th2 cells produce IL-4, IL-5, IL-6, and IL-10, and these are the main effectors of antibody-mediated humoral responses. The third T helper cell population are Th0 cells which are precursor cells which can be converted to either Th1- or Th2-type cells and can produce both Th1 and Th2 cytokines as well as TNF-α and granulocyte–macrophage colony-stimulating factor (GM-CSF).

Th1 AND Th2 CYTOKINES AND RECURRENT MISCARRIAGE

Studies in rodents carried out in the early 1990s provided strong evidence that successful pregnancy outcome is associated with a predominant Th2 cytokine profile and that Th1 cytokines are detrimental to pregnancy outcome.[10] These studies were carried out on matings between 2 specific strains of mice that have been used extensively in the study of repeated pregnancy loss. Matings between CBA/J female and DBA/2 male mice result in a high number of abortions, whereas matings between CBA/J and BALC/C mice result in normal pregnancy outcomes. Placental production of the Th1 cytokines IFN-γ, TNF-α and IL-2 is greater in the CBA/J $\times$ DBA/2 mice than in the CBA/J $\times$ BALB/C mice and peripheral blood lymphocytes from the abortion-prone mice produce more IFN-γ, TNF-α, and IL-2 when challenged than similarly challenged cells from the non-abortion-prone mice. Injection of TNF-α, IFN-γ, or IL-2 into non-abortion-prone mice results in increased abortion rates,[10] whereas injection of IL-10 (a Th2 cytokine) into abortion-prone mice decreases abortion rates.[11] These results are summarized in Figure 5.1.

More recently, however, many investigators (including one of the original contributors) have questioned the validity of such a simple hypothesis, even in animals.[12] They point out that injection of IL-10 in a series of non-abortion-prone matings has no effect on pregnancy outcome. In addition, experiments with IL-10 and IL-4 double-deficient mice have shown that neither maternal nor fetoplacental deficiency of these cytokines is crucial for fetal or neonatal survival,[13] thus suggesting that the results of the original experiments were dependent on the strain of mice used. However, the simplicity of the original hypothesis was attractive to many investigators and has led to numerous studies in humans.

Th1 AND Th2 CYTOKINES IN HUMANS

The observation that cell-mediated autoimmune diseases such as rheumatoid arthritis, which are

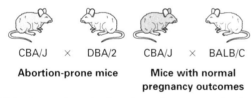

| CBA/J | × | DBA/2 | CBA/J | × | BALB/C |

Abortion-prone mice   **Mice with normal pregnancy outcomes**

High placental production of IL-2, IFN-γ, and TNF-α

Low placental production of IL-2, IFN-γ, and TNF-α

Production of IL2-, IFN-γ, and TNF-α by stimulated peripheral blood leukocytes

Low production of IL-2, IFN-γ, and TNF-α stimulated peripheral blood leukocytes

Injection of IL-10 decreases abortion rate

Injection of IL-2, IFN-γ, and TNF-α increases abortion rate

Figure 5.1 Summary of experiments in abortion-prone and normal mice, providing evidence for a role for Th1 and Th2 cytokines in pregnancy outcome.

driven by a Th1 cytokine response, are ameliorated during pregnancy, while antibody-mediated diseases such as malaria or systemic lupus erythematosus (driven by a Th2 cytokine response) are increased, suggests that pregnancy results in an increase in the ratios of Th2/Th1 cytokines.[10] Direct support for this observation has come from a recent study that showed increased production of IL-10 and IL-4 and decreased production of IFN-γ and TNF-α by stimulated peripheral blood mononuclear cells (PBMCs) from pregnant women compared with non-pregnant women.[14]

The evidence supporting a role for Th2 cytokines in preventing pregnancy loss in humans is more controversial. Studies from one group have shown that PBMCs obtained from women with unexplained RM at the time of miscarriage and stimulated with trophoblast cell extracts produce decreased amounts of IL-6 and IL-10 and increased amounts of IFN-γ compared with stimulated PBMCs obtained at the time of delivery in fertile women with no history of RM.[3] They have also shown decreased production of IL-4, IL-5, IL-6, and IL-10, and increased production of IFN-γ, IL-2, TNF-α, and TNF-β, by PMA (phorbol 12-myristate 13-acetate)-stimulated PBMCs obtained from women with RM at the time of miscarriage compared with stimulated PBMCs obtained during the first trimester of ongoing pregnancies in fertile women.[15] However, these studies involved comparing results from blood samples taken with and without miscarriage and at different times during pregnancy, both of which are likely to affect cytokine production.

Other studies on samples taken either from non-pregnant women, or from pregnant women prior to miscarriage, have also produced conflicting results. PBMCs taken before pregnancy from women with RM produce TNF-α and IFN-γ in response to stimulation from trophoblast cell extracts, whereas cells from non-pregnant fertile women and men produce IL-10 in response to incubation with trophoblast cell extracts. This abnormal Th-1 type response is not seen in women with RM with chromosomally abnormal fetuses or in women with a uterine structural abnormality.[2] Unstimulated

PBMCs isolated from non-pregnant women with unexplained RM have also been shown to produce more IL-2 than either unstimulated PBMCs from women with no history of reproductive failure or normal males.[16] Two other studies have shown increased production of IFN-γ by stimulated PBMCs[17] or increased plasma levels[18] in non-pregnant RM women compared with non-pregnant controls. In addition, increased levels of IFN-γ during the first trimester of pregnancy in RM women who subsequently miscarried were seen compared with pregnant fertile women.[19] Another study has shown opposite effects, with increased IL-4 and IL-10 and decreased IFN-γ and TNF-α production by stimulated PMBCs taken from RM women during early pregnancy (prior to miscarriage) compared with samples taken from gestationally age-matched fertile women.[14]

The differences in these results may be due to whether the cytokine is measured directly in plasma, or after incubation of unstimulated or stimulated peripheral blood cells. Levels of cytokines in the plasma are very low and are near the detection limit for most of the assays used, which is why there is a tendency to use incubated cells. However, the levels in the plasma may better reflect the biological potential of the cytokine.

The numbers of peripheral blood CD4+ and CD8+ T cells producing Th1 and Th2 cytokines has also been compared in RM and control women. Increased ratios of TNF-α/IL-10- and TNF-α/IL-4-producing CD4+ T cells and an increase in the ratio of TNF-α/IL-4-producing CD8+ cells in blood taken prior to pregnancy from women with RM compared with controls has been reported,[20] although when the individual cell numbers are considered (rather than the ratio of cells) the only difference seen was a small decrease in IL-10-producing CD8+ cells in women with RM. In another study, no differences were seen in the number of CD4+ or CD8+ IL-4-, IL-10-, TNF-α-, or IFN-γ-producing cells in blood from RM and control women taken during the first trimester of pregnancy.[21]

These previous studies have concentrated on levels of cytokines in the maternal blood. Although

these cytokines will have access to the syncytiotrophoblast, they will have less access to the villous and extravillous trophoblast cells than cytokines produced by placental cells. However, there are very few reports of studies on the production of cytokines by fetoplacental cell populations in women with RM, probably because of the difficulties in obtaining the required tissue. Differences in Th1 and Th2 cytokine production by T-cell clones derived from the decidua of RM women and decidua from women undergoing terminations have been reported.[7] Significantly lower levels of IL-4 and IL-10 were produced by isolated decidual CD4+ and CD8+ T-cell clones obtained during miscarriage from RM women after stimulation with PMA and CD3 antibody compared with stimulated CD4+ and CD8+ clones isolated from decidua from women undergoing terminations. However, these cells underwent considerable in-vitro manipulations (cloning and artificial stimulation) before cytokine measurement. In addition, the T-cell population from which these clones were derived only makes up a small percentage of cytokine-producing cells in the decidua.

Th1 and Th2 cytokine mRNA expression in the endometrium of normal fertile women and RM women during the peri-implantation phase of the menstrual cycle has also been investigated.[5] This study showed that fewer women with RM had detectable levels of IL-6 in their endometrium, but more had detectable levels of TNF-β, IFN-γ, IL-2, and IL-12, compared with fertile women. In this study, mRNA was extracted from intact endometrial biopsies, so that levels will reflect cytokine production by all endometrial cells, including stromal and epithelial cells. Other studies have shown a decrease in the number of IFN-γ- and TNF-α-producing CD4+ cells in the endometrium of women with RM compared with controls.[22] In this study, only CD4+ cells were considered. Cytokines are produced by many other cells in the endometrium, and this might account for the differences in the results seen.

Various studies have been carried out comparing the genotype and allele distributions of gene polymorphisms for the Th1 and Th2 cytokines in RM and control women. The rationale for such studies is that the presence of a particular genotype may influence the production and levels of that cytokine in the body. Once again, the results of these studies have been inconclusive. No significant associations have been found between RM and alleles at the −308 and −863 positions of the *TNF-α* gene[23–25] or between RM and the variable number of tandem repeat polymorphism in the *IL-4* gene.[26] Some studies have shown an increased frequency of allele T at +874 of the IFN-γ gene,[23,27] whereas others have shown no difference.[25] Similarly, for IL-10, one study has shown increased frequency of the G/G genotype at the −1082 position of the *IL-10* gene,[23] whereas others have shown no differences in RM women.[25,27]

PROINFLAMMATORY CYTOKINES

The proinflammatory family of cytokines includes IL-1, TNF-α, IL-6, and LIF. There is considerable confusion in the literature about the role of this family of cytokines in implantation and placental development. Many authors have suggested that all proinflammatory cytokines are detrimental to pregnancy outcome. However, many studies have shown that leukemia inhibitory factor (LIF) is not detrimental to pregnancy outcome (see later section), and IL-6 has been considered as a Th2 cytokine in some studies. There is also considerable evidence supporting a role for IL-1 in implantation and placental development. This further illustrates the need to extend our thinking beyond the constraints of the Th1/Th2 hypothesis.

IL-1

Several studies have suggested the importance of IL-1 in reproduction. Addition of IL-1 receptor antagonist (IL-1ra), which prevents IL-1 binding to its receptor, to mice prevents blastocyst implantation.[28] IL-1β and IL-1ra are produced by the human endometrium and blastocyst.[29] IL-1 receptors are present on endometrial and trophoblast cells and IL-1 has been shown to stimulate production of factors known to be important in the implantation process, such as matrix metalloproteinases,[30] integrins,[29] and other cytokines such as LIF.[31]

Numerous studies have investigated the presence of various *IL-1* gene polymorphisms in women with recurrent miscarriage; these are summarized in Table 5.1. Many of these polymorphisms have been associated with proinflammatory diseases and are thought to affect IL-1 production.[32] Although some studies have shown differences in allele and genotype distributions in RM women, overall there is no consistent pattern. Moreover, the study by Helfer et al[33] showed no correlation between serum IL-1β levels and the G/A +3594 *IL1-β* polymorphisms in either normal fertile or women with RM, suggesting that the polymorphism has little effect on IL-1β production in vivo.

Decreased expression of IL-1β protein and mRNA in the endometrium of non-pregnant RM women has also been shown.[38]

Table 5.1 Comparison of polymorphisms of the *IL-1* family of genes in women with recurrent miscarriage (RM) and controls

Gene	Polymorphism	Result	Reference
IL-1β	G/A at +3594 in exon 5	No difference	24, 33, 34
IL-1β	C/T at −511 in promoter	Increased frequency of C in RM women	34
IL-1β	C/T at −511 in promoter	No difference	35
IL-1β	C/T at −31 in promoter	Increased frequency of T in RM women	34
IL-1RN	Tandem repeat in intron 2	Increased frequency of 2 repeats in RM women	36
IL-1RN	Tandem repeat in intron 2	No difference	34
IL-1RN	Tandem repeat in intron 2	Increased frequency of 5 repeats in RM women	37

LIF AND IL-11

LIF and IL-11 belong to the same family of cytokines which also includes IL-6. These cytokines share a similar structure, but also act via receptors that use gp130 to signal within the cell and thus might be expected to have similar effects on cell function.

Studies in mice have suggested the importance of LIF and IL-11 in successful pregnancy outcome.[39,40] Implantation does not occur in LIF knockout mice, although transfer of homozygous LIF-negative blastocysts to pseudopregnant, wild-type mice results in normal implantation and pregnancy outcome.[39] Female mice with either an inactive or null mutation for the IL-11 receptor α chain (IL-11Rα) are fertile and their blastocysts implant. However, only small decidua form and then subsequently degrade to result in pregnancy loss.[40] Decreased expression of LIF in the endometrium of non-pregnant RM women has been shown,[41] and isolated decidual CD4+ T-cell clones obtained during miscarriage from RM women after stimulation with PMA and CD3 antibody produced less LIF than similarly stimulated CD4+ T-cell clones from women undergoing terminations,[42] suggesting that LIF may be important in preventing pregnancy loss. In contrast, other studies have shown that high levels of endometrial LIF are associated with pregnancy failure after in vitro fertilization (IVF).[43] However, in this study, LIF was measured in endometrial flushings obtained on day 26 of the menstrual cycle, which is at a time when LIF levels are normally decreasing;[31] therefore, high LIF may indicate endometrial dysfunction, and this may be the cause of unsuccessful pregnancy outcome. Despite the similarity between the pregnancy outcomes in the IL-11Rα knockout mice and women with recurrent miscarriage, there are few studies looking at IL-11 in women with RM. One study has shown decreased expression of epithelial cell IL-11, but not IL-11Rα in the endometrium of RM women compared with controls.[44]

IL-18 AND IL-12

IL-18 is a proinflammatory cytokine with structural similarities with the IL-1 family of proteins. It functions to promote a Th1 response through induction of IFN-γ production. High levels were therefore expected to be associated with pregnancy loss. However, studies in mice have shown that the placentas from abortion-prone matings (CBA/J × DBA/2) produce less IL-18 than those from non-abortion-prone matings (CBA/J × BALB/C).[12] Studies in women have suggested that abnormal endometrial expression of IL-18 is associated with infertility[45] and that plasma levels of IL-18 are lower in non-pregnant women with RM than in non-pregnant fertile women.[18] However, in another study by the same group, serum levels of IL-18 during the first trimester of pregnancy were higher in RM women who subsequently miscarried than in those who had a live birth.[19]

IL-12 is another proinflammatory cytokine that is thought to be detrimental to pregnancy outcome, by increasing Th1 cytokine (particularly IFN-γ) production. IL-12 is produced by the murine fetal placental unit, and coinjection of IL-12 and IL-18 into mice induces abortion.[12] Abnormal endometrial IL-12 production is also associated with infertility.[43] Higher plasma levels of IL-12 have also been shown in non-pregnant RM women compared with controls,[18] whereas another study has shown increased levels of IL-12 in RM women who subsequently miscarried compared with fertile pregnant women.[19] By contrast, a study from a different group has shown no differences between serum IL-12 levels in women undergoing terminations and those undergoing spontaneous miscarriage, and IL-12 production by both peripheral and decidual mononuclear cells was decreased in the women undergoing spontaneous abortion.[46]

OTHER CYTOKINES

Studies using knockout mice have also suggested that GM-CSF and colony-stimulating factor-1 (CSF-1; also known as M-CSF) are important in successful pregnancy outcome.[47,48] Implantation is compromised in CSF-1 mutant mice (op/op mice), which have both a lower rate of implantation and fetal viability, both of which are restored to normal by administration of exogenous CSF-1.[47] Decreased CSF-1 production by PMA and CD3 antibody-stimulated decidual CD4+ T-cell clones obtained during miscarriage from women with RM compared with similarly stimulated decidual CD4+ clones from women undergoing terminations has also been reported.[42] Abnormal placental function and development have also been reported in GM-CSF deficient mice,[48] and a recent study has suggested that there is an increase in plasma GM-CSF levels during pregnancy in normal fertile women, but that this increase is not seen in women with RM.[49]

Plasma levels of transforming growth factor-β_1 (TGF-β_1) in women with RM at the time of miscarriage are reported as being significantly higher than plasma levels of gestational weeks' matched normal women. In addition, levels of TGF-β_1 in women with RM were approximately threefold higher than non-pregnant controls.[50] In contrast to increased peripheral TGF-β_1 blood levels, a deficiency in decidual lymphoid cells which produce TGF-β_2-suppressing activity is reported in a subset of women with RM.[6]

LIMITATIONS OF CYTOKINE STUDIES

Many studies have concentrated on production of cytokines by immune cells and, in particular, T cells. However, cytokines are also produced by epithelial and stromal cells of the endometrium and the decidual and cytotrophoblast cells of the placenta. This is particularly pertinent to their potential role in reproductive failure, as T cells are only a minor population within the secretory endometrium and first-trimester placental tissue and therefore may not be the main source of cytokines in the fetoplacental unit. In addition, cytokines are designed to act locally. Once in the plasma they are rapidly inactivated, either by binding to protein, or by dilution in the systemic blood. Therefore, measurements of amounts present in the fetoplacental unit postimplantation are of greater significance than measurements

in peripheral blood or measurements prior to implantation.

POSSIBLE MECHANISMS OF PREGNANCY FAILURE AS A RESULT OF ABNORMAL CYTOKINE PRODUCTION

Abnormal production of cytokines is postulated to bring about pregnancy loss in two different ways: either by activation of uterine natural killer (uNK) cells or by affecting trophoblast cell growth and function.

The receptors for various cytokines, including IL-1, IL-2, and TNF-α, are found on uNK cells.[51,52] It was originally proposed that the way in which Th1 cytokines brought about miscarriage was via activation of uNK cells by binding to these receptors.[10] In humans, IL-2 has been shown in vitro to increase expression of CD16 on uNK cells[53] and induce cytotoxicity against trophoblasts.[54] IL-4 has been shown to inhibit the expression of IL-2Rα, IL-2Rβ, and IL2-Rγ by decidual NK cells, thus preventing them reacting to IL-2.[55]

The receptors for numerous cytokines – including those for IL-1, IFN-γ, TNF-α, TGF-β, CSF-1, GM-CSF, LIF, IL-4 and IL-6 – are present on human trophoblast cells,[28,51,56] showing that cytokines have the potential to directly affect human trophoblast cell growth and function. Various studies have shown that TNF-α and IFN-γ can inhibit human trophoblast cell growth and metabolic activity and stimulate apoptosis in vitro.[57] IL-4, IL-6, and LIF stimulate human chorionic gonadotropin (hCG) secretion by trophoblast cells,[58,59] and LIF may also drive differentiation of cytotrophoblast cells away from syncytiotrophoblasts towards a non-invasive extravillous trophoblast type with decreased production of matrix metalloproteinases (MMPs).[60] IL-1, TNF-α, and IL-6 can increase cytotrophoblast MMP-2 and MMP-9 production and activity.[30,61] TGF-β is known to affect growth and differentiation of trophoblast cells and to inhibit cellular activity of these cells.[61,62] Both CSF-1 and GM-CSF have also been shown to stimulate differentiation of cytotrophoblast cells into syncytium in vitro and to stimulate hCG and MMP production by these cells.[30,60,63]

IMMUNE CELL POPULATIONS IN WOMEN WITH RECURRENT MISCARRIAGE

The human endometrium and decidua contain a unique population of lymphocytes, which consists mainly of uNK cells, macrophages, and T cells. The majority of uNK cells are different to those in the peripheral blood in that they express large amounts of CD56, but are CD16 negative (i.e. are CD56+ CD16−). However, there is also a small population of CD16+ cells which express small amounts of CD56, and these are sometimes referred to as CD56^{dim} CD16+ cells. Whereas the number of macrophages and T cells in the endometrium and decidua remain fairly constant, the numbers of CD56+ CD16– cells increase dramatically in the secretory phase of the menstrual cycle and during the first trimester of pregnancy.[64]

CD56+ CELLS

Because of their name, the fact that they show cytolytic activity, and that there are high numbers present in the fetoplacental unit of abortion-prone mice, it is often assumed that there will be high numbers of NK cells in women with RM and that they are the cause of miscarriage. However, although there is some evidence to support this supposition, at present the relationship between CD56+ cells and RM is not conclusive.[65]

Several studies have shown increased numbers of CD56+ NK cells in the peripheral blood of women with RM either prior to or during pregnancy compared with non-pregnant or pregnant controls.[66,67] Studies have also shown that levels of peripheral blood CD56+ cells both prior to and during pregnancy can predict pregnancy outcome in women with RM.[68,69] In contrast to fertile women, where peripheral CD56+ NK cell activity decreases during the first trimester of pregnancy, CD56+ NK cell activity remains high in women with RM.[67] Other studies have shown that the high CD56+ NK cell number and activity is only seen in pregnant RM women with chromosomally normal fetuses, thus suggesting that the presence of high CD56+ levels are a cause rather than effect of recurrent miscarriage.[9,69] However, another study has shown no differences in the levels of peripheral blood CD56+ cells in women undergoing missed miscarriage with chromosomally normal and abnormal fetuses.[70]

Although NK cells in the blood will have contact with the syncytiotrophoblast cells, they will have less contact with the developing fetus than cells within the decidua, and therefore uNK cells may be more important in determining pregnancy outcome. In contrast to the increased numbers of CD56+ cells in peripheral blood, a decreased number of decidual CD56+ NK cells are reported in the miscarried placental tissue in RM women compared with tissue from spontaneous miscarriages in women without RM and women requesting terminations.[8,71] A decreased cytotoxic capability of decidual CD56+ NK cells in placental tissue from spontaneous aborters has also been shown,[72] although women with RM were not included in this study.

Two separate studies have shown increased numbers of CD56+ cells in the non-pregnant endometrium of women with RM,[4,73] and lower numbers were seen in women with RM who subsequently had a live birth compared with those who miscarried.[4] This is in contrast to a number of other studies which show similar numbers of CD56+ cells in the endometrium of women with RM and control subjects.[22,74,75] In one of these studies, however, the women with RM did have increased numbers of endometrial CD56^{dim} CD16+ cells compared with control subjects.[74]

Taken together, these results suggest that there are alterations in the CD56+ population of leukocytes in women with RM; however, whether these are increased or decreased depends on whether peripheral blood, first-trimester decidua, or peri-implantation endometrium is analyzed. CD56+ cells constitute <10% of peripheral blood leukocytes, and therefore these changes may not be significant to total peripheral blood cellular activity. The fact that there appears to be decreased numbers of CD56+ cells in the decidua and possibly increased numbers in the endometrium is more difficult to explain, but may be due to the presence of two different populations of CD56+ cells, either CD16+ or CD16–. Far more studies are required to determine the role of decidual and endometrial NK cells in recurrent pregnancy loss and to define normal levels of these cells before treatments can be considered.[65] Studies on whether endometrial and/or decidual NK cell numbers are predictive of pregnancy outcome in a larger number of patients would be extremely useful. If they are found to be predictive, the effects of NK cell number or activity modulation on pregnancy outcome in women with high NK cell numbers would also be needed.

POSSIBLE ROLE OF uNK CELLS IN PREGNANCY FAILURE

Two potential roles for uNK cells have been proposed: cytolysis and cytokine production. In common with peripheral blood NK cells, uNK cells are able to lyse cells with low or absent HLA (human leukocyte antigen) expression, but not when the cells are transfected with HLA class 1 genes. It has also been shown that trophoblast cells which express HLA class 1 molecules are not susceptible to lysis.[76] It is possible that uNK cells in women with pregnancy failure have increased cytolytic activity compared with those from normal fertile women; this activity may also be affected by cytokine levels. uNK cells themselves are also known to produce numerous cytokines, including CSF-1, TNF-α, IFN-γ, IL-1α, TGF-β, LIF, and GM-CSF.[51,52] Increased or decreased numbers of uNK cells may therefore alter cytokine levels, which may affect trophoblast cell growth and function (see above).

CD3+ T CELLS

The second most abundant population of leukocytes within the endometrium and decidua are CD3+ T cells. Numerous studies have shown no differences in the numbers of CD3+ T cells in either the peripheral blood or the endometrium prior to pregnancy[4,67,74,75] or in the decidua in early pregnancy[8,71] in control and RM women. However,

one study has shown a significantly decreased number of CD3+ T cells in the peripheral blood during pregnancy in women with RM who subsequently miscarried compared with those who had a live birth and normal pregnant controls.[67] Two recent studies have investigated a subpopulation of CD3+ T cells that also express the CD56+ uNK cell marker, and shown a decrease in the number of CD56+ CD3+ cells in the peripheral blood prior to pregnancy and in first-trimester decidua of women with RM compared with controls.[71,77]

T cells can also be classified according to protein components of their CD3 receptor. The majority of T cells express $\alpha\beta$ receptor components, but some may express $\gamma\delta$. Large numbers of $\gamma\delta$ T cells are found in the decidua of abortion-prone mice, and injection of monoclonal antibodies to $\gamma\delta$TCR decreased the number of stress-induced abortions in these mice.[78] The ratio of specific subpopulations of peripheral blood $\gamma\delta$ T cells (Vγ1,Vδ1 to Vγ9Vδ2) is reported to be different in pregnant women with a history of RM compared with controls. There are a number of reports suggesting the presence and importance of $\gamma\delta$ T cells in the human decidua.[79] However, other work has shown that most human decidual T cells are $\alpha\beta$ positive, with only 5–10% of T cells expressing $\gamma\delta$.[80]

The balance between the CD4+ and CD8+ T-cell subsets has also been investigated, and studies have shown a shift towards a higher CD4+/CD8+ ratio in endometrial biopsies from women with RM.[4,74]

Thus although there appears to be no differences in the total T-cell numbers in women with RM, there may be differences in subpopulations of T cells, which may be important.

MACROPHAGES

No significant difference has been found in the number of macrophages in first-trimester decidua from women with RM either with chromosomally normal and abnormal fetuses or in first-trimester decidua from spontaneous abortions and controls.[8] However, an increase in the number of macrophages in the non-pregnant endometrium of women with RM, together with an increased number of endometrial macrophages in RM women who subsequently miscarried, compared with those who had a live birth has also been reported.[4]

CELL ACTIVATION MARKERS

Differences in the absolute numbers of leukocytes may not reflect differences in the activity and therefore the function of the cells. Perhaps a better understanding of the role of these cells in RM would be obtained from the measurement of their activities. The activation status of both T cells and CD56+ cells has been investigated by measurement of expression of the CD25 (IL-2Rα) and CD69 activation markers. An increased number of CD25+ cells have been shown in the first-trimester decidua of women with RM with chromosomally normal fetuses compared with decidua from elective terminations and women with RM with chromosomally abnormal fetuses.[8] An increased number of CD25+ cells have also been shown in the first-trimester decidua of women undergoing spontaneous abortion compared with decidua from elective terminations.[81] In a study of a small number of women, levels of IL-2Rα in peripheral blood obtained from women with RM in the first trimester of pregnancy were higher than those of fertile pregnant and nonpregnant women.[82] Increased expression of CD69 on peripheral blood CD56+ (both CD56[bright] and CD56[dim]) cells of women with unexplained RM compared with normal controls has also been reported.[83] Increased intracellular CD69+ expression is also seen on both peripheral and endometrial CD3+ T cells from RM women compared with controls.[84] Further work is required on the activity of these cells in women with recurrent miscarriage, not only with respect to the activation markers but also with regard to investigation of functional parameters such as cytolysis and secretory activity.

DIFFERENCES IN HLA AND NK RECEPTOR EXPRESSION IN RM WOMEN

The activation status of NK cells is determined by the interaction of HLA molecules with inhibiting and activating receptors on the NK cells, and this has led to the suggestion that recurrent pregnancy loss may be due to abnormal interactions between trophoblastic HLA molecules and maternal decidual NK cell receptors. Although this is pure speculation at present, there are a few studies comparing expression of these molecules in women with RM. A recent study has shown decreased expression of HLA-G immunostaining in extravillous and endovascular cytotrophoblast tissue obtained after miscarriage compared with cytotrophoblast staining in tissue obtained from healthy pregnancies.[85]

Although polymorphisms of the HLA-G are limited, a number have been described and their presence in populations of women with RM has been studied. Three polymorphisms have been described which result in changes in amino acid sequences. The *0103 polymorphism results in a thr to ser substitution at codon 31, whereas the *0104 polymorphisms results in a leu to ile replacement at codon 110. These are relatively conservative amino acid substitutions with respect to amino acid polarity and would not be expected to interfere with HLA-G structure and function. The *0105 polymorphism is a frame shift mutation due to a single base deletion at codon 130 and leads to instability of HLA-G1 due to the loss of a disulfide bridge between residues 101 and 164.[86] The presence of these various isoforms is associated with differences in levels of soluble HLA-G, which is considered a useful indicator of HLA-G expression. The *0103 and *0105 polymorphisms are associated with decreased HLA-G levels, whereas the presence of *0104 is associated with increased expression.[86] Although earlier studies on small populations suggested that there are no differences in HLA-G polymorphisms in women with RM,[87] more recent studies have shown an association of the HLA-G*0105N,[86,88] the HLA-G*0104,[88] and the HLA-G*0103,[89] with repeated pregnancy loss in populations of women with RM.

Studies on the expression of NK receptors in women with RM are very limited, but two independent studies have shown either a more limited expression of the KIR (killer immunoglobulin-like receptor) inhibitory receptors (2DL1, 2DL2, or 2DL3)[90] or, specifically, decreased expression of the

2DL1 inhibitory receptor, but not the 2DL2 or 2DL3 receptor,[91] on peripheral blood NK cells from women with RM compared with controls. In further studies, expression of these inhibitory receptors on decidual NK cells was investigated: 60% of the women with RM did not express all three inhibitory receptor types compared with 6.6% in controls. In this study, HLA-Cw typing of the corresponding trophoblast tissue was also carried out, and it was shown that in 33% of women with RM no epitope matching existed between the maternal inhibitory receptors and trophoblastic HLA-Cw, which compared with 0% in the control group.[90]

IMMUNOSUPPRESSIVE MOLECULES AND RECURRENT PREGNANCY LOSS

The lack of response of the maternal immune system to paternal antigens on the developing fetus has also been postulated to be due to the presence of immunosuppressive molecules, which inhibit such responses. Glycodelin (also known as placental protein 14 or PP14) and progesterone-induced blocking factor (PIBF) are examples of potential immunosuppressive factors.

Glycodelin is a major product of the endometrium. It is produced exclusively by endometrial epithelial cells and is stimulated both in vivo and in vitro by progesterone.[92,93] Endometrial levels of glycodelin increase dramatically during the secretory phase of the cycle and can reach levels of 10 μg/ml or more.[94] Plasma levels are also increased at this time and remain high during the first trimester of pregnancy.[93] The exact role for glycodelin is uncertain, but it is thought to have immunosuppressive properties; it has been shown to suppress both lymphocyte and NK cell activity in vitro.[95,96] Both endometrial and plasma levels of glycodelin are decreased in women with RM during the mid–late luteal phase of the cycle.[97,98] In addition, endometrial glycodelin levels were decreased in women with RM who subsequently miscarried compared with women with RM who went on to have a live birth.[99]

PIBF is a 34 kDa protein produced by peripheral blood and decidual lymphocytes. The major sources of PIBF are γδ T cells. During pregnancy, there is an increased expression of progesterone receptors by these cells, and progesterone therefore increases production of PIBF at this time. PIBF appears to have an inhibitory effect on a number of immunological functions. It has been shown to increase the production of the Th2 cytokines IL-3, IL-4, and IL-10 by activated lymphocytes in mice; in the same experiments, production of IFN-γ (a Th1 cytokine) was unaltered.[100] PIBF has also been shown to alter cytokine production by human and mouse NK cells in a similar manner and to decrease mouse NK cell activity.[101] Decreased numbers of peripheral blood PIBF-positive lymphocytes are reported in women undergoing spontaneous pregnancy termination at the time of sampling and those showing symptoms of pre-mature pregnancy termination;[102] however, this study was not limited to women with RM.

AUTOIMMUNITY AND RECURRENT MISCARRIAGE

Autoimmunity is an immune reaction to self that is caused by a loss of tolerance to self-tissue. The increased levels of autoantibodies associated with autoimmunity may, in some cases, result in pathological damage to the tissue. Certain autoimmune abnormalities have been associated with RM, including antiphospholipid antibodies, lupus coagulant, and antithyroid antibodies. In contrast to the disorders that result from abnormal embryo implantation, the diagnosis and treatment of women with autoimmune disease is much more established.

ANTIPHOSPHOLIPID SYNDROME AND RECURRENT MISCARRIAGE

Antiphospholipid syndrome (APS) is a form of autoimmune condition characterized by the presence of antiphospholipid antibodies (aPLs) and/or lupus anticoagulant. It is a well-recognized cause of

RM and has been reported in 7–42% of women.[1] In contrast to women with unexplained or other causes of RM, where pregnancy loss occurs predominantly in the first trimester, pregnancy loss in women with APS not uncommonly occurs in the second or third trimester.[103] The antibodies present may be of IgG, IgM, and/or IgA isotypes, and are usually directed against negatively charged phospholipids. The most commonly detected antibodies are those against lupus coagulant and anticardiolipin antibody (aCL). β_2-Glycoprotein-1 (β_2GP-1) is a protein involved in binding aPLs to phospholipid surfaces and is a cofactor for the binding of aPLs to cardiolipin.[103,104] Antibodies against β_2GP-1 may also be present in women with RM.

The diagnosis of APS in recurrent miscarriage women requires fulfilment of at least one of the following three clinical criteria:[105]

- three or more unexplained consecutive spontaneous abortions before the 10th week of gestation with maternal anatomic or hormonal abnormalities and paternal and maternal chromosomal abnormalities excluded
- one or more explained deaths of a morphologically normal fetus (determined by ultrasound or direct examination of the fetus) at or beyond the 10th week of gestation.
- one or more premature births of a morphologically normal neonate at or before the 34th week of gestation because of severe pre-eclampsia or eclampsia or severe placental insufficiency.

In addition to the clinical data, laboratory tests must show the presence of lupus coagulant (detected by coagulation-based assays) and/or aCL IgG or IgM – detected by enzyme-linked immunosorbent assay (ELISA) – when measured at least twice, 6 weeks apart.

The exact mechanism of recurrent pregnancy loss in women with APS is still unclear. One possible mechanism is that aPLs interact with platelets to produce a prothrombotic state, which results in increased likelihood of first- and second-trimester loss. The excellent response of APS to anticoagulant therapy, including low-dose aspirin and heparin, supports the hypothesis that microvascular thrombosis plays an important part in the pathogenesis of recurrent pregnancy loss in APS.[106] Another possible mechanism is a direct action of aPLs on trophoblastic cell growth and function. Human aPLs have been shown to bind to cytotrophoblast cells and to inhibit the release of hCG from placental explants[104] and aCLs have been shown to inhibit trophoblast proliferation.[107] In addition, Simone et al[108] have shown that aPLs are associated with reduced integrin expression in trophoblast cells in culture and postulated that this may in turn lead to abnormal trophoblast invasion.

ANTITHYROID ANTIBODIES AND RECURRENT PREGNANCY LOSS

Autoimmune thyroid disorders are characterized by the presence of antithyroglobulin and antithyroid peroxidase. The association between these thyroid antibodies and RM has been examined in a number of studies. An increased prevalence of antithyroglobulin and/or antithyroid peroxidase in RM women compared with controls has been reported in a number of studies. Typically, prevalence is reported to be between 20 and 30% in women with RM compared with between 10 and 20% in control women.[104,109,110] The association between RM and thyroid antibodies may be a result of either a direct effect of these autoantibodies on fetal tissue or the presence of thyroid antibodies indicating a more generalized defect in autoimmunity.

In an earlier study among women with RM known to be positive for antithyroid peroxidase, those who miscarried again in a subsequent pregnancy had a significantly higher antibody titer than those who had a live birth,[105] which suggests that antibody titer is of prognostic value. Moreover, in those pregnancies which continued to term, the titer and avidity declined as pregnancy progressed. However, a more recent study suggested that the presence of thyroid autoantibodies does not affect the future pregnancy outcome of women with a history of RM.[111] The prognostic value of thyroid autoantibodies remains uncertain and two separate reports have suggested that routine screening for thyroid antibodies in women with RM is not warranted.[103,112]

INFECTION AND PREGNANCY LOSS

Infections do not appear to play a significant role in first-trimester RM. Associations between RM and high titers of IgG antibody to chlamydia have been reported,[113] although later studies have refuted this connection.[114] Other authors have concluded that infection is an occasional cause of sporadic spontaneous abortion and, consistent with statistical probability, RM due to infection must be rare.[115] Most patients with a history of RM will not benefit from an extensive infection work-up. Charles and Larsen also concluded that it is very unlikely that maternal infection causes recurrent miscarriage.[116] In our unit, we have recently ceased to carry out TORCH (*t*oxoplasmosis, *o*ther agents, *r*ubella, *c*ytomegalovirus, *h*erpes simplex) screening, and intrauterine swabs for chlamydia, after our own internal audit had shown that there were no positive results among 200 patients over a 5-year period. A recent guideline published by the Royal College of Obstetricians and Gynaecologists (RCOG) on recurrent miscarriage[112] also stated that TORCH screening should be abandoned in women presenting with recurrent pregnancy loss.

Bacterial vaginosis (BV) is a condition associated with a complex (quantitative) alteration in vaginal flora involving *Mobiluncus* spp, *Bacteroides* spp, peptostreptococci, and *Mycoplasma hominis*, in addition to *Gardnerella vaginalis*. These changes are accompanied by a depletion in vaginal lactobacilli. Unlike other infections that depend primarily on bacteriological study, the diagnosis of BV is based on composite criteria,[117] in which three out of four of the following should be present:

- vaginal pH >4.5
- a grey homogeneous (malodorous, fishy-smelling) vaginal discharge
- the presence of clue cells in a wet mount preparation of vaginal fluid
- the amine test, in which fishy odor is released

after the addition of 10% potassium hydroxide to vaginal fluid.

Although BV is associated with second-trimester loss, preterm premature rupture of membranes, and preterm labour,[118] and is generally considered to be unrelated to first-trimester RM, a more recent study[119] showed that BV was associated with an increased risk of miscarriage in the first trimester in women undergoing IVF treatment.

CONCLUSION

The major ways in which inflammation may cause recurrent miscarriage is via autoimmunity (mainly aPLs) and abnormal embryo implantation. The diagnosis and treatment of autoimmune disease for women with RM is well established. However, the immune cell interactions which occur during implantation and which may be abnormal in women with unexplained RM are still not clearly understood. One of the problems in this field is the amount of contradictory findings: some of this variation occurs due to the difficulties in obtaining the optimum tissue, whereas other problems may result from differences in study design. Factors that might account for differences are the compartments (peripheral blood, endometrium, or decidua) in which the cells and molecules are measured. The measurement of factors such as cytokines (which are known to act locally) in peripheral blood may have little significance, as this compartment has less contact with the trophoblast than the endometrium or decidua. In addition, the peripheral blood cell population is considerably different to that of the endometrium and decidua. The timing of sampling is also important, both with respect to the point in the menstrual cycle and pregnancy and whether it is at the time or just after miscarriage, as both of these factors will affect the expression of cytokines and cell number and activity.

The fact that recurrent miscarriage is distressing to the patient, and that for over half of cases the cause is unknown, makes it extremely difficult to treat. Ideally, treatments should be based on scientific evidence. However, at present, we have to accept that the available data are very contradictory and that further rigorous research in this area is required.

REFERENCES

1. Li TC, Makris M, Tomsu M et al. Recurrent miscarriage: aetiology management and prognosis. Hum Reprod Update 2002; 5:463–481.

2. Hill JA, Polgar K, Anderson DJ. T-helper 1-type immunity to trophoblast in women with recurrent spontaneous abortion. JAMA 1995; 273:1933–1936.

3. Raghupathy R, Makhseed M, Azizieh F et al. Maternal Th1 and Th2-type reactivity to placental antigens in normal human pregnancy and unexplained recurrent spontaneous abortions. Cell Immunol 1999; 196:122–130.

4. Quenby S, Bates M, Doig T et al. Pre-implantation endometrial leukocytes in women with recurrent miscarriage. Hum Reprod 1999; 14:2386–2391.

5. Lim KJH, Odukoya OA, Ajjan RA et al. The role of T-helper cytokines in human reproduction. Fertil Steril 2000; 73:136–142.

6. Lea RG, Underwood J, Flanders KC et al. A subset of patient with recurrent spontaneous abortion is deficient in transforming growth factor β-2 producing 'suppressor cells' in uterine tissue near the placental attachment site. Am J Reprod Immunol 1995; 34:52–64.

7. Piccinni M, Beloni L, Livi C et al. Defective production of both leukemia inhibitory factor and type 2 T-helper cytokines by decidual T cells in unexplained recurrent abortions. Nat Med 1998; 4:1020–1024.

8. Quack KC, Vassiliadou N, Pudney J et al. Leukocyte activation in the decidua of chromosomally normal and abnormal fetuses from women with recurrent abortion. Hum Reprod 2001; 16:949–955.

9. Yamada H, Kato HE, Kobashi G et al. High NK cell activity in early pregnancy correlates with subsequent abortion with normal chromosomes in women with recurrent abortion. Am J Reprod Immunol 2001; 46:132–136.

10. Wegmann TG, Lin H, Guilbert L, Mosmann TR. Bidirectional cytokine interactions in the maternal–fetal relationship: is successful pregnancy a TH2 phenomenon? Immunol Today 1993; 14:353–356.

11. Chaouat G, Assal Meliani A, Martal J et al. IL-10 prevents naturally occurring fetal loss in the CBA × DBA/2 mating combination, and local defect in IL-10 production in this abortion-prone combination is corrected by in vivo injection of IFN-tau. J Immunol 1995; 154:4261–4268.

12. Chaouat G, Ledee-Bataille N, Dubanchet S et al. Reproductive immunology 2003: reassessing the Th1/Th2 paradigm. Immunol Lett 2004; 92:207–214.

13. Svensson L, Arvola M, Sallstrom M, Holmdahl R, Mattsson R. The Th2 cytokines IL-4 and IL-10 are not crucial for completion of allogenic pregnancy in mice. J Reprod Immunol 2001; 51:3–7.

14. Bates MD, Quenby S, Takakuwa K et al. Aberrant cytokine production by peripheral blood mononuclear cells in recurrent pregnancy loss? Hum Reprod 2002; 17:2439–2444.

15. Raghupathy R, Makhseed M, Azizieh F et al. Cytokine production by maternal lymphocytes during normal pregnancy and in unexplained recurrent spontaneous abortion. Hum Reprod 2000; 15:713–718.

16. Hamai Y, Fuji T, Kozuma S et al. Secretion of interleukin 2 from unstimulated peripheral blood mononuclear cells is a possible pathogenic mechanism in recurrent abortion. Am J Reprod Immunol 1998; 40:63–64.

17. Dahar S, Denardi K, Blotta M et al. Cytokines in recurrent pregnancy loss. J Reprod Immunol 2004; 62:151–157.

18. Wilson R, Jenkins C, Miller H et al. Abnormal cytokine levels in non-pregnant women with a history of recurrent miscarriage. Eur J Obstet Gynecol 2004; 115:51–54.

19. Wilson R, Moor J, Jenkins C et al. Abnormal first trimester serum IL18 levels are associated with a poor outcome in women with a history of recurrent miscarriage. Am J Reprod Immunol 2004; 51:156–159

20. Kwak-Kim JYH, Chung-Bang HS, Ng SC et al. Increased Th1 cytokine responses by circulating T cells are present in women with recurrent pregnancy losses and in infertile women with multiple implantation failures. Hum Reprod 2003; 18:767–773.

21. Ng SC, Gilman-Sachs A, Thaker P et al. Expression of intracellular Th1 and Th2 cytokines in women with recurrent spontaneous abortion, implantation failure after IVF/ET or normal pregnancy. Am J Reprod Immunol 2002; 48:77–86.

22. Shimada S, Hirayama K, Morikawa M et al. No difference in natural killer or natural killer T-cell population, but aberrant T-helper cell population in the endometrium of women with repeated miscarriage. Hum Reprod 2004; 19:1018–1024.

23. Dahar S, Shulzhenko N, Morgun A et al. Associations between cytokine gene polymorphisms and recurrent pregnancy loss. J Reprod Immunol 2003; 58:69–77.

24. Reid JG, Simpson NAB, Walker RG et al. The carriage of pro-inflammatory cytokine gene polymorphisms in recurrent pregnancy loss. Am J Reprod Immunol 2001; 45:35–40.

25. Babbage SJ, Arkwright PD, Vince GS et al. Cytokine promoter gene polymorphisms and idiopathic recurrent pregnancy loss. J Reprod Immunol 2001; 51:21–27.

26. Saijo Y, Sata F, Yamada H et al. Interleukin-4 gene polymorphism is not involved in the risk of recurrent pregnancy loss. Am J Reprod Immunol 2004; 52:143–146.

27. Prigoshin N, Tambutti M, Larriba J et al. Cytokine gene polymorphisms in recurrent pregnancy loss of unknown cause. Am J Reprod Immunol 2004; 52:35–41.

28. Simon C, Frances A, Piquette GN. Embryonic implantation in mice is blocked by interleukin-1 receptor antagonist (IL-1ra). Endocrinology 1994; 134:521–528.

29. Simon C, Gimeno MJ, Mercader A et al. Embryonic regulation of integrins β3, α4 and α1 in human endometrial epithelial cells in vitro. J Clin Endocrinol Metab 1997; 82:2607–2616.

30. Meisser A, Chardonnens D, Campana A, Bischof P. Effects of TNFα, ILα, M-CSF and TGFβ on trophoblastic matrix metalloproteinases. Mol Hum Reprod 1999; 5:252–260.

31. Laird SM, Tuckerman E, Dalton CF et al. The production of leukaemia inhibitory factor (LIF) by human endometrium: presence in uterine flushings and production by cells in culture. Hum Reprod 1997; 12:569–574.

32. Santilla S, Savinainen K, Hurme M. Presence of IL-1ra allele 2 (IL1RN-2) is associated with enhanced IL-1β production in vitro. Scand J Immunol 1998; 27:195–198.

33. Helfer LA, Tempfer CB, Unfried G et al. A polymorphism of the interleukin 1β gene and idiopathic recurrent miscarriage. Fertil Steril 2001; 76:2377–2379.

34. Wang ZC, Yunis E, De los Santos MJ et al. T helper 1-type immunity to trophoblast antigens in women with a history of recurrent pregnancy loss is associated with polymorphism of the IL1B promoter region. Genes Immun 2002; 3:38–42.

35. Hefler LA, Tempfer CB, Bashford MT et al. Polymorphisms of the angiotensinogen gene, the endothelial nitric oxide synthase gene and

the interleukin-1β gene promoter in women with idiopathic recurrent miscarriage. Mol Hum Reprod 2002; 8:95–100.

36. Unfied G, Tempfer C, Schneeberger C et al. Interleukin 1 receptor antagonist polymorphism in women with idiopathic recurrent miscarriage. Fertil Steril 2001; 75:683–687.

37. Karhukorpi J, Laitinen T, Kivela H et al. IL1 receptor antagonist gene polymorphism in recurrent spontaneous abortion. J Reprod Immunol 2003; 58:61–67.

38. Von Wolff M, Thaler CJ, Strowitzki T et al. Regulated expression of cytokines in human endometrium throughout the menstrual cycle: dysregulation in habitual abortion. Mol Hum Reprod 2000; 6:627–634.

39. Stewart CL, Kasper P, Brunet LJ et al. Blastocyst implantation depends on maternal expression of leukaemia inhibitory factor. Nature 1992; 359:76–79.

40. Cork BA, Tuckerman EM, Warren MA et al. Expression of LIF and IL6 in endometrial epithelial cells of normal fertile women and women who suffer recurrent miscarriage. Hum Reprod 1999; 14:P174.

41. Robb L, Li R, Hartley L et al. Infertility in female mice lacking the receptor for interleukin 11 is due to a defective uterine response to implantation. Nat Med 1998; 4:303–308.

42. Piccinni M, Scaletti C, Vultaggio A et al. Defective production of LIF, M-CSF and Th2-type cytokines by T cells at fetomaternal interface is associated with pregnancy loss. J Reprod Immunol 2001; 52:35–43.

43. Ledee-Bataille N, Lappree-Delage G, Taupin JL et al. Concentrations of leukaemia inhibitory factor in uterine flushing fluid is highly predictive of embryo implantation. Hum Reprod 2001; 10:2073–2078.

44. Linjawi S, Tuckerman EM, Blakemore AIF et al. Expression of IL11 and IL11Rα in the endometrium of women with recurrent miscarriage. J Reprod Immunol 2004; 64:145–155.

45. Ledee-Bataille N, Dubanchet S, Bonnet K et al. A new role for natural killer cells IL12 and IL18 in repeated implantation failure. Fertil Steril 2003; 81:59–65.

46. Zenclussen AC, Fest S, Busse P et al. Questioning the Th1/Th2 paradigm in reproduction: peripheral levels of IL-12 are down-regulated in miscarriage patients. Am J Reprod Immunol 2002; 48:245–251.

47. Pollard JW, Hunt JS, Wiktor-Jedrzejczak W. A pregnancy defect in the osteopetrotic (op/op) mouse demonstrates the requirement for CSF-1 in female fertility. Dev Biol 1991; 148:273–278.

48. Robertson SA, Roberts CT, Farr KL et al. Fertility impairment in GM-CSF deficient mice. Biol Reprod 1999; 60:251–261.

49. Perricone R, De Carolis C, Giacomelli R et al. GM-CSF and pregnancy: evidence of significantly reduced blood concentrations in unexplained recurrent abortion efficiently reverted by intravenous immunoglobulin treatment. Am J Reprod Immunol 2003; 50: 232–237.

50. Ogasawara MS, Aoki K, Aoyama T et al. Elevation of TGFβ1 is associated with recurrent miscarriage. J Clin Immunol 2000; 20:453–457.

51. Jokhi PP, King A, Loke YW. Cytokine production and cytokine receptor expression by cells of the human first trimester placental uterine interface. Cytokine 1997; 9:126–137.

52. Saito S, Nishikawa K, Morii T et al. Cytokine production by CD16–CD56 bright natural killer cells in the human early pregnancy decidua. Int Immunol 1993; 5:559–563.

53. King A, Wheeler R, Carter NP et al. The response of human decidual leucocytes to IL2. Cell Immunol 1992; 141:409–421.

54. Ferry BL, Sargent IL, Starky PM, Redman CWG. Cytotoxic activity against trophoblast and choriocarcinoma cells of large granular lymphocytes from human early pregnancy decidua. Cell Immunol 1991; 132:140–149.

55. Saito S, Umekage H, Nishikawa K et al. Interleukin 4 blocks the IL2-induced increases in natural killer activity and DNA synthesis off decidual CD16–CD56bright NK cells by inhibiting expression of the IL-2Rα, β and γ. Cell Immunol 1996; 170:71–77.

56. Laird SM, Tuckerman EM, Cork BA et al. A review of immune cells and molecules in women with recurrent miscarriage. Hum Reprod Update 2003; 9:163–174.

57. Yui J, Garcia-Lloret M, Wegmann TG, Guilbert LJ. Cytotoxicity of TNFα and IFNγ against primary human placental trophoblasts. Placenta 1994; 15:819–835.

58. Sawai K, Matsuzaki N, Kameda T et al. Leukemia inhibitory factor produced at the fetomaternal interface stimulates chorionic gonadotrophin production: its possible implication during pregnancy, including implantation period. J Clin Endocrinol Metab 1995; 80:1449–1456.

59. Saito S, Harada N, Ishii N et al. Functional expression on human trophoblasts of IL 4 and IL 7 receptor complexes with common γ chain. Biochem Biophys Res Commun 1997; 231:429–434.

60. Nachtigall MJ, Kliman HJ, Feinberg RF et al. The effect of leukemia inhibitory factor (LIF) on trophoblast differentation: a potential role in human implantation. J Clin Endocrinol Metab 1996; 81:801–806.

61. Meisser A, Cameo P, Islami D et al. Effects of interleukin 6 on cytotrophoblast cells. Mol Hum Reprod 1999; 5:1055–1058.

62. Morrish DW, Bhardwaj D, Paras MT. TGFβ1 inhibits placental differentiation and hCG and human placental lactogen secretion. Endocrinology 1991; 129:22–26.

63. Garcia-Lloret MI, Morrish DW, Wegmann TG et al. Demonstration of functional cytokine-placental interactions: CSF-1 and GM-CSF stimulate human cytotrophoblast differentiation and peptide hormone secretion. Exp Cell Res 1994; 214:46–54.

64. Bulmer JN. Cellular constituents of human endometrium in the menstrual cycle and early pregnancy. In: Bronson RA, Alexander NJ, Anderson D et al, eds. Reproductive Immunology. Oxford: Blackwell Science; 1996: 212–239.

65. Moffett A, Regan L, Braude P. Natural killer cells, miscarriage, and infertility. BMJ 2004; 329:1283–1285.

66. Aoki K, Kajiura S, Matsumoto Y et al. Preconceptional natural killer cell activity as a predictor of miscarriage. Lancet 1995; 345: 1340–1342.

67. Kwak JYH, Beaman KD, Gilman-Sachs A et al. Up-regulated expression of CD56+, CD56+/CD16+, and CD19+ cells in peripheral blood lymphocytes in pregnant women with recurrent pregnancy loss. Am J Reprod Immunol 1995; 34:93–99.

68. Emmer PM, Nelen WL, Steegers EA et al. Peripheral natural killer cytotoxicity and CD56+CD16+ cells increase during early pregnancy in women with a history of recurrent spontaneous abortion. Hum Reprod 2000; 15:1163–1169.

69. Coulam CB, Goodman C, Roussev RG et al. Systemic CD56+ cells can predict pregnancy outcome. Am J Reprod Immunol 1995; 33: 40–46.

70. Yamamoto T, Takahashi Y, Kase N, Mori H. Role of decidual natural killer (NK) cells in patients with missed abortion: differences between cases with normal and abnormal chromosome. Clin Exp Immunol 1999; 116:449–452.

71. Yamamoto T, Takahashi Y, Kase N, Mori H. Proportion of CD56+3+ T cells in decidual and peripheral lymphocytes of normal pregnancy and spontaneous abortion with and without history of recurrent abortion. Am J Reprod Immunol 1999; 42:355–360.

72. Vassiliadou N, Bulmer JN. Functional studies of human decidua in spontaneous early pregnancy loss: effect of soluble factors and purified CD56+ lymphocytes on killing of natural killer and

lymphokine-activated-killer-sensitive targets. Biol Reprod 1998; 58:982–987.

73. Clifford K, Flanagan AM, Regan L. Endometrial natural killer cells in women with recurrent miscarriage: a histomorphometric study. Hum Reprod 1999; 14:2727–2730.

74. Lachapelle M, Miron P, Hemmings R, Roy DC. Endometrial T, B and NK cells in patients with recurrent spontaneous abortion. J Immunol 1996; 156:4027–4034.

75. Michimata T, Ogasawara MS, Tsuda H et al. Distributions of endometrial NK cells, B cells, T cells and Th2/Tc2 cells fail to predict pregnancy outcome following recurrent abortion. Am J Reprod Immunol 2002; 47:196–202.

76. Loke YW, King A. Decidual natural-killer-cell inactivation with trophoblast: cytolysis or cytokine production? Biochem Soc Trans 2000; 28:196–198.

77. Yahata T, Kurabayashi T, Honda A et al. Decrease in the proportion of granulated CD56+ T-cells in patients with a history of recurrent abortion. J Reprod Immunol 1998; 38:63–73.

78. Arck PC, Ferrick DA, Steele-Norwood D, Croitoru K, Clark DA. Regulation of abortion by γδ T cells. Am J Reprod Immunol 1997; 37:87–93.

79. Szekeres-Bartho J, Barakonyi A, Miko E, Polgar B, Palkovics T. The role of γ/δ T cells in the feto-maternal relationship. Semin Immunol 2001; 13:229–233.

80. Vassiliadou N, Bulmer, JN. Characterisation of endometrial T lymphocyte subpopulations in spontaneous early loss. Hum Reprod 1998; 13:44–47.

81. Vassiliadou N, Searle RF, Bulmer JN. Elevated expression of activation molecules by decidual lymphocytes in women suffering early spontaneous loss. Hum Reprod 1999; 14:1194–1200.

82. MacLean MA, Wilson R, Jenkins C et al. Interleukin-2 receptor concentrations in pregnant women with a history of recurrent miscarriage. Hum Reprod 2002; 17:221–227.

83. Ntrivalas EI, Kwak-Kim JYH, Gilman-Sachs A et al. Status of peripheral blood natural killer cells in women with recurrent spontaneous abortions and infertility of unknown aetiology. Hum Reprod 2001; 16:855–861.

84. Ramhorst R, Garcia V, Agriello E et al. Intracellular expression of CD69 in endometrial and peripheral T cells represents a useful marker in women with recurrent miscarriage: modulation after allogeneic leukocyte immunotherapy. Am J Reprod Immunol 2003; 49:149–158.

85. Emmer PM, Steegers EAP, Kerstens HMJ et al. Altered phenotype of HLA-G expressing trophoblast and decidual natural killer cells in pathological pregnancies. Hum Reprod 2002; 17:1072–1080.

86. van der Ven K, Pfeiffer K, Skrablin S. HLA-G polymorphisms and molecule function – questions and more questions – a review. Placenta 2000; 21:S86–S92.

87. Karhukorpi J, Laitinen T, Tiilikainen AS. HLA-G polymorphism in Finnish couples with recurrent spontaneous miscarriage. Br J Obstet Gynaecol 1997; 104:1212–1214.

88. Aldrich CL, Stephenson MD, Karrison T et al. HLA-G genotypes and pregnancy outcome in couples with unexplained recurrent miscarriage. Mol Hum Reprod 2001; 7:1167–1172.

89. Pfeiffer KA, Fimmers R, Engels G et al. The HLA-G genotype is potentially associated with idiopathic recurrent spontaneous abortion. Mol Hum Reprod 2001; 7:373–378.

90. Varla-Leftherioti M. Role of KIR/HLA-C allorecognition system in pregnancy. J Reprod Immunol 2004; 62:19–27.

91. Yamada H, Shimada S, Kato EH et al. Decrease in a specific killer cell immunoglobulin-like receptor on peripheral NK cells in women with recurrent spontaneous abortion of unexplained etiology. Am J Reprod Immunol 2004; 51:241–247.

92. Laird SM, Li TC, Bolton AE. The production of placental protein 14 and interleukin 6 by human endometrial cells in culture. Hum Reprod 1993; 8:795–798.

93. Seppala M, Koistinen R, Rutanen EM. Uterine endocrinology and paracrinology – IGFBP-1 and PP14 revisited. Hum Reprod 1994; 9(Suppl 2):96–106.

94. Li TC, Ling E, Dalton C et al. Concentrations of endometrial protein PP14 in uterine flushings throughout the menstrual cycle. Br J Obstet Gynaecol 1993; 100:460–464.

95. Pockley AG, Mowles EA, Stoker RJ et al. Suppression of in vitro lymphocyte reactivity to phytohaemagglutinin by PP14. J Reprod Immunol 1988; 13:31–39.

96. Okamoto N, Uchida A, Takakura K et al. Suppression by human PP14 of natural killer cell activity. Am J Reprod Immunol 1991; 26:137–142.

97. Dalton CF, Laird SM, Serle E et al. The measurement of CA 125 and placental protein 14 in uterine flushings; correlation with endometrial morphology. Hum Reprod 1995; 10:2680–2684.

98. Tulppala M, Julkunen M, Titinen A et al. Habitual abortion is accompanied by low serum levels of PP14 in the luteal phase of the fertile cycle. Fertil Steril 1995; 63:792–795.

99. Dalton CF, Laird SM, Estdale S et al. Levels of endometrial proteins PP14 and CA125 in flushings from women who suffer recurrent miscarriage; comparison with endometrial morphology and correlation with pregnancy outcome. Hum Reprod 1998; 13: 3197–3202.

100. Szekeres-Bartho J, Wegmann TG. A progesterone-dependent immunomodulatory protein alters the Th1/Th2 balance. J Reprod Immunol 1996; 31:81–95.

101. Szekeres-Bartho J, Barakonyi A, Par G et al. Progesterone as an immunomodulatory molecule. Int Immunopharmacol 2001; 1: 1037–1048.

102. Szekeres-Bartho J, Faust Z, Varga P. The expression of a progesterone-induced immunomodulatory protein in pregnancy lymphocytes. Am J Reprod Immunol 1995; 34:342–348.

103. Fausett MB, Branch DW. Autoimmunity and pregnancy loss. Semin Reprod Med 2000; 50:379–392.

104. Kutteh WH, Ghazeeri GS. Autoimmune factors and their influence on assisted reproduction. Immunol All Clin N Am 2002; 22: 643–661.

105. Wilson WA, Gharavi AE, Koike T et al. International consensus statement on preliminary classification criteria for definite antiphospholipid syndrome: report of an international workshop. Arthritis Rheum 1999; 42:1309–1311.

106. Rai R, Cohen H, Dave M, Regan L. Randomised controlled trial of aspirin and aspirin plus heparin in pregnant women with recurrent miscarriage associated with phospholipid antibodies (or antiphospholipid antibodies). BMJ 1997; 314:253–257.

107. Chamley LW, Duncalf AM, Mitchell MD, Johnson PM. Action of anticardiolipin and antibodies to β2-glycoprotein-1 on trophoblast proliferation as a mechanism for fetal death. Lancet 1998; 352:1037–1038.

108. Di Simone N, Castellani R, Caliandro D, Caruso A. Antiphospholipid antibodies regulate the expression of trophoblast cell adhesion molecules. Fertil Steril 2002; 77:805–811.

109. Pratt DE, Kaberlein G, Dudkiewicz A et al. The association of antithyroid antibodies in euthyroid non-pregnant women with recurrent first trimester abortions in next pregnancy. Fertil Steril 1993; 60:1001–1005.

110. Bussen S, Steck T. Thyroid autoantibodies in euthyroid non-pregnant women with recurrent spontaneous abortions. Hum Reprod 1995; 10:2938–2940.

111. Rushworth FH, Backos M, Rai R et al. Prospective pregnancy outcome in untreated recurrent miscarriages with thyroid autoantibodies. Hum Reprod 2000; 15:1647–1639.

112. The investigation and treatment of couples with recurrent miscarriage. Guideline 17, published by the Royal College of Obstetricians and Gynaecologists. London 2003.

113. Daya S. Issues in the aetiology of recurrent spontaneous abortion. Curr Opin Obstet Gynaecol 1994; 6:153–159.

114. Osser S, Presson K. Chlamydial antibodies in women who suffer miscarriage. Br J Obstet Gynaecol 1996; 103:137–141.

115. Summers PR. Microbiology relevant to recurrent miscarriage. Clin Obstet Gynecol 1994; 37:722–729.

116. Charles D, Larsen B. Spontaneous abortion as a result of infection. In: Huisjes HB, Lind T, eds. Early Pregnancy Failure. Edinburgh: Churchill Livingstone; 1990: 161–176.

117. Hillier SL. Diagnosis microbiology of bacterial vaginosis. Am J Obstet Gynecol 1993; 169:776–778.

118. Hay PE, Lamont RF, Taylor-Robinson D et al. Abnormal bacterial colonisation of the genital tract and subsequent pre-term delivery and late miscarriage. BMJ 1994; 308:295–298.

119. Ralph SG, Rutherford AJ, Wilson JD. Influence of bacterial vaginosis on conception and miscarriage in the first trimester: cohort study. BMJ 1999; 319:220–223.

6. Inflammation and normal labor

Murray D Mitchell and Jeffrey A Keelan

INTRODUCTION

Inflammation is an integral aspect of parturition.[1] Leukocyte infiltration/activation of the extraplacental membranes (amnion, chorion, and decidua), cervix, and uterus occurs prior to, and during, term labor and is accompanied by increased cytokine expression, eicosanoid production, and extracellular matrix degradation. These processes are propagated during labor to ensure progression through to delivery, and in normal parturition they occur in concert and in a timely fashion to effect cervical ripening, membrane rupture, and sustained uterine contractions. In contrast, pathological intrauterine inflammation (most frequently diagnosed by the presence of histological chorioamnionitis) appears to be a causative factor in a significant proportion of preterm births. The presence of an infective organism in the amniotic cavity is confirmed in about half of pregnancies delivered preterm with chorioamnionitis, but in the remainder the cause of the excessive inflammatory response remains undetermined. Hence, there is some uncertainty whether precocious initiation of inflammatory changes, or abnormal inflammatory activation, is the cause of preterm birth or its sequela. Despite such controversies, there is widespread appreciation that inflammatory processes play central roles in multiple aspects of both term and preterm parturition.

PLACENTAL CYTOKINES

The placenta and its associated membranes produce a wide variety of cytokines throughout normal gestation; these are listed in Table 6.1. Production of cytokines and cytokine distribution within the tissues of pregnancy varies with gestational age and probably reflects specific functions within these tissues. Indeed, it is realized that within the placenta,

as in other organs, cytokines often have pleiotropic functions and perform homeostatic or regulatory roles independent of their more widely recognized immune-related functions. Cytokines are produced by the resident cells of normal healthy placental tissues, as well as by infiltrating leukocytes. The realization that non-immune tissues have the ability to express and secrete cytokines was an important advance in the context of understanding inflammatory mechanisms of parturition. Cytokine receptors are expressed in placental tissues, indicating that they are both sources and targets of these important biological mediators.

INFLAMMATORY CYTOKINES

In the first trimester of pregnancy, messenger RNA (mRNA) for tumor necrosis factor-α (TNF-α), interleukins IL-1α, IL-1β, IL-6, and macrophage migration inhibitory factor (MIF) have been found in placenta/trophoblast and decidua (see Table 6.1). Placental trophoblasts are major producers of the inflammatory cytokines; however, inflammatory cytokines are also secreted by macrophages (Hofbauer cells) and stromal cells in the placenta.[2–4] In first-trimester decidua, mRNA and protein for IL-1α, IL-1β, IL-6, and TNF-α have been localized to cells of immune origin,[5–8] but are also produced by other decidual cell types.[2,6,9] Immunodetectable MIF has also been identified in first-trimester decidua.[10]

At term, mRNA for TNF-α, IL-1α, IL-1β, and IL-6 have been identified in placenta/trophoblast and decidua, and these cytokines are produced and secreted by both tissue types (see Table 6.1). In the fetal membranes it has been reported that the chorion contains mRNA for TNF-α, IL-1β, and IL-6, but expresses protein for only IL-1β and IL-6,[11,12] whereas amnion expresses all three proteins.[11,12] IL-1β is produced by both trophoblasts and placental

Table 6.1 Cytokines produced by human gestational tissues during normal pregnancy

Cytokine	Tissue		
	Placenta	Decidua	Fetal membranes
Inflammatory cytokines			
IL-1α/β	Throughout gestation, localized to trophoblast and Hofbauer cells	Throughout gestation	Term, amnion and chorion
IL-6	Throughout gestation, localized to trophoblast and Hofbauer cells	Throughout gestation (choriodecidua included)	1st trimester and term, amnion and chorion
IL-12	3rd trimester	3rd trimester and term	3rd trimester and term[a]
IL-16	Not assessed	3rd trimester and term[a]	3rd trimester and term[a]
IL-18	1st trimester trophoblast	1st and 3rd trimester	3rd trimester (chorion)
TNF-α/β	Throughout gestation, localized to trophoblast and Hofbauer cells	1st trimester and term, including leukocytes	Term, amnion and chorion
MIF	1st trimester, trophoblast	1st trimester and term	Term, amnion and chorion
PBEF	Throughout gestation	Throughout gestation	Throughout gestation, amnion and chorion
Anti-inflammatory cytokines			
IL-4	Throughout gestation, placenta including trophoblast	Throughout gestation, also associated with leukocytes	1st trimester and term, amnion and chorion
IL-10	Throughout gestation, trophoblast and Hofbauer cells	1st trimester and term	Term, chorion (including decidua)
IL-13	Throughout gestation (1st trimester mainly)	1st trimester (weak)	Not assessed
IL-1RA	Throughout gestation, including Hofbauer cells	1st trimester and term	Term, amnion and chorion
Other cytokines			
IL-11	1st trimester, chorionic villi	1st trimester and term[a]	3rd trimester and term[a]
Oncostatin M	Not assessed	3rd trimester and term[a]	3rd trimester and term[a]
TRAIL	Throughout gestation, trophoblast and stromal cells	3rd trimester and term	3rd trimester and term
TWEAK	Throughout gestation	3rd trimester and term[a]	3rd trimester and term[a]
G-CSF	Throughout gestation, mostly term	3rd trimester	Term labor[a]
GM-CSF	Term	3rd trimester and term	3rd trimester and term[a]
Chemokines			
IL-8	Throughout gestation, trophoblast	Throughout gestation, found associated with immune cells	Amnion and chorion, 3rd trimester and term
ENA-78	Not assessed	3rd trimester and term	Term, amnion and chorion[a]
RANTES	Not assessed	3rd trimester and term	Chorion, 3rd trimester and term
MIP-1α/β	Not assessed	3rd trimester and term	Chorion, 3rd trimester and term amnion with labor[a]
MIP-3α	Not assessed	Not detected (cDNA array)	Term and amnion[a]
MCP-1/2/3/4	Trophoblast, throughout gestation	3rd trimester and term	Amnion, 3rd trimester and term
MPIF-1	Not assessed	3rd trimester and term[a]	3rd trimester and term[a]
PREF-1	Not assessed	3rd trimester and term[a]	3rd trimester and term[a]
Fractalkine	Not assessed	1st trimester	2nd and 3rd trimester, amnion and chorion

[a]Expression detected by cDNA array analysis of 3rd-trimester labored and non-labored amnion and choriodecidual tissues;[47] no other supporting evidence.
Abbreviated, updated, and modified from Bowen et al.[174]

macrophages,[13] and trophoblasts also release IL-1α.[13] IL-1α and IL-1β production by trophoblast has been detected during the first trimester and at term, declining over the course of gestation.[14] IL-6 staining intensity and production rates in the placenta are increased at term compared with early pregnancy. IL-6 is the only villous placental cytokine whose production has been shown to be up-regulated with the onset of labor.[15]

ANTI-INFLAMMATORY CYTOKINES

Inflammatory activation can both be stimulated and resolved by cytokines, and several potent anti-inflammatory cytokines have been characterized and studied in the context of pregnancy and parturition. Indeed, it has been suggested that successful pregnancy requires a withdrawal of the effects of anti-inflammatory cytokines, as well as an augmentation of the effects of proinflammatory mediators.[16]

Messenger RNA and protein for IL-4 and IL-10 have been located in placenta/trophoblast and decidua throughout pregnancy. Reports of IL-10 production in the fetal membranes have been inconsistent. The chorion appears to secrete small quantities of IL-10 at term, whereas amnion production is low or undetectable.[17–19] Immunohistochemical results indicate that placental abundance of IL-4 and IL-10 decreases with increasing gestational age, whereas decidual production of these cytokines increases.[20] In contrast, Roth et al[21] found that secretion of IL-10 by trophoblasts in culture was stable over gestation.

IL-10,[22] IL-4,[22,23] and IL-1ra (interleukin-1 receptor antagonist)[24] have been detected in amniotic fluid collected at term. Increases in amniotic fluid concentrations of both IL-10[25] and IL-1ra[26,27] have been observed between the second trimester and term. Interestingly, amniotic fluid concentrations of IL-1ra in late pregnancy are additionally elevated in pregnancies where a female fetus is present.[26,27] IL-1ra in the amniotic fluid may derive from the amnion and chorion, which are reported to produce this cytokine at term.[28] IL-1ra is also produced by first-trimester trophoblasts,[2,29] first-trimester decidua,[2] and term decidual cultures.[28] IL-13

mRNA has been identified in placental trophoblasts from all stages of gestation, but IL-13 immunoreactivity has only been identified in first-trimester placenta.[30,31]

CHEMOKINES

The two major chemokine subfamilies are distinguished structurally according to the presence of an amino acid (X) between the characteristic cysteine residues found near the amino terminus. The CXC chemokine most commonly discussed with regard to pregnancy is IL-8, which is produced constitutively by all the tissues of gestation in the later stages of pregnancy (Tables 6.1 and 6.2). Production of IL-8 by the placenta has been reported to increase towards term, although expression of mRNA for this chemokine does not appear to change.[32] Amniotic fluid contains detectable levels of IL-8[33–35] and another CXC chemokine, GRO-α,[36] throughout gestation, and concentrations of both these chemokines increase with advancing gestational age.[35,36] Similarly, the CXC chemokine ENA-78, which, like IL-8, is a neutrophil attractant, has also been detected in amniotic fluid and is produced by gestational membranes in vitro.[37] Amnion tissue levels of ENA-78 were found to be increased following term labor, but not amniotic fluid concentrations,

Table 6.2 Cytokines and chemokines expressed in human gestational membranes in increased amounts with normal labor, as determined by cDNA array

Tissue	Cytokines	Chemokines	Others
Amnion	IL-1α	IL-8	G-CSF
	IL-6	GRO-α/β/γ	LIF
	IL-11	IP-10	ST2
	PBEF	MIP-1α/1β	
		MIP-3α	
Choriodecidua	IL-1α	IL-8	G-CSF
	IL-6	GRO-α/β/γ	GM-CSF
	IL-11	MPIF-1	LIF
	IL-12		Oncostatin M
	IL-16		ST2
	PBEF		Activin βA

Adapted from Keelan et al[47] and Marvin et al.[48]

although amniotic fluid ENA-78 concentrations were positively correlated with gestational age at sampling. In contrast, amniotic fluid concentrations of the chemokine IL-16 decline from mid-gestation to term.[38]

The CC β-chemokine family contains a number of well-characterized chemokines, including the monocyte chemoattractant proteins (MCPs), RANTES (regulated on activation, normal T cells expressed and secreted), and the macrophage inflammatory proteins (MIPs). These chemokines primarily activate monocytes, lymphocytes, basophils, and eosinophils. MCP-1 mRNA is present in mid-trimester and term decidua[39] and the placenta throughout gestation, with increased expression in the third trimester coinciding with an increase in production of MCP-1 protein.[40] Secretion of MCP-1 from third-trimester decidua, chorion, and amnion has also been reported, and this cytokine is also present in amniotic fluid.[17] Of the other CC chemokines, mRNA for MCP-2 has been detected in placenta[41] and RANTES is secreted from the chorion, decidua, and placenta at term.[17]

RANTES is also detectable in amniotic fluid in the second and third trimesters and concentrations of this chemokine decrease with advancing gestational age.[42] MIP-1α has also been detected in amniotic fluid at mid gestation and term,[43] although it is present in only a proportion of women in the absence of labor.[44] Constitutive secretion of MIP-1α from gestational tissues has not been reported; however, cultured human chorionic[45] and decidual[46] cells from term pregnancies produce this chemokine when stimulated with inflammatory cytokines or bacterial products.

CHANGES IN CYTOKINE ELABORATION WITH LABOR

Production of mRNA or protein for many cytokines has been shown to change during normal labor and parturition. These alterations may play a significant role in the processes that culminate in successful delivery (Figure 6.1). Concentrations of inflammatory cytokines in amniotic fluid, for example,

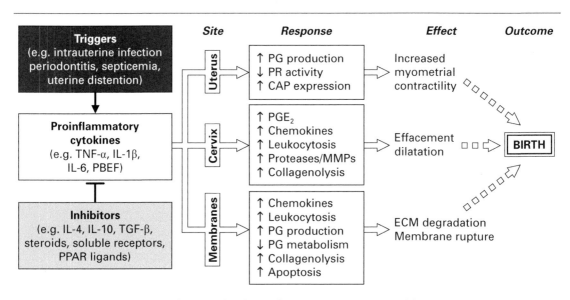

Figure 6.1 Cytokines, chemokines, and eicosanoids: roles in inflammatory processes in parturition. PR, progesterone receptor; CAP, contractile associated protein; ECM, extracellular matrix; TNF-α, tumor necrosis factor-α; IL-1β, IL-4, IL-6, IL-10, interleukins; TGF-β, transforming growth factor-β; PG, prostaglandin; PGE₂, prostaglandin E₂, MMPs, matrix metalloproteinases; PPAR, peroxisome proliferator activated receptor; PBEF, pre-B-cell colony enhancing factor.

increase towards term in normal pregnancies, and play a regulatory role in parturition by stimulating the local production of chemokines, prostaglandins, and collagenases.

INFLAMMATORY CYTOKINES

Array studies of cytokine gene expression in extra-placental membranes have identified a significant number of cytokines and chemokines that are up-regulated at term following spontaneous labor and vaginal delivery[47,48] (see Table 6.2). There was reasonable agreement and consistency in this study between gene expression changes in amnion compared with choriodecidua. These expression data support measurements of IL-1β, IL-6, and IL-8 by ELISA (enzyme-linked immunosorbent assay) in the same set of tissue samples, showing increased abundance of these proteins in the membranes with labor.[49] Exposure to labor at term results in increases in IL-1α production by the placenta,[13,50] amnion,[50] choriodecidua,[50] and unseparated fetal membranes.[51] Expression of IL-1β mRNA is also increased with labor in the amnion, chorion, and isolated decidua.[15]

Synthesis and release of IL-6 also appears to be increased by labor in gestational tissues,[52,53] although in-vitro production by amnion explants[49,54] and isolated decidual cultures[55] is not increased. Term labor is reportedly associated with strong immunoreactive staining for both IL-1β and IL-6 in endothelial cells of the placenta.[56] These authors earlier reported an increase in IL-6 production by the placenta following the onset of spontaneous term labor[55] which they attributed to placental endothelial cell production.[4] However, other studies have reported that exposure to labor does not increase IL-6 release from placental cultures[53,57] or IL-1β and IL-6 tissue content.[49] Messenger RNA for TNF-α is increased in amnion, chorion, and decidua with labor at term,[15] although release from decidual cell cultures is not affected by labor.[55] Release of TNF-α from placental cultures, in contrast, is increased following exposure to term labor,[55] apparently originating from placental macrophages.[4]

Many studies have measured cytokines in amniotic fluids, but only a few of these have identified changes in cytokine concentrations with onset of normal term labor (Table 6.3). Amniotic fluid IL-1β,[51,58,59] IL-6,[34,51,53,59–62] and TNF-α[59,63] concentrations are all reported to increase during labor. Concentrations of these cytokines in amniotic fluid appear to correlate with the amount of granulocyte infiltration observed in the placentae.[64] Of those cytokines found to be present in increased amounts with term labor, most have been shown to be up-regulated at the mRNA level in fetal membranes (see Table 6.2), suggesting that these tissues are the major source of the cytokines found in amniotic fluid. Fetal leukocytes and tissues (such as the lung) may also be contributing sources.

TNF-α, IL-1α, IL-6, and IL-8 can also be detected in cervicovaginal fluids before labor in the third trimester of pregnancy, particularly in women with bacterial vaginosis or who deliver preterm with associated intra-amniotic infection.[65–68] Concentrations of inflammatory cytokines in cervicovaginal secretions increase during spontaneous term labor[69] (see Table 6.3), peaking at the time of complete cervical dilation.

ANTI-INFLAMMATORY CYTOKINES

With term labor, there are no consistent reports of increased expression or production of anti-inflammatory cytokines, in marked contrast to the data on proinflammatory cytokines (see Table 6.2).

Table 6.3 Cytokines and chemokines measured in amniotic and cervicovaginal fluids in increased amounts with term labor

Fluid	Cytokines	Chemokines	Others
Amniotic	IL-1β IL-2 IL-6 TNF-α	IL-8 MCP-1 MIP-1α MIF RANTES	G-CSF
Cervicovaginal	IL-1α/β IL-6 TNF-α	IL-8 MCP-1	G-CSF

Derived and adapted from Bowen et al,[175] Jetta et al,[176] and Zicari et al.[177]

Whereas exposure to labor has been reported to *decrease* secretion of IL-10 from choriodecidua,[19] other clinicians have reported no change in amniotic fluid IL-10 levels[22,25,70] or in decidual IL-10 production[22] with labor. Amniotic fluid IL-4 concentrations are only rarely elevated following normal term labor.[71] IL-1 receptor antagonist (IL-1ra) is present in extremely high concentrations in amniotic fluid in mid to late gestation, but there is no evidence of an increase associated with parturition.[72] Decidual IL-1ra expression is similarly unaffected by labor[73] as are cord blood levels.[74] Only maternal plasma levels of IL-1ra have been reported to be elevated with labor.[75] Transforming growth factor-β (TGF-β) and the related molecule MIC-1 (macrophage inhibitory cytokine-1) are present in amniotic fluid at term,[76,77] but there are no changes in MIC-1 concentrations in amniotic fluid with parturition.[78]

CHEMOKINES

Expression of several chemokine genes in gestational membranes is up-regulated with term labor, as revealed by cDNA array analysis[47,48] (see Table 6.2). Levels of various chemokines in amniotic fluid are also increased following labor (see Table 6.3), including RANTES[42] and the ubiquitous IL-8.[35,79] Some studies report increased IL-8 production from placental explants[80] and increased IL-8 concentrations in tissue extracts of amnion and choriodecidual tissue[49] following spontaneous labor. Levels of IL-8 in the lower uterine segment are also elevated with labor.[81,82] Amniotic fluid concentrations of the chemokines GRO-α and IL-16 do not appear to alter in response to this stimulus,[36,38] despite increases in their mRNA expression in amnion (see Table 6.2).

LEUKOCYTE INFILTRATION AND ACTIVATION IN PARTURITION

The concept that leukocyte recruitment and activation is a key process in the mechanisms of parturition is now well established, particularly in the context of cervical ripening (reviewed by Yellon et al).[83] In the cervix, neutrophil recruitment and activation occurs in response to chemoattractants such as IL-8 and – in combination with local release of proinflammatory cytokines, prostaglandins, and MMPs (matrix metalloproteinases) – plays a crucial role in cervical ripening.[84–87] Leukocyte subpopulations (T cells, macrophages, and neutrophils) increase markedly in the cervix in late pregnancy, with additional increases after labor onset.[88] The factors responsible for the prelabor initiation of cervical leukocytosis are not known, but prostaglandins, cytokines, and steroids – such as dehydroepiandrosterone (DHEA) – are all possibilities that have been explored. Cervical leukocytosis is accompanied by increased expression of cytokines in the cervix and myometrium.[89] Macrophages are also a significant source of prostaglandins and nitric oxide (in addition to cytokines and MMPs), both of which are promoters of cervical ripening.

A recent study[90] quantified infiltrating inflammatory cells in myometrium with onset of normal term labor. Leukocytosis was greatest in the lower uterus, suggesting a degree of regionality exists in this process (an appreciation of which has been lacking in many studies). Elevated expression of adhesion molecules has also been documented in the myometrium and cervix, which at least in part is likely to be a consequence of leukocytic infiltration.[91] In myometrium from pregnancies with advanced cervical dilation, extensive leukocyte infiltration was recently documented after ruptured fetal membranes, with minimal changes detectable before parturition.[92] Leukocytes in myometrium (mainly neutrophils and macrophages) were immunostained for cytokines IL-1β, IL-6, IL-8, and TNF-α,[93] suggesting that they contribute to the proinflammatory milieu associated with parturition. Such findings suggest that leukocytosis of the myometrium is more associated with the progression and sequelae of labor than its initiation.

Within the membranes, although extensive leukocyte infiltration is commonly seen in pregnancies with intra-amniotic infection (i.e. chorioamnionitis), in normal pregnancies inflammatory cells in the gestational membranes are relatively rare prior to labor. Modest infiltration of the decidua is relatively common after onset of labor, however, correlating with cervical dilation.[94] The fetal membranes, on the other hand, show minimal infiltration either before or after labor. However, the importance of regionality should not be underestimated, particularly in light of the findings of Malak and Bell, who showed marked histological and structural changes in the region of membranes overlying the cervical os, the so-called 'zone of altered morphology' (ZAM).[95] The interrelationship between leukocytosis, inflammatory activation, and the formation of the ZAM has not yet been clarified, although the findings of a recently presented paper did not support the concept of a region-specific increase in leukocyte infiltration or cytokine expression in association with term labor.[96]

CYTOKINE REGULATION OF MYOMETRIAL CONTRACTILITY

INFLAMMATORY SIGNALING AND UTERINE QUIESCENCE

The uterine smooth muscle remains quiescent throughout pregnancy, primarily as a result of progesterone-induced suppression of contractile associated proteins (CAPs). Initiation of myometrial contractions requires conversion of the myometrium from a quiescent to an activated tissue. Changes in local concentrations of several uterotonins (e.g. prostaglandins) and their receptors have been implicated in this transition (reviewed by Keelan et al[97]), and this has been at the forefront of research over the past 20 years (detailed below). Cytokines have been investigated for their role in modulating prostaglandin (PG) biosynthesis and receptor activity in pregnant uterus. Most recently, the amnion-derived cytokine PBEF (pre-B-cell colony enhancing factor) has been reported to be a direct activator of human myometrium in vitro.[98] Expression of this cytokine in the fetal membranes[99,100] was identified as being up-regulated

with term and preterm labor, and able to increase local PG biosynthesis. These more recent findings of direct actions in the myometrium support claims that this cytokine may be of pivotal importance in human parturition.

Recent discoveries relating to the expression and activity of uterine progesterone receptors (PRs) have identified a role of cytokines and inflammation in the withdrawal of progesterone-mediated uterine quiescence at term.[101] This exciting development expands the sphere of influence of inflammatory processes in parturition (see Figure 6.1). The intracellular nexus for inflammatory signaling is the transcription factor NF-κB (nuclear factor-κB). Many parturition-related genes have NF-κB response elements in their promoters and their expression is up-regulated by NF-κB activation. Proinflammatory cytokines and so-called pathogen-associated molecular patterns (PAMPs) such as bacterial lipopolysaccharide (LPS) are potent activators of the NF-κB signaling pathway. Inhibitors of NF-κB can suppress inflammatory cytokine production by gestational tissues in vitro.[102,103] In amnion, labor is associated with NF-κB activation, which drives the expression of COX-2 (cyclo-oxygenase-2), the enzyme responsible for the increased prostaglandin production during labor.[104] PR activity is repressed by NF-κB activation in this tissue.[104] There is also evidence that PR expression is down-regulated in response to prostaglandins.[105] Similarly, in myometrium, term labor is associated with increased NF-κB activity[106] and increased expression of PRA (progesterone receptor A). PRA acts as a dominant negative, resulting in an increase in the PRA/PRB (progesterone receptor A/progesterone receptor B) ratio,[81,82] effectively reducing activity at the site of the PR promoter. Further effects on PR activity appear to be mediated by changes in coactivator expression,[107] although the significance of inflammatory signaling in this phenomenon is unknown. Finally, Dong et al described increased expression of a novel corepressor of PR action called PSF. Cytokines are known to increase the levels of expression of this protein in mammalian cells, and it is speculated that this could provide an additional mechanism linking inflammation with functional progesterone withdrawal.[108]

PROSTAGLANDINS

Prostaglandins E_2 and $F_{2\alpha}$ are potent stimulators of myometrial contractility and have long been appreciated to be critical factors in the initation of labor. Production of prostaglandins by cells from the amnion,[109–111] chorion,[112] decidua,[113] and myometrium[114–119] is enhanced by the inflammatory cytokines IL-1 and TNF-α, probably through increased expression of prostaglandin H synthase-2.[120] IL-6 has also been shown to stimulate prostaglandin production by the amnion and decidua at high doses,[121] whereas MIP-1α stimulates amnion and chorion cell prostaglandin production.[122]

Prostaglandin concentrations can also be modulated through regulation of metabolic inactivation. The enzyme that catabolizes prostaglandins to inactive metabolites, 15-hydroxy prostaglandin dehydrogenase (PGDH), is abundant in the chorion, placental trophoblast, and (to a lesser extent) the decidua.[123–125] Its activity is believed to prevent prostaglandins in the amniotic fluid from acting upon the myometrium. PGDH expression and activity in gestational membranes and cultured chorionic trophoblast is decreased by IL-1β and TNF-α.[126,127] PGDH protein and activity in chorionic trophoblast of the lower uterine segment has been shown to decrease with term labor, possibly contributing to the activation of the myometrium.[128]

Cytokines can also act to decrease prostaglandin production by gestational tissues. TGF-β₁ decreases basal and cytokine-stimulated prostaglandin production from amnion and decidual cells,[109] whereas IL-1ra and TGF-β₁ both suppress IL-1-induced PG production in the myometrium.[116] IL-4 decreases prostaglandin production from decidual cells while increasing production of IL-1ra,[109] and decreases inflammatory cytokine-stimulated prostaglandin production by placenta/trophoblast cultures, as does IL-10.[129,130] However, both IL-4 and IL-10 have also been reported to *stimulate* the release of prostaglandins and inflammatory cytokines by

some gestational tissues,[16,131] whereas IL-1ra has been found to increase prostaglandin production by decidual cells.[132] This has led to the hypothesis that term labor is associated with a withdrawal or reversal of anti-inflammatory agents as part of an evolutionary adaptation to accelerate inflammatory processes necessary for successful labor and delivery.[19]

MEMBRANE REMODELING AND RUPTURE

Rupture of the fetal membranes is an essential part of normal parturition. Cytokines may be involved in the initiation and progression of processes involved in rupture of the membranes at term and preterm (see Figure 6.1), particularly when associated with intrauterine infection and chorioamnionitis. Morphological examination of the amnion suggests that the membrane does not undergo a widespread process of degeneration at term; rather, localized weakening of the membrane, with reduced cytotrophoblast and decidual thickness, may occur at a specific rupture point overlying the cervix.[133,134]

Digestion of extracellular matrix of the fetal membranes occurs at term and is carried out largely by locally produced MMPs, the activity of which is negatively regulated by a family of inhibitory proteins, tissue inhibitors of metalloproteinases (TIMPs). Changes in activity of plasminogen activator, MMPs, and TIMPs in amniotic fluid and gestational tissues are associated with the onset of labor and rupture of the fetal membranes.[135–139] Cytokines drive the increased levels of MMP expression and activity in the membranes associated with rupture. Intrauterine infection has been associated with higher MMP-9 concentrations in amniotic fluid, whether or not membrane rupture occurred.[140] This increase in MMP-9 may reflect an increase in leukocyte colonization of the amniotic fluid. TNF-α, IL-1β, IL-6, and M-CSF (macrophage colony-stimulating factor) have all been shown to increase MMP gelatinase secretion by first trimester trophoblast.[141,142] TNF-α stimulates production of MMPs (MMP-1 and MMP-3) and plasminogen activator by chorion, and decreases the production of TIMP, whereas IL-1α increases synthesis of MMP-1 by cultured chorionic cells.[143] Treatment of amniochorion explants with LPS, a stimulator of cytokine release, also results in an increase in synthesis and release of MMP-2 and a decrease in the synthesis and release of its tissue inhibitor.[144] Relaxin, a hormone well-known for its ability to remodel extracellular matrix and accelerate membrane rupture, has recently been shown to superinduce cytokine (IL-1β and IL-6) expression in fetal membranes.[145] Concentrations of IL-8, a chemoattractant for leukocytes, have been significantly correlated with those of MMP-9 in the amnion and chorion during the later stages of cervical dilation.[81,82] IL-8 production in chorion and amnion is stimulated by IL-1β and TNF-α.[146–148] Interestingly, both IL-8 production and collagenase activity in the fetal membranes are increased by mechanical stretching,[149] pointing to an indirect mechanism of action for these cytokines in the remodeling of the extracellular matrix.

In addition to digestion of the extracellular matrix, there is some evidence that apoptosis contributes to weakening of the fetal membranes prior to rupture, particularly in the chorion layer at the site of rupture.[150,151] Apoptotic cell death may be a reaction to the destruction of extracellular matrix in the membranes or a significant and separate part of membrane thinning and rupture. TNF-α, in concert with interferon-γ (IFN-γ), induces trophoblast apoptosis.[152,153] TNF-α and other family members such as TRAIL (tumor necrosis factor-related apoptosis-inducing ligand)[37] may thus be involved in the normal rupture of fetal membranes at term, through induction of apoptosis.

CERVICAL RIPENING

The processes of cervical ripening are similar to those involved in induction of membrane rupture, including changes in extracellular matrix composition, invasion of neutrophils, and tissue remodeling by proteolytic enzymes.[86,87,154] Cytokines, particularly IL-8, have been implicated in this process (see Table 6.3). IL-8 synthesis and secretion is greatly increased in the cervix with labor, and concentrations of IL-8 in the cervix and lower uterine segment increase with cervical ripening.[84,155,156] The increase in IL-8 during cervical ripening correlates with increases in leukocyte infiltration and concentrations of MMPs in the tissue.[86,87,157,158] Concentrations of IL-1β, TNF-α, and IL-6 in the lower uterine segment also increase with cervical dilation[156,159] and have been shown to affect production of TIMPs and MMPs by human cervical fibroblasts and smooth muscle cells.[160–163] Increases in IL-6, G-CSF (granulocyte colony-stimulating factor), and MCP-1 – cytokines which affect proliferation and activation of immune cells – also occur with cervical ripening.[155,164]

Whereas the majority of cytokine effects on cervical ripening are likely to be induced by locally produced cytokines, it is possible that cytokines secreted by the placenta and membranes may have an indirect effect. IL-1β has been shown to induce IL-8 secretion by human cervical fibroblasts in vitro, alone and in concert with TGF-β$_1$ and growth factors.[165,166] Prostaglandin E$_2$ (PGE$_2$), the secretion of which is influenced by many cytokines, also stimulates IL-8 release from cervical tissue,[17,89,167,168] affects proteolytic enzyme activity,[17,89,167,168] and induces cervical ripening (reviewed by Kelly et al[169]). Hence, cytokines – acting through release of PGE$_2$, chemokines, and MMP activation – are potent drivers of cervical ripening.

FINAL COMMENTS

Is parturition an inflammatory reaction or process? We can summarize with some studies from key investigators. Studies from Trudinger and colleagues have demonstrated elegantly that inflammatory reactions occur within the gestational tissues and fetus with parturition.[170] Other studies from Osman and colleagues have described findings consistent with this viewpoint, and have extended their datasets to include myometrium.[17,89,167,168] Other clinicians, including Calder and coworkers, have extended significantly the information supporting the view that cervical ripening has elements in common with an inflammatory reaction.[17,167] Although we have focused on changes in cytokine expression and actions as evidence of parturition as an inflammatory reaction, there are also data from changes in expression and actions of many other mediators (e.g. nitric oxide, MMPs, etc.)[171-173] to support this view. Hence, we may conclude with confidence that parturition can be regarded as a process in which specialized forms of inflammation are fundamental to a successful outcome.

REFERENCES

1. Mitchell MD, Ellwood DA, Brennecke SP. Prostaglandins and parturition in sheep. In: MacDonald PC, Porter JC, eds. Initiation of Parturition: Prevention of Prematurity. Columbus: Ross Laboratories; 1983: 34–41.

2. Simon C, Frances A, Piquette G et al. Interleukin-1 system in the materno-trophoblast unit in human implantation: immunohistochemical evidence for autocrine/paracrine function. J Clin Endocrinol Metab 1994; 78:847–854.

3. Vince G, Shorter S, Starkey P et al. Localization of tumour necrosis factor production in cells at the materno/fetal interface in human pregnancy. Clin Exp Immunol 1992; 88:174–180.

4. Steinborn A, von Gall C, Hildenbrand R, Stutte HJ, Kaufmann M. Identification of placental cytokine-producing cells in term and preterm labor. Obstet Gynecol 1998; 91:329–335.

5. Saito S, Nishikawa K, Morii T et al. Cytokine production by CD16–CD56bright natural killer cells in the human early pregnancy decidua. Int Immunol 1993; 5:559–563.

6. Jokhi PP, King A, Loke YW. Cytokine production and cytokine receptor expression by cells of the human first trimester placental-uterine interface. Cytokine 1997; 9:126–137.

7. Jokhi PP, King A, Sharkey AM, Smith SK, Yung Wai L. Screening for cytokine messenger ribonucleic acids in purified human decidual lymphocyte populations by the reverse-transcriptase polymerase chain reaction. J Immunol 1994; 153:4427–4435.

8. Simon C, Moreno C, Remohi J, Pellicer A. Cytokines and embryo implantation. J Reprod Immunol 1998; 39:117–131.

9. Montes MJ, Tortosa CG, Borja C et al. Constitutive secretion of interleukin-6 by human decidual stromal cells in culture – regulatory effect of progesterone. Am J Reprod Immunol 1995; 34: 188–194.

10. Arcuri F, Ricci C, Ietta F et al. Macrophage migration inhibitory factor in the human endometrium: expression and localization during the menstrual cycle and early pregnancy. Biol Reprod 2001; 64:1200–1205.

11. Menon R, Swan KF, Lyden TW, Rote NS, Fortunato SJ. Expression of inflammatory cytokines (interleukin-1beta and interleukin-6) in amniochorionic membrane. Am J Obstet Gynecol 1995; 172: 493–500.

12. Fortunato SJ, Menon R, Swan KF. Expression of TNF-alpha and TNFR p55 in cultured amniochori. Am J Reprod Immunol 1994; 32:188–193.

13. Taniguchi T, Matsuzaki N, Kameda T et al. The enhanced production of placental interleukin-1 during labor and intrauterine infection. Am J Obstet Gynecol 1991; 165:131–137.

14. Librach CL, Feigenbaum SL, Bass KE et al. Interleukin-1 beta regulates human cytotrophoblast metalloproteinase activity and invasion in vitro. J Biol Chem 1994; 269:17125–17131.

15. Dudley DJ, Collmer D, Mitchell MD, Trautman MS. Inflammatory cytokine mRNA in human gestational tissues: implications for term and preterm labor. J Soc Gynecol Invest 1996; 3:328–335.

16. Mitchell MD, Simpson KL, Keelan JA. Paradoxical proinflammatory actions of interleukin-10 in human amnion: potential roles in term and preterm labor. J Clin Endocrinol Metab 2004; 89:4149–4152.

17. Denison FC, Kelly RW, Calder AA, Riley SC. Cytokine secretion by human fetal membranes, decidua and placenta at term. Hum Reprod 1998; 13:3560–3565.

18. Dudley DJ. Pre-term labor: an intra-uterine inflammatory response syndrome? J Reprod Immunol 1997; 36:93–109.

19. Simpson KL, Keelan JA, Mitchell MD. Labor-associated changes in interleukin-10 production and its regulation by immunomodulators in human choriodecidua. J Clin Endocrinol Metab 1998; 83: 4332–4337.

20. Chaouat G, Cayol V, Mairovitz V, Dubanchet S. Localization of the Th2 cytokines IL-3, IL-4, IL-10 at the fetomaternal interface during human and murine pregnancy and lack of requirement for Fas/Fas ligand interaction for a successful allogeneic pregnancy. Am J Reprod Immunol 1999; 42:1–13.

21. Roth I, Corry DB, Locksley RM et al. Human placental cytotrophoblasts produce the immunosuppressive cytokine interleukin 10. J Exp Med 1996; 184:539–548.

22. Jones CA, Finlay-Jones JJ, Hart PH. Type-1 and type-2 cytokines in human late-gestation decidual tissue. Biol Reprod 1997; 57:303–311.

23. Dudley DJ, Collmer D, Mitchell MD, Trautman MS. Inflammatory cytokine mRNA in human gestational tissues: implications for term and preterm labor. J Soc Gynecol Invest 1996; 3:328–335.

24. Baergen R, Benirschke K, Ulich TR. Cytokine expression in the placenta: the role of interleukin 1 and interleukin 1 receptor antagonist expression in chorioamnionitis and parturition. Arch Pathol Lab Med 1994; 118:52–55.

25. Greig PC, Herbert WNP, Robinette BL, Teot LA. Amniotic fluid interleukin-10 concentrations increase through pregnancy and are elevated in patients with preterm labor associated with intrauterine infection. Am J Obstet Gynecol 1995; 173:1223–1227.

26. Romero R, Gomez R, Galasso M et al. The natural interleukin-1 receptor antagonist in the fetal, maternal, and amniotic fluid compartments: the effect of gestational age, fetal gender, and intrauterine infection. Am J Obstet Gynecol 1994; 171:912–921.

27. Bry K, Teramo K, Lappalainen U, Waffarn F, Hallman M. Interleukin-1 receptor antagonist in the fetomaternal compartment. Acta Paediatr 1995; 84:233–236.

28. Fidel PL Jr, Romero R, Ramirez M et al. Interleukin-1 receptor antagonist (IL-1ra) production by human amnion, chorion, and decidua. Am J Reprod Immunol 1994; 32:1–7.

29. Kelly RW, Carr GG, Elliott CL, Tulppala M, Critchley HOD. Prostaglandin and cytokine release by trophoblastic villi. Hum Reprod 1995; 10:3289–3292.

30. Dealtry GB, Clark DE, Sharkey A, Charnock-Jones DS, Smith SK. Expression and localization of the Th2-type cytokine interleukin-13 and its receptor in the placenta during human pregnancy. Am J Reprod Immunol 1998; 40:283–290.

31. Williams JA, Pontzer CH, Shacter E. Regulation of macrophage interleukin-6 (IL-6) and IL-10 expression by prostaglandin E2: the

role of p38 mitogen-activated protein kinase. J Interferon Cytokine Res 2000; 20:291–298.

32. Shimoya K, Matsuzaki N, Taniguchi T et al. Human placenta constitutively produces interleukin-8 during pregnancy and enhances its production in intrauterine infection. Biol Reprod 1992; 47: 220–226.

33. Denison FC, Riley SC, Wathen NC et al. Differential concentrations of monocyte chemotactic protein-1 and interleukin-8 within the fluid compartments present during the first trimester of pregnancy. Hum Reprod 1998; 13:2292–2295.

34. Olah KS, Vince GS, Neilson JP, Deniz G, Johnson PM. Interleukin-6, interferon-gamma, interleukin-8, and granulocyte-macrophage colony stimulating factor levels in human amniotic fluid at term. J Reprod Immunol 1996; 32:89–98.

35. Laham N, Rice GE, Bishop GJ, Ransome C, Brennecke SP. Interleukin 8 concentrations in amniotic fluid and peripheral venous plasma during human pregnancy and parturition. Acta Endocrinol 1993; 129:220–224.

36. Cohen J, Ghezzi F, Romero R et al. GRO alpha in the fetomaternal and amniotic fluid compartments during pregnancy and parturition. Am J Reprod Immunol 1996; 35:23–29.

37. Lonergan M, Aponso D, Marvin KW et al. Tumor necrosis factor-related apoptosis-inducing ligand (TRAIL), TRAIL receptors, and the soluble receptor osteoprotegerin in human gestational membranes and amniotic fluid during pregnancy and labor at term and preterm. J Clin Endocrinol Metab 2003; 88:3835–3844.

38. Athayde N, Romero R, Maymon E et al. Interleukin 16 in pregnancy, parturition, rupture of fetal membranes, and microbial invasion of the amniotic cavity. Am J Obstet Gynecol 2000; 182: 135–141.

39. Arici A, MacDonald PC, Casey ML. Regulation of monocyte chemotactic protein-1 gene expression in human endometrial cells in cultures. Mol Cell Endocrinol 1995; 107:189–197.

40. Shimoya K, Matsuzaki N, Sawai K et al. Regulation of placental monocyte chemotactic and activating factor during pregnancy and chorioamnionitis. Mol Hum Reprod 1998; 4:393–400.

41. Van Coillie E, Fiten P, Nomiyama H et al. The human MCP-2 gene (SCYA8) – cloning, sequence analysis, tissue expression, and assignment to the CC chemokine gene contig on chromosome 17q11.2. Genomics 1997; 40:323–331.

42. Athayde N, Romero R, Maymon E et al. A role for the novel cytokine RANTES in pregnancy and parturition. Am J Obstet Gynecol 1999; 181:989–994.

43. Srivastava MD, Lippes J, Srivastava BIS. Cytokines of the human reproductive tract. Am J Reprod Immunol 1996; 36:157–166.

44. Mazor M, Chaim W, Horowitz S, Romero R, Glezerman M. The biomolecular mechanisms of preterm labor in women with intrauterine infection. Israel J Med Sci 1994; 30:317–322.

45. Dudley DJ, Edwin SS, Dangerfield A, Van Waggoner J, Mitchell MD. Regulation of cultured human chorion cell chemokine production by group B streptococci and purified bacterial products. Am J Reprod Immunol 1996; 36:264–268.

46. Dudley DJ, Spencer S, Edwin S, Mitchell MD. Regulation of human decidual cell macrophage inflammatory protein-1alpha (MIP-1alpha) production by inflammatory cytokines. Am J Reprod Immunol 1995; 34:231–235.

47. Keelan JA, Blumenstein M, Helliwell RJ et al. Cytokines, prostaglandins and parturition – a review. Placenta 2003; 24 (Suppl A):S33–46.

48. Marvin KW, Keelan JA, Eykholt RL, Sato TA, Mitchell MD. Use of cDNA arrays to generate differential expression profiles for inflam-

matory genes in human gestational membranes delivered at term and preterm. Mol Hum Reprod 2002; 8:399–408.

49. Keelan JA, Marvin KW, Sato TA et al. Cytokine abundance in placental tissues: evidence of inflammatory activation in gestational membranes with term and preterm parturition. Am J Obstet Gynecol 1999; 181:1530–1536.

50. Laham N, Brennecke SP, Bendtzen K, Rice GE. Labor-associated increase in interleukin-1-alpha release in vitro by human gestational tissues. J Endocrinol 1996; 150:515–522.

51. Gunn L, Hardiman P, Tharmaratnam S, Lowe D, Chard T. Measurement of interleukin-1-alpha and interleukin-6 in pregnancy-associated tissues. Reprod Fertil Dev 1996; 8:1069–1073.

52. Keelan JA, Marvin KW, Sato TA et al. Cytokine abundance in placental tissues: evidence of inflammatory activation in gestational membranes with term and preterm parturition. Am J Obstet Gynecol 1999; 181:1530–1536.

53. Laham N, Brennecke SP, Bendtzen K, Rice GE. Differential release of interleukin-6 from human gestational tissues in association with labor and in vitro endotoxin treatment. J Endocrinol 1996; 149: 431–439.

54. Simpson KL, Keelan JA, Mitchell MD. Labor-associated changes in the regulation of production of immunomodulators in human amnion by glucocorticoids, bacterial lipopolysaccharide and pro-inflammatory cytokines. J Reprod Fertil 1999; 116:321–327.

55. Steinborn A, Gunes H, Roddiger S, Halberstadt E. Elevated placental cytokine release, a process associated with preterm labor in the absence of intrauterine infection. Obstet Gynecol 1996; 88:534–539.

56. Steinborn A, Niederhut A, Solbach C et al. Cytokine release from placental endothelial cells, a process associated with preterm labor in the absence of intrauterine infection. Cytokine 1999; 11:66–73.

57. Matsuzaki N, Taniguchi T, Shimoya K et al. Placental interleukin-6 production is enhanced in intrauterine infection but not in labor. Am J Obstet Gynecol 1993; 168:94–97.

58. Romero R, Parvizi ST, Oyarzun E et al. Amniotic fluid interleukin-1 in spontaneous labor at term. J Reprod Med 1990; 35:235–238.

59. Opsjon SL, Wathen NC, Tingulstad S et al. Tumor necrosis factor, interleukin-1, and interleukin-6 in normal human pregnancy. Am J Obstet Gynecol 1993; 169:397–404.

60. Romero R, Avila C, Santhanam U, Sehgal PB. Amniotic fluid interleukin 6 in preterm labor. Association with infection. J Clin Invest 1990; 85:1392–1400.

61. Saito S, Kasahara T, Kato Y, Ishihara Y, Ichijo M. Elevation of amniotic fluid interleukin 6 (IL-6), IL-8 and granulocyte colony stimulating factor (G-CSF) in term and preterm parturition. Cytokine 1993; 5:81–88.

62. Santhanam U, Avila C, Romero R et al. Cytokines in normal and abnormal parturition: elevated amniotic fluid interleukin-6 levels in women with premature rupture of membranes associated with intrauterine infection. Cytokine 1991; 3:155–163.

63. Romero R, Mazor M, Sepulveda W et al. Tumor necrosis factor in preterm and term labor. Am J Obstet Gynecol 1992; 166:1576–1587.

64. Halgunset J, Johnsen H, Kjollesdal AM et al. Cytokine levels in amniotic fluid and inflammatory changes in the placenta from normal deliveries at term. Eur J Obstet Gynecol Reprod Biol 1994; 56: 153–160.

65. Inglis SR, Jeremias J, Kuno K et al. Detection of tumor necrosis factor-alpha, interleukin-6, and fetal fibronectin in the lower genital tract during pregnancy: relation to outcome. Am J Obstet Gynecol 1994; 171:5–10.

66. Mattsby-Baltzer I, Platz-Christensen JJ, Hosseini N, Rosen P. IL-1-beta, IL-6, TNF-apha, fetal fibronectin, and endotoxin in the lower

genital tract of pregnant women with bacterial vaginosis. Acta Obstet Gynecol Scand 1998; 77:701–706.

67. Rizzo G, Capponi A, Rinaldo D et al. Interleukin-6 concentrations in cervical secretions identify microbial invasion of the amniotic cavity in patients with preterm labor and intact membranes. Am J Obstet Gynecol 1996; 175:812–817.

68. Wennerholm UB, Holm B, Mattsby-Baltzer I et al. Interleukin-1-alpha, interleukin-6 and interleukin-8 in cervico/vaginal secretion for screening of preterm birth in twin gestation. Acta Obstet Gynecol Scand 1998; 77:508–514.

69. Cox SM, King MR, Casey ML, MacDonald PC. Interleukin-1 beta, -1 alpha, and -6 and prostaglandins in vaginal/cervical fluids of pregnant women before and during labor. J Clin Endocrinol Metab 1993; 77:805–815.

70. Dudley DJ, Edwin SS, Dangerfield A, Jackson K, Trautman MS. Regulation of decidual cell and chorion cell production of interleukin-10 by purified bacterial products. Am J Reprod Immunol 1997; 38:246–251.

71. Dudley DJ, Hunter C, Varner MW, Mitchell MD. Elevation of amniotic fluid interleukin-4 concentrations in women with preterm labor and chorioamnionitis. Am J Perinatol 1996; 13:443–447.

72. Romero R, Sepulveda W, Mazor M et al. The natural interleukin-1 receptor antagonist in term and preterm parturition. Am J Obstet Gynecol 1992; 167:863–872.

73. Ammala M, Nyman T, Salmi A, Rutanen EM. The interleukin-1 system in gestational tissues at term – effect of labor. Placenta 1997; 18:717–723.

74. Hata T, Kawamura T, Inada K et al. Cord blood cytokines and soluble adhesion molecules in vaginal and cesarean delivered neonates. Gynecol Obstet Invest 1996; 42:102–104.

75. Austgulen R, Lien E, Liabakk N, Jacobsen G, Arntzen KJ. Increased levels of cytokines and cytokine activity modifiers in normal pregnancy. Eur J Obstet Gynecol Reprod Biol 1994; 57:149–155.

76. Lang AK, Searle RF. The immunomodulatory activity of human amniotic fluid can be correlated with transforming factor-beta 1 (TGF-beta1) and beta2 activity. Clin Exp Immunol 1994; 97: 158–163.

77. Moore AG, Brown DA, Fairlie WD et al. The transforming growth factor-ss superfamily cytokine macrophage inhibitory cytokine-1 is present in high concentrations in the serum of pregnant women. J Clin Endocrinol Metab 2000; 85:4781–4788.

78. Keelan JA, Wang K, Chaiworapongsa T et al. Macrophage inhibitory cytokine 1 in fetal membranes and amniotic fluid from pregnancies with and without preterm labor and premature rupture of membranes. Mol Hum Reprod 2003; 9:535–540.

79. Saito S, Nishikawa K, Morii T et al. Cytokine production by CD16–CD56bright natural killer cells in the human early pregnancy decidua. Int Immunol 1993; 5:559–563.

80. Elliott CL, Kelly RW, Critchley HO, Riley SC, Calder AA. Regulation of interleukin 8 production in the term human placenta during labor and by antigestagens. Am J Obstet Gynecol 1998; 179: 215–220.

81. Mesiano S, Chan EC, Fitter JT et al. Progesterone withdrawal and estrogen activation in human parturition are coordinated by progesterone receptor A expression in the myometrium. J Clin Endocrinol Metab 2002; 87:2924–2930.

82. Pieber D, Allport VC, Hills F, Johnson M, Bennett PR. Interactions between progesterone receptor isoforms in myometrial cells in human labor. Mol Hum Reprod 2001; 7:875–879.

83. Yellon SM, Mackler AM, Kirby MA. The role of leukocyte traffic and activation in parturition. J Soc Gynecol Invest 2003; 10:323–338.

84. Sennstrom MKB, Brauner A, Lu Y et al. Interleukin-8 is a mediator of the final cervical ripening in humans. Eur J Obstet Gynecol Reprod Biol 1997; 74:89–92.

85. Osmers RGW, Blaser J, Kuhn W, Tschesche H. Interleukin-8 synthesis and the onset of labor. Obstet Gynecol 1995; 86:223–229.

86. Osmers RGW, Adelmann-Grill BC, Rath W et al. Biochemical events in cervical ripening dilatation during pregnancy and parturition. J Obstet Gynecol 1995; 21:185–194.

87. Winkler M, Oberpichler A, Tschesche H et al. Collagenolysis in the lower uterine segment during parturition at term: correlations with stage of cervical dilatation and duration of labor. Am J Obstet Gynecol 1999; 181:153–158.

88. Bokstrom H, Brannstrom M, Alexandersson M, Norstrom A. Leukocyte subpopulations in the human uterine cervical stroma at early and term pregnancy. Hum Reprod 1997; 12:586–590.

89. Osman I, Young A, Ledingham MA et al. Leukocyte density and pro-inflammatory cytokine expression in human fetal membranes, decidua, cervix and myometrium before and during labor at term. Mol Hum Reprod 2003; 9:41–45.

90. Thomson AJ, Telfer JF, Young A et al. Leukocytes infiltrate the myometrium during human parturition: further evidence that labor is an inflammatory process. Hum Reprod 1999; 14:229–236.

91. Ledingham MA, Thomson AJ, Jordan F et al. Cell adhesion molecule expression in the cervix and myometrium during pregnancy and parturition. Obstet Gynecol 2001; 97:235–242.

92. Keski-Nisula LT, Aalto ML, Kirkinen PP, Kosma VM, Heinonen ST. Myometrial inflammation in human delivery and its association with labor and infection. Am J Clin Pathol 2003; 120:217–224.

93. Young A, Thomson AJ, Ledingham M et al. Immunolocalization of proinflammatory cytokines in myometrium, cervix, and fetal membranes during human parturition at term. Biol Reprod 2002; 66:445–449.

94. Keski-Nisula L, Aalto ML, Katila ML, Kirkinen P. Intrauterine inflammation at term: a histopathologic study. Hum Pathol 2000; 31:841–846.

95. Malak TM, Bell SC. Structural characteristics of term human fetal membranes: a novel zone of extreme morphological alteration within the rupture site. Br J Obstet Gynaecol 1994; 101:375–386.

96. Osman I, Young A, Jordan F, Greer IA, Norman JE. Leukocyte density and proinflammatory cytokine expression in human preterm myometrium. J Soc Gynecol Invest 2005; 12:257A.

97. Keelan JA, Coleman M, Mitchell MD. The molecular mechanisms of term and preterm labor: recent progress and clinical implications. Clin Obstet Gynecol 1997; 40:460–478.

98. Betancourt A, Ognjanovic S, Wentz M et al. Pre-B-cell colony enhancing factor (PBEF) stimulates spontaneous contractile activity of uterine tissues from pregnant women at term. J Soc Gynecol Invest 2005; 12:251A.

99. Ognjanovic S, Bao S, Yamamoto SY et al. Genomic organization of the gene coding for human pre-B-cell colony enhancing factor and expression in human fetal membranes. J Mol Endocrinol 2001; 26:107–117.

100. Ognjanovic S, Bryant-Greenwood GD. Pre-B-cell colony-enhancing factor, a novel cytokine of human fetal membranes. Am J Obstet Gynecol 2002; 187:1051–1058.

101. Henderson D, Wilson T. Reduced binding of progesterone receptor to its nuclear response element after human labor onset. Am J Obstet Gynecol 2001; 185:579–585.

102. Lappas M, Permezel M, Rice GE. N-Acetyl-cysteine inhibits phospholipid metabolism, proinflammatory cytokine release, protease activity, and nuclear factor-kappaB deoxyribonucleic acid-binding

activity in human fetal membranes in vitro. J Clin Endocrinol Metab 2003; 88:1723–1729.

103. Yosaatmadja F, Mitchell MD, Keelan JA. The NF-kappaB inhibitor sulfasalazine is an effective anti-inflammatory drug in an ex-vivo model of intrauterine infection. Perinatal Society of Australia and New Zealand 8th Annual Congress Sydney; 2004.

104. Allport VC, Pieber D, Slater DM et al. Human labor is associated with nuclear factor-kappaB activity which mediates cyclo-oxygenase-2 expression and is involved with the 'functional progesterone withdrawal'. Mol Hum Reprod 2001; 7:581–586.

105. Goldman S, Weiss A, Almalah I, Shalev E. Progesterone receptor expression in human decidua and fetal membranes before and after contractions: possible mechanism for functional progesterone withdrawal. Mol Hum Reprod 2005; 11:269–277.

106. Chapman NR, Europe-Finner GN, Robson SC. Expression and deoxyribonucleic acid-binding activity of the nuclear factor kappaB family in the human myometrium during pregnancy and labor. J Clin Endocrinol Metab 2004; 89:5683–5693.

107. Condon JC, Jeyasuria P, Faust JM, Wilson JW, Mendelson CR. A decline in the levels of progesterone receptor coactivators in the pregnant uterus at term may antagonize progesterone receptor function and contribute to the initiation of parturition. Proc Natl Acad Sci USA 2003; 100:9518–9523.

108. Dong X, Shylnova O, Challis JRG, Lye SJ. Identification and characterization of the protein-associated splicing factor as a negative co-regulator of the progesterone receptor. J Biol Chem 2005; 280:13329–13340.

109. Bry K, Hallman M. Transforming growth factor-beta opposes the stimulatory effects of interleukin-1 and tumor necrosis factor on amnion cell prostaglandin E2 production: implication for preterm labor. Am J Obstet Gynecol 1992; 167:222–226.

110. Romero R, Durum S, Dinarello CA et al. Interleukin-1 stimulates prostaglandin biosynthesis by human amnion. Prostaglandins 1989; 37:13–22.

111. Romero R, Manogue KR, Mitchell MD et al. Infection and labor. IV. Cachectin-tumor necrosis factor in the amniotic fluid of women with intraamniotic infection and preterm labor. Am J Obstet Gynecol 1989; 161:336–341.

112. Lundin-Schiller S, Mitchell MD. Prostaglandin production by human chorion laeve cells in response to inflammatory mediators. Placenta 1991; 12:353–363.

113. Mitchell MD, Edwin S, Romero RJ. Prostaglandin biosynthesis by human decidual cells: effects of inflammatory mediators. Prostaglandins Leukot Essent Fatty Acids 1990; 41:35–38.

114. Hertelendy F, Romero R, Molnar M, Todd H, Baldassare JJ. Cytokine-initiated signal transduction in human myometrial cells. Am J Reprod Immunol 1993; 30:49–57.

115. Molnar M, Romero R, Hertelendy F. Interleukin-1 and tumor necrosis factor stimulate arachidonic acid release and phospholipid metabolism in human myometrial cells. Am J Obstet Gynecol 1993; 169:825–829.

116. Todd HM, Dundoo VL, Gerber WR et al. Effect of cytokines on prostaglandin E2 and prostacyclin production in primary cultures of human myometrial cells. J Matern Fetal Med 1996; 5:161–167.

117. Pollard JK, Mitchell MD. Intrauterine infection and the effects of inflammatory mediators on prostaglandin production by myometrial cells from pregnant women. Am J Obstet Gynecol 1996; 174:682–686.

118. Pollard JK, Mitchell MD. Effects of gestational age on prostaglandin production and its regulation in human myometrial cells. J Matern Fetal Med 1996; 5:93–98.

119. Grammatopoulos DK, Hillhouse EW. Basal and interleukin-1beta-stimulated prostaglandin production from cultured human myometrial cells: differential regulation by corticotropin-releasing hormone. J Clin Endocrinol Metab 1999; 84:2204–2211.

120. Rauk PN, Chiao JP. Interleukin-1 stimulates human uterine prostaglandin production through induction of cyclooxygenase-2 expression. Am J Reprod Immunol 2000; 43:152–159.

121. Mitchell MD, Dudley DJ, Edwin SS, Schiller SL. Interleukin-6 stimulates prostaglandin production by human amnion and decidual cells. Eur J Pharmacol 1991; 192:189–191.

122. Dudley DJ, Edwin SS, Mitchell MD. Macrophage inflammatory protein-I alpha regulates prostaglandin E2 and interleukin-6 production by human gestational tissues in vitro. J Soc Gynecol Invest 1996; 3:12–16.

123. Germain AM, Smith J, Casey ML, MacDonald PC. Human fetal membrane contribution to the prevention of parturition: uterotonin degradation. J Clin Endocrinol Metab 1994; 78:463–470.

124. Cheung PY, Walton JC, Tai HH, Riley SC, Challis JR. Localization of 15-hydroxy prostaglandin dehydrogenase in human fetal membranes, decidua, and placenta during pregnancy. Gynecol Obstet Invest 1992; 33:142–146.

125. Erwich JJ, Keirse MJ. Placental localization of 15-hydroxy-prostaglandin dehydrogenase in early and term human pregnancy. Placenta 1992; 13:223–229.

126. Brown NL, Alvi SA, Elder MG, Bennett PR, Sullivan MH. Interleukin-1beta and bacterial endotoxin change the metabolism of prostaglandins E2 and F2alpha in intact term fetal membranes. Placenta 1998; 19:625–630.

127. Mitchell MD, Goodwin V, Mesnage S, Keelan JA. Cytokine-induced coordinate expression of enzymes of prostaglandin biosynthesis and metabolism: 15-hydroxyprostaglandin dehydrogenase. Prostaglandins Leukot Essent Fatty Acids 2000; 62:1–5.

128. Van Meir CA, Ramirez MM, Matthews SG et al. Chorionic prostaglandin catabolism is decreased in the lower uterine segment with term labor. Placenta 1997; 18:109–114.

129. Pomini F, Caruso A, Challis JR. Interleukin-10 modifies the effects of interleukin-1beta and tumor necrosis factor-alpha on the activity and expression of prostaglandin H synthase-2 and the NAD$^+$-dependent 15-hydroxyprostaglandin dehydrogenase in cultured term human villous trophoblast and chorion trophoblast cells. J Clin Endocrinol Metab 1999; 84:4645–4651.

130. Goodwin VJ, Sato TA, Mitchell MD, Keelan JA. Anti-inflammatory effects of interleukin-4, interleukin-10, and transforming growth factor-beta on human placental cells in vitro. Am J Reprod Immunol 1998; 40:319–325.

131. Adamson S, Edwin SS, LaMarche S, Mitchell MD. Actions of interleukin-4 on prostaglandin biosynthesis at the chorion–decidual interface. Am J Obstet Gynecol 1993; 169:1442–1447.

132. Mitchell MD, Edwin SS, Silver RM, Romero RJ. Potential agonist action of the interleukin-1 receptor antagonist protein: implications for treatment of women. J Clin Endocrinol Metab 1993; 76: 1386–1388.

133. Malak TM, Bell SC. Structural characteristics of term human fetal membranes: a novel zone of extreme morphological alteration within the rupture site. Br J Obstet Gynaecol 1994; 101:375–386.

134. McLaren J, Malak TM, Bell SC. Structural characteristics of term human fetal membranes prior to labor: identification of an area of altered morphology overlying the cervix. Hum Reprod 1999; 14:237–241.

135. Koay ES, Bryant-Greenwood GD, Yamamoto SY, Greenwood FC. The human fetal membranes: a target tissue for relaxin. J Clin Endocrinol Metab 1986; 62:513–521.

136. Bryant-Greenwood GD, Yamamoto SY. Control of peripartal collagenolysis in the human chorion-decidua. Am J Obstet Gynecol 1995; 172:63–70.

137. Draper D, McGregor J, Hall J et al. Elevated protease activities in human amnion and chorion correlate with preterm premature rupture of membranes. Am J Obstet Gynecol 1995; 173: 1506–1512.

138. Vadillo-Ortega F, Gonzalez-Avila G, Furth EE et al. 92-kd type IV collagenase (matrix metalloproteinase-9) activity in human amnio-chorion increases with labor. Am J Pathol 1995; 146:148–156.

139. Vadillo-Ortega F, Hernandez A, Gonzalez-Avila G et al. Increased matrix metalloproteinase activity and reduced tissue inhibitor of metalloproteinases-1 levels in amniotic fluids from pregnancies complicated by premature rupture of membranes. Am J Obstet Gynecol 1996; 174:1371–1376.

140. Athayde N, Edwin SS, Romero R et al. A role for matrix metalloproteinase-9 in spontaneous rupture of the fetal membranes. Am J Obstet Gynecol 1998; 179:1248–1253.

141. Meisser A, Chardonnens D, Campana A, Bischof P. Effects of tumour necrosis factor-alpha, interleukin-1 alpha, macrophage colony stimulating factor and transforming growth factor beta on trophoblastic matrix metalloproteinases. Mol Hum Reprod 1999; 5:252–260.

142. Meisser A, Cameo P, Islami D, Campana A, Bischof P. Effects of interleukin-6 (IL-6) on cytotrophoblastic cells. Mol Hum Reprod 1999; 5:1055–1058.

143. Katsura M, Ito A, Hirakawa S, Mori Y. Human recombinant interleukin-1 alpha increases biosynthesis of collagenase and hyaluronic acid in cultured human chorionic cells. FEBS Lett 1989; 244:315–318.

144. Fortunato SJ, Menon R, Lombardi SJ. Amniochorion gelatinase–gelatinase inhibitor imbalance in vitro: a possible infectious pathway to rupture. Obstet Gynecol 2000; 95:240–244.

145. Bryant-Greenwood G, Yamamoto S, Lowndes K. Relaxin causes proinflammatory response in the fetal membranes but is uninvolved in the infection-mediated cytokine response. J Soc Gynecol Invest 2005; 12:267A.

146. Ito A, Nakamura T, Uchiyama T et al. Stimulation of the biosynthesis of interleukin 8 by interleukin 1 and tumor necrosis factor α in cultured human chorionic cells. Biol Pharm Bull 1994; 17: 1463–1467.

147. Trautman MS, Dudley DJ, Edwin SS, Collmer D, Mitchell MD. Amnion cell biosynthesis of interleukin-8: regulation by inflammatory cytokines. J Cell Physiol 1992; 153:38–43.

148. Keelan JA, Sato T, Mitchell MD. Interleukin (IL)-6 and IL-8 production by human amnion: regulation by cytokines, growth factors, glucocorticoids, phorbol esters, and bacterial lipopolysaccharide. Biol Reprod 1997; 57:1438–1444.

149. El Maradny E, Kanayama N, Halim A, Maehara K, Terao T. Stretching of fetal membranes increases the concentration of interleukin-8 and collagenase activity. Am J Obstet Gynecol 1996; 174:843–849.

150. Runic R, Lockwood CJ, LaChapelle L et al. Apoptosis and Fas expression in human fetal membranes. J Clin Endocrinol Metab 1998; 83:660–666.

151. McLaren J, Taylor DJ, Bell SC. Increased incidence of apoptosis in non-labor-affected cytotrophoblast cells in term fetal membranes overlying the cervix. Hum Reprod 1999; 14:2895–2900.

152. Yui J, Garcia-Lloret M, Wegmann TG, Guilbert LJ. Cytotoxicity of tumour necrosis factor-alpha and gamma-interferon against primary human placental trophoblasts. Placenta 1994; 15:819–835.

153. Garcia-Lloret MI, Yui J, Winkler-Lowen B, Guilbert LJ. Epidermal growth factor inhibits cytokine-induced apoptosis of primary human trophoblasts. J Cell Physiol 1996; 167:324–332.

154. Liggins GC. Cervical ripening as an inflammatory reaction. In: Ellwood DA Anderson ABM, eds. The Cervix in Pregnancy and Labour, Clinical and Biochemical Investigations. Edinburgh: Churchill Livingstone; 1981: 1–9.

155. Sennstrom MB, Ekman G, Westergren-Thorsson G et al. Human cervical ripening, an inflammatory process mediated by cytokines. Mol Hum Reprod 2000; 6:375–381.

156. Winkler M, Fischer DC, Hlubek M et al. Interleukin-1beta and interleukin-8 concentrations in the lower uterine segment during parturition at term. Obstet Gynecol 1998; 91:945–949.

157. Osmers RGW, Blaser J, Kuhn W, Tschesche H. Interleukin-8 synthesis and the onset of labor. Obstet Gynecol 1995; 86:223–229.

158. Winkler M, Fischer DC, Ruck P et al. Parturition at term: parallel increases in interleukin-8 and proteinase concentrations and neutrophil count in the lower uterine segment. Hum Reprod 1999; 14:1096–1100.

159. Winkler M, Fischer DC, Ruck P et al. Cytokine concentrations and expression of adhesion molecules in the lower uterine segment during parturition at term: relation to cervical dilatation and duration of labor. Z Geburtshilfe Neonatol 1998; 202:172–175.

160. Ito A, Sato T, Iga T, Mori Y. Tumor necrosis factor bifunctionally regulates matrix metalloproteinases and tissue inhibitor of metalloproteinases (TIMP) production by human fibroblasts. FEBS Lett 1990; 269:93–95.

161. Ito A, Leppert PC, Mori Y. Human recombinant interleukin-1 alpha increases elastase-like enzyme in human uterine cervical fibroblasts. Gynecol Obstet Invest 1990; 30:239–241.

162. Sato T, Ito A, Mori Y. Interleukin 6 enhances the production of tissue inhibitor of metalloproteinases (TIMP) but not that of matrix metalloproteinases by human fibroblasts. Biochem Biophys Res Commun 1990; 170:824–829.

163. Ogawa M, Hirano H, Tsubaki H, Kodama H, Tanaka T. The role of cytokines in cervical ripening: correlations between the concentrations of cytokines and hyaluronic acid in cervical mucus and the induction of hyaluronic acid production by inflammatory cytokines by human cervical fibroblasts. Am J Obstet Gynecol 1998; 179:105–110.

164. Denison FC, Riley SC, Elliott CL et al. The effect of mifepristone administration on leukocyte populations, matrix metalloproteinases and inflammatory mediators in the first trimester cervix. Mol Hum Reprod 2000; 6:541–548.

165. Winkler M, Ruck P, Horny HP et al. Expression of cell adhesion molecules by endothelium in the human lower uterine segment during parturition at term. Am J Obstet Gynecol 1998; 178: 557–561.

166. Winkler M, Rath W, Fischer DC, van de Leur E, Haubeck H. Regulation of interleukin-8 synthesis in human lower uterine segment fibroblasts by cytokines and growth factors. Obstet Gynecol 2000; 95:584–588.

167. Denison FC, Calder AA, Kelly RW. The action of prostaglandin E2 on the human cervix: stimulation of interleukin 8 and inhibition of secretory leukocyte protease inhibitor. Am J Obstet Gynecol 1999; 180:614–620.

168. Osman I, Crawford M, Jordan F et al. Expression and localization of cell adhesion molecules in human fetal membranes during parturition. J Reprod Immunol 2004; 63:11–21.

169. Kelly RW. Inflammatory mediators and cervical ripening. J Reprod Immunol 2002; 57:217–224.

170. Wang X, Athayde N, Trudinger B. A proinflammatory cytokine response is present in the fetal placental vasculature in placental insufficiency. Am J Obstet Gynecol 2003; 189: 1445–1451.

171. Athayde N, Romero R, Gomez R et al. Matrix metalloproteinases-9 in preterm and term human parturition. J Matern Fetal Med 1999; 8:213–219.

172. Bartlett SR, Bennett PR, Campa JS et al. Expression of nitric oxide synthase isoforms in pregnant human myometrium. J Physiol 1999; 521:705–716.

173. Roh C, Oh W, Yoon B, Lee J. Up-regulation of matrix metalloproteinase-9 in human myometrium during labor: a cytokine-mediated process in uterine smooth muscle cells. Mol Hum Reprod 2000; 6:96–102.

174. Bowen JM, Chamley L, Mitchell MD, Keelan JA. Cytokines of the placenta and extra-placental membranes: biosynthesis, secretion and roles in establishment of pregnancy in women. Placenta 2002; 23:239–256.

175. Bowen JM, Chamley L, Keelan JA, Mitchell MD. Cytokines of the placenta and extra-placental membranes: roles and regulation during human pregnancy and parturition. Placenta 2002; 23: 257–273.

176. Ietta F, Todros T, Ticconi C et al. Macrophage migration inhibitory factor in human pregnancy and labor. Am J Reprod Immunol 2002; 48:404–409.

177. Zicari A, Ticconi C, Pasetto N et al. Interleukin-2 in human amniotic fluid during pregnancy and parturition: implications for prostaglandin E2 release by fetal membranes. J Reprod Immunol 1995; 29:197–208.

7. Role of inflammatory mediators in preterm premature rupture of fetal membranes

Ramkumar Menon and Stephen J Fortunato

INTRODUCTION

Spontaneous preterm delivery (PTD) (less than 37 weeks of gestation), prematurity, and low birth weight due to prematurity account for a large proportion of neonatal morbidity and mortality (85%). PTD arises from multiple etiological pathways and these can be grouped mainly into four categories: infectious, idiopathic, preterm premature rupture of the membranes (preterm PROM), and other medical and obstetrical complications. Premature rupture of the membranes (PROM) at term occurs in approximately 10% of all pregnancies and, in most cases, the latency between PROM and delivery is less than 24 hours. Preterm PROM (from hereon referred as pPROM) occurs in approximately 1–4% of women before 37 weeks of gestation. This condition is directly antecedent to one-third of all preterm births and complicates 120 000 pregnancies annually in the United States.[1] A number of major etiological factors have been linked to the onset of PROM. Weakening of the amniochorion extracellular matrix (ECM) by collagen degradation is one of the key events predisposing to rupture. Both endogenous and exogenous factors activate collagen degradation. The endogenous factors include a local variation in membrane thickness and a reduction in collagen content. The exogenous factors include effects of bacterial metabolism or the host or fetal inflammatory response. Although bacterial collagenases are detected in the amniotic fluid (AF) during PROM, they are neither specific nor produced in sufficient quantities to degrade human collagens. Infection-induced activation of metalloproteinase (MMPs) has recently been shown to be associated with excessive collagen turnover and membrane weakening leading to rupture. Increased concentrations of active forms of MMPs have been documented in the AF and in the membranes after PROM. Traditional tests (e.g. fern tests, funneling, nitrazine, pooling, etc.) are used to confirm and diagnose PROM after it has occurred; however, no tests exist to predict PROM before its occurrence, partly because the underlying mechanisms that lead to pPROM are still unclear. In this chapter, we review the structure of the membranes and discuss the latest biochemical and molecular findings suggesting that pPROM is an endogenous autotoxic disease mediated by the maternal–fetal inflammatory response.

FETAL MEMBRANE STRUCTURE AND FUNCTIONS

Human fetal membrane consists of amnion and chorion connected by an ECM (Figure 7.1).[2] The amniotic epithelium is the innermost layer and it is in direct contact with the AF. The ECM is made of

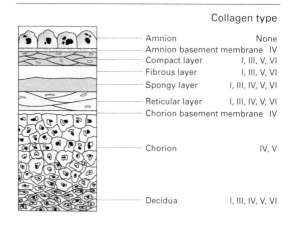

Collagen type

Amnion	None
Amnion basement membrane	IV
Compact layer	I, III, V, VI
Fibrous layer	I, III, V, VI
Spongy layer	I, III, IV, V, VI
Reticular layer	I, III, IV, V, VI
Chorion basement membrane	IV
Chorion	IV, V
Decidua	I, III, IV, V, VI

Figure 7.1 Amniochorion extracellular matrix (ECM) structure and major collagen types associated with each region.

fibrous proteins embedded in a polysaccharide gel and it forms the architectural framework of amniochorion.[3] The tensile strength of the membrane depends on the type of collagen that makes up the ECM. Collagens form the major structural framework of the fetal membrane ECM.[4–10] The major tensile strength is provided by interstitial collagen types I and III, together with small amounts of types V, VI, and VII. Type III collagen is the interstitial collagen and forms the collagen architecture that provides the structural integrity to the membranes. Type IV collagen of the basement membrane (the amnion and chorion are connected to the ECM region by a basement) provides the scaffold for the assembly of other non-collagen structural proteins (laminin, entacin, and proteoglycan). This collagen plays a major role in the development and maintenance of the ECM.[6] Types V and VII are minor fibrillar collagens, and they provide an additional anchoring function for the basement membrane along with type IV collagen. Types VI and VII are present in smaller quantities in the fetal membrane ECM; however, along with types III and I they form an anchoring fibrillar structure. Other non-collagenous components of the ECM include laminin, elastin, proteoglycan, microfibrils, fibronectin, decorin, plasminogen, and integrins.[6–8] The ECM collagens undergo constant turnover throughout the pregnancy to accommodate the increasing volume and tension as gestation progresses.[11] This is shown by a decrease in collagen content of the amnion over the last 8 weeks of pregnancy.[11]

FETAL MEMBRANE COLLAGENOLYSIS IN PRETERM PREMATURE RUPTURE OF THE MEMBRANES

Many studies have identified a major change in the collagen content or collagen network that distorts the structural framework of the membranes in pPROM and leads to membrane weakening and pPROM. As in the case of membranes at term, Skinner and colleagues[11] found that membranes collected from women with pPROM had significantly lower collagen content compared with samples from patients without ROM, suggesting a collagenolytic process in fetal membranes associated with pPROM. This was supported by findings from Vadillo-Ortega et al, in which they documented increased collagenolytic activity, collagen solubility, and a decrease in collagen synthesis in amniotic membranes from pPROM subjects.[12] Kanayama and colleagues analyzed the ratio between major collagen types (I and III to total collagen) and found that in pPROM the ratios of III/I, III/V, and III/total collagen were significantly lower than those from membranes with no ROM. There was no change in the ratios between other collagen types. This indicates a major decrease in type III collagen content in amnion associated with weakening of the membranes.[13,14]

ZONE OF ALTERED MORPHOLOGY AND PRETERM PREMATURE RUPTURE OF THE MEMBRANES

The zone of altered morphology (ZAM), as described by Malak and Bell in their study of the membranes collected from the rupture site after term delivery, showed extensive distortion of the ECM and disintegration of the basement membrane.[15] ZAM included marked disruption of the connective tissue layers and marked reduction of the thickness, and hence cellularity, of both the cytotrophoblast and decidual layers Given the structural features of the ZAM and its restricted localization to an area within the rupture line, it has been proposed that the ZAM may represent the site of initial fetal membrane rupture in response to the increased intra-amniotic pressures experienced during labor.[16] A ZAM was also found by Malak's group in membranes lying over the cervix collected from women before labor, indicating a developing site of rupture during active labor. Extensive structural damage was also detected by this group in membranes collected after pPROM. It has been documented that there is a 35% decrease in the membrane thickness at the rupture site with massive degradation of the type IV collagen-rich basement membrane.[17,18]

PREMATURE RUPTURE OF THE MEMBRANES AND BACTERIAL PROTEASES

Various epidemiological and clinical factors are considered precursors to pPROM.[19] Intra-amniotic infection and histological chorioamnionitis – inflammation of the amniochorion diagnosed by more than 4 polymorphonuclear leukocytes (neutrophils)/high power field – has been associated with more than 50% of pPROM.[20] Epidemiological, clinical, histological, microbiological, and molecular biological data suggest that focal infection or inflammation may play primary or secondary roles in the pathogenesis of pPROM.[19–22] Of note, there is an increasing incidence of chorioamnionitis with decreasing gestational age at the time of pPROM.[22–24] Histological studies show that infection of the intra-amniotic cavity and infection or inflammation of the fetal membranes frequently precedes pPROM. Histological evidence of inflammatory changes is more often noted adjacent to the putative site of membrane rupture.[5]

Bacterial toxins and ECM-degrading enzymes produced by bacteria have been proposed as causative agents in pPROM.[25] Bacterial strains frequently isolated from lower genital tract infections of women with pPROM and preterm labor were tested for their effect on fetal membranes. McGregor et al suggested that protease production by cervico/vaginal microorganisms may alter or inactivate a variety of proteins important in host defense and the structural–functional integrity of collagen-containing chorioamniotic membranes and of the uterine cervix.[26] Additionally, host tissues may be made more susceptible to other organisms' virulence factors by protease-producing members of local genital tract flora.[26] In-vitro exposure of fetal membranes to bacterial collagenase and collagenase-producing microorganisms significantly reduced the tensile strength and elasticity of the membrane.[27–29] These factors can lead to rupture of the membranes in a dose-dependent manner. This effect was not noticed in controls exposed to organisms that did not produce collagenase.[27,29]

Even though many bacterial toxins have been associated with pPROM, the concentration of bacterial products required to produce the deleterious effect seen in vitro are not achieved in AF. Moreover, these enzymes are not specific for human amniochorion ECM substrates.[29] It also appears that the host resistance and antibiotic therapy can limit the damage these toxins produce in the body.[29] Additionally, pPROM is seen in women with intra-amniotic infection due to organisms that do not produce proteases, and pPROM can occur after effective antibacterial therapy. It appears that aggressive antibacterial treatment does not reduce the risk of pPROM.[29] Many investigators now believe that bacterial infection may be an initiator, whereas the host inflammatory response is the true causative agent in premature labor and pPROM.[30, 31] It is hypothesized that pPROM is an endogenous autotoxic disease in which the host inflammatory response activates ECM-specific enzymes (MMPs). Endogenous activation of MMPs may lead to ECM degradation and weakening, predisposing to rupture.

It is clear that several of the MMPs are overexpressed during pPROM. Our studies have shown that collagenases and stromelysins are most likely involved in membrane remodeling, as their expression is constitutive. Gelatinases are overexpressed in the amniotic fluid of women with pPROM, whereas collagenases and stromelysins are not increased when compared with term or preterm labor. A review of the literature and our own laboratory's immunohistochemical analysis of type IV collagen staining in pPROM membranes (unpublished data) suggest that basement membrane (BM) degradation is essential for ECM weakening, which eventually leads to membrane rupture. Type IV collagen-rich BM degradation requires specific enzymatic action.

MATRIX METALLOPROTEINASES AND TISSUE INHIBITORS OF METALLOPROTEINASES IN PRETERM PREMATURE RUPTURE OF THE MEMBRANES

A programmed collagenolytic remodeling process exists in amniochorion during gestation to allow accommodation of the membranes to the increasing uterine pressure and volume as gestation progresses.[32,33] This controlled collagenolytic process is mediated by MMPs, each of which degrades a type-specific substrate.[33,34] There are a number of regulatory mechanisms that can influence the ultimate impact of an MMP on ECM degradation. Regulation occurs at the transcriptional level, translational level, post-translational (activation of zymogen forms of MMPs) level, and in addition at the tissue level by specific regulators known as the tissue inhibitors of metalloproteinases (TIMPs). A balanced activity between MMPs and TIMPs has been documented during tissue remodeling in several systems.[34] There are 28 members of the MMP family of proteins cloned and sequenced so far, along with four members of the TIMP family. The role of MMPs and collagenolysis in human labor and pPROM has been a subject of considerable study over the past several years.[35–37] Increased collagenolysis, a drop in the collagen content of the membranes, and activation of MMPs have been documented during active labor.[35–38] Several other non-MMPs, such as serine proteases, cystine proteases, and ADAMs (a disintegrin and metalloproteinases), can also break down amniochorion ECM substrates; however, this chapter will focus on the role of MMPs. Several lines of evidence have documented the significance of MMPs in pPROM. Some of these findings are listed below:

1. Zymogram studies have reported increased gelatinolytic activity in fetal membranes collected from women with PROM (compared with those from women in preterm and term labor).[35]
2. Increased MMP activity and reduced TIMP activity are present in the AF of women with PROM.[39]
3. Increased expression of MMP2 and induction of MMP9 are seen in infected fetal membranes.[40]
4. Fetal membranes express all four of the MMP inhibitors (the TIMPs).[41]
5. Infection creates an imbalance in the MMP/TIMP molar ratio, creating increased bioavailability of MMPs in the intra-amniotic cavity and at the level of the membranes. In vitro, amniochorion shows an imbalance in the levels of MMPs and TIMPs in response to bacterial toxins similar to that seen in vivo in PROM.[42,43]
6. An increased concentration of active MMP9 is documented in the AF of women with PROM.[44]
7. A specific regional induction of pro-MMP9 has been noted in the fetal membranes close to the cervical area before labor and may play a role in 'programming' this area for subsequent rupture after an infection or during labor.[45]
8. An increased molar ratio of MMP9 to TIMP1 is related to a decreased tensile strength of human fetal membranes in uncomplicated labor.[46]

Tables 7.1 and 7.2 provide a list of MMP family members screened in amniotic fluid, expression of MMP mRNA in amniochorionic membranes, and their relevance to pPROM. These data demonstrate that a fully functional MMP/TIMP system exists in human fetal membranes and plays a role both during labor and in pPROM. Although no studies have clearly documented the exact role of the MMPs during pPROM, it is clear that some MMPs are involved in tissue remodeling[47] during membrane and placental growth and some of them are involved in pPROM. Based on the evidence described herein, it can be summarized that inappropriate MMP activity constitutes part of the pathogenic mechanism associated with pPROM and that pPROM is a result of the host inflammatory response to stimuli that result in the endogenous activation of the MMP cascade causing ECM degradation and rupture.

PROGRAMMED CELL DEATH OR APOPTOSIS DURING PRETERM PREMATURE RUPTURE OF THE MEMBRANES

Apoptosis is defined as a deliberate attempt by an unwanted cell in a multicellular organ system programming itself to die, in contrast to necrosis, which results from acute tissue injury. Apoptosis is initiated by certain stimuli – infection, injury

Table 7.1 Matrix metalloproteinase (MMP) expression pattern in amniochorion and its significance during preterm premature rupture of the membrane (pPROM) in the amniotic fluid compared with term

MMP No.[a]	Family	mRNA expression in amniochorion		Amniotic fluid levels in pPROM[b]
		Amnion	Chorion	
MMP1	Collagenase 1	+	+	↑
MMP2	Gelatinase A	+	+	↑
MMP3	Stromelysin 1	+	+	↑
MMP7	Matrilysin	−	−	No data
MMP8	Neutrophil collagenase	−	−	↑
MMP9	Gelatinase B	+	+	↑
MMP10	Stromelysin 2	+	+	No data
MMP11	Stromelysin 3	+	+	No data
MMP12	Macrophage elastase	−	−	No data
MMP13	Collagenase 3	+	+	No change
MMP14/MT1-MMP[c]	Membrane-type MMP1	+	+	No data

[a] MMP4–6 do not exist.
[b] ↑, Amniotic fluid levels increased when compared with normal gestational age-matched controls or samples collected from women at term regardless of the labor status.
[c] Expression of MT1-MMP mRNA increases in membranes.

Table 7.2 MMP screening in human amniochorionic membranes

MMP No.[a]	Family	pPROM	Term labor
MMP15	MT-MMP	+	+
MMP16	MT-MMP	−	−
MMP17	MT-MMP	−	+
MMP19	RASI	+	+
MMP20	Enamelysin	−	−
MMP23	?	+	+
MMP24	MT-MMP	−	+/−
MMP25	MT-MMP	−	−
MMP26	Matrilysin	−	−

[a] These MMPs have been screened in human fetal membranes collected from women after preterm premature rupture of the membrane (pPROM) or after term labor. Amniotic fluid levels of these MMPS during pPROM or during labor are not available due to the lack of commercially available assay reagents.
  Data on MMP 21, 22, and 27 in human fetal membranes are not available.

beyond repair, stress such as starvation, DNA damage initiated by ionization radiation or chemotherapy – and it is carried out by coordinated and tightly regulated events, which eventually results in cell death. Apoptosis often follows classic morphological changes characterized by nuclear chromatin condensation, cytoplasmic shrinking, dilated endoplasmic reticulum, and membrane blebbing; none of these changes are seen in necrosis.[48,49]

Two major apoptotic pathways exist, either of which can play a role in pPROM. These may be initiated by infection, genotoxic agents, or other unknown factors.[50] First, there are the tumor necrosis factor (TNF) receptor 1 (TNFR1)- and Fas-mediated pathways. These receptor proteins bind to their respective ligands, TNF and Fas L, which initiate signal transduction through two docking proteins, TRADD (TNFR-associated death domain) and FADD (FAS-associated death domain) – Figure 7.2. These death domain-containing proteins activate a group of proteases known as caspases. Activation of the caspase cascade can result in proteolysis of three major groups of substrates:

- mainly proteins that play a role in the homeostatic response to stress stimuli, notably PARP (poly (ADP-ribose) polymerase), a DNA damage repair enzyme, and DNA-dependent protein kinase (DNA PKcs)
- structural proteins that maintain the integrity of the cytoskeleton or nuclear matrix (β-actin, lamin)
- several proteins of unknown function.[51]

Caspases are normally present in the cell as inactive proenzymes that are activated by proteolytic

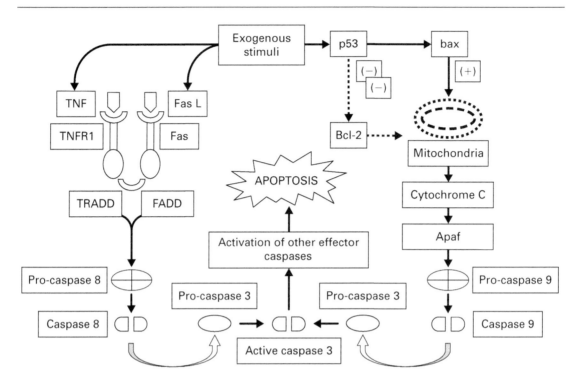

Figure 7.2 Two major apoptotic pathways may exist in PROM which can be initiated by infection or unknown factors. (1) TNFR–FAS-mediated pathway – these receptor proteins bind to their respective ligands TNF and Fas L which initiate signal transduction through two docking proteins, TRADD (TNFR-associated death domain) and FADD (FAS-associated death domain). These death domain proteins activate pro-caspase 8 to active caspase 8. (2) The p53-mediated pathway is initiated by DNA fragmentation. DNA damage increases transactivator protein p53 in the cell. p53 transactivates bax, which causes damage to the mitochondrial membrane, resulting in the release of cytochrome C. Cytochrome C activates Apaf (apoptosis protease activating factor), which converts pro-caspase 9 to the active form. p53 also suppresses Bcl-2, a factor that stops mitochondrial membrane damage. Active caspase 8 or 9 can initiate a cascade of effector caspase activation, which will cause proteolysis of structural proteins, proteins of homeostasis, and several other proteins, and program the cell to death. Solid arrows, activation; broken arrows, inhibition.

cleavage at Asp residues. Caspases are divided into two groups: initiators or effectors of apoptosis. Initiators are a group of caspases that initiate a cascade of proteolysis, whereas effectors are a group of caspases whose activity eventually results in apoptosis.[52] TRADD and FADD independently activate pro-caspase 8 to active caspase 8.[53–60]

The second pathway is initiated by p53. An increase in p53, a transactivator protein for many genes in the cell, can induce the expression of bax, which causes damage to the mitochondrial membrane, resulting in the release of cytochrome C.

Cytochrome C activates Apaf (apoptosis protease activating factor), which converts pro-caspase 9 to its active form. p53 also suppresses Bcl-2, a factor that inhibits mitochondrial membrane damage. Active caspase 8 or 9 generated from either one of these pathways can initiate effecter caspase activation. Caspases 3, 7, and 6 are activated sequentially, causing proteolysis of structural proteins, proteins of homeostasis, and several other proteins. They program the cell to die. These pathways crossover at several points. p53 can induce Fas in some tissue types. Caspase 8 is a known suppressor of Bcl-2 and activator of 'bid', which also causes cytochrome release. Redundancy exists in that caspase 8 can also activate caspase 9 if Apaf is absent in the system.[61,62]

Preliminary experimental data from our laboratory and other researchers indicates that apoptosis may initiate membrane weakening and rupture. Reports by Lei et al have described that amnion epithelial cells undergo a process of programmed cell death associated with orchestrated ECM degradation which begins before the onset of active labor in animal models.[63] This suggests that fetal membrane rupture is likely to be the result of biochemical changes as well as physical forces. We have conducted comprehensive studies to determine the fetal membrane pathway leading to apoptosis. Proto-oncogene p53 is a vital step in the apoptosis pathway. Fetal membranes collected from women with pPROM indeed show increased expression of p53 compared with gestational age-matched controls (membranes collected from women with preterm labor (PTL) with no ROM; see Table 7.5). p53 triggers apoptosis by regulating the expression of the Bcl family of proteins, namely, Bcl-2 (antiapoptotic) and bax (proapoptotic).[50] The p53 downregulates Bcl-2 and induces the expression of bax, which leads to the activation of a cascade of events that eventually results in apoptosis.

Both Bcl-2 and bax expressions were studied in fetal membranes during pPROM (Table 7.3). Bcl-2 expression was lower, whereas bax expression was higher, in pPROM membranes compared with membranes from PTL with no ROM. Normal cell functioning requires a 1:1 ratio between these proteins. An increased expression of one or the other can tilt this balance towards either cell proliferation (increased Bcl-2) or apoptosis (increased bax).[64,65] Increased DNA fragmentation and TUNEL-positive cells were also seen in pPROM membranes, indicating apoptotic activity.[66]

The p53 increase seen in pPROM can stimulate MMP2 expression and lead to activation of the gelatinases. Hence, it is possible that both of the molecular pathways (apoptosis and MMP activation) are coexistent in pPROM.[67] Our laboratory has made supportive observations. Fetal membrane infection in vitro – lipopolysaccharide (LPS) stimulation of cultured amniochorion – induces many of the apoptotic pathway genes. Table 7.4 documents the induction of apoptotic pathway genes in response to an infectious process. Fas, Caspase 8, and other initiator (2, 9) and effecter (6, 7 and 10) caspases are induced in response to an in-vitro infection compared with unstimulated control tissue, suggesting a role for apoptosis during intra-amniotic infection (IAI). These in-vitro findings are similar to observations in PROM membranes.[68] These findings are supportive of an association between MMP activation and apoptosis in fetal membranes with pPROM.

Table 7.3 Quantitative expression of apoptotic factors during preterm premature rupture of the membranes (pPROM)

	pPROM (n = 10) Median	PTL (n = 10) Median	p
p53	60	3	0.001
Bax	486.5	32	0.003
Bcl-2	2.8	58	0.05

Comparison was made between pPROM membranes and preterm labor (PTL) with no rupture of the membranes (ROM). Data presented as number of transcripts/0.5 μg of total RNA.

Table 7.4 Induction of apoptosis pathway genes in fetal membranes in response to an in-vitro infection (lipoolysaccharide stimulation)[a]

Gene name	Stimulated membranes	Unstimulated controls
Fas	+	−
Fas ligand	−	−
Caspase 2	+	−
Caspase 3	+	+/−
Caspase 4	+	+
Caspase 6	+	+
Caspase 7	+	−
Caspase 8	+	−
Caspase 9	+	−
Caspase 10	+	+/−

[a] Gene expression studies documented by RT-PCR (reverse transcription–polymerase chain reaction) and multiplex PCR experiments: +, induction of gene; +/−, 50% of tissues showed expression; −, no expression.

FETAL MEMBRANE AS A SITE OF INFLAMMATORY CYTOKINE PRODUCTION

One of the most reproducible findings in preterm labor and in pPROM is the increased concentration of proinflammatory cytokines in the amniotic fluid and membranes regardless of the infectious status. An amniochorion organ explant system developed in our laboratory in the early 1990s documented the fetal membrane cytokine response to an in-vitro model of IAI.[69] The organ explant system was developed to preserve the integrity of the amniochorion and allow the investigation of this tissue as a functional unit. Amniochorion was found to be a source of virtually all the inflammatory cytokines in our in-vitro culture system.[70–73] Immunomodulatory cytokine expression was not seen in amniochorion, except for interleukin (IL)-10, which was present at the time of collection and disappeared in response to culture conditions. The expression pattern of mRNA – as detected by polymerase chain reaction (PCR) – for the proinflammatory and immunomodulatory cytokines in cultured amniochorion, as well as in amniochorion collected from women with PTD (with documented IAI as reported by positive amniotic fluid culture for microorganisms), is shown in Table 7.5. The amniochorion cytokine release pattern in response to LPS stimulation in vitro mirrored that noted in amniotic fluid during IAI. IL-6 and IL-8 levels were in the nanogram ranges and IL-1 and TNF levels were in the picogram range in both culture media and amniotic fluid.[74] IL-6 levels were much higher compared with the levels of IL-8 consistent with the predicted association of IL-6 with PTD. These findings agreed with previous reports examining decidual and amniotic fluid concentrations of these mediators, suggesting that IL-6 and IL-8 are key marker cytokines associated with IAI. These cytokines exhibit similar patterns of expression in amniochorion and display differential response to distinct infectious stimuli.[75] Inflammatory cytokines initiate a vicious cycle of events which can lead to increased prostaglandin production, resulting in PTD.

These data support the theory that fetal membranes are an essential part of the host response to IAI or microbial invasion of the intra-amniotic cavity and that the membranes are integral in determining the outcome of pregnancy in these cases. Further data supporting this theory come from Kent and colleagues, who reported that intact fetal membranes act as a barrier to cytokines produced by the decidua.[76] Decidual cytokines do not cross intact membranes and therefore do not significantly contribute to the amniotic fluid cytokine pool. It has also been documented that separating the membranes and culturing them individually or as a cell culture reduces the capacity of the immune response.

In summary, intact fetal membranes in association with membrane neutrophils/macrophages are the primary originators of the immune response in the amniotic cavity. The inflammatory cytokine network interactions, MMP activation, MMP/TIMP imbalance, and activation of the

Table 7.5 Inflammatory cytokine mRNA expression in amniochorion in culture at various time points and in membranes from preterm delivery (PTD) with documented (intra-amniotic infection)

Cytokine	In vitro					In vivo	
	0 h	24 h	48 h	LPS	Control	Infected amniochorion (PTD)	Non-infected term control membranes
IL-1β	+	+	+	++	−	+++	+
TNF-α	+	+	+	+	−	+++	+
IL-6	−	+	+	+++	−	+++	−
IL-8[a]	−	+	+	+++	+	+++	−
IL-15	+	+	+	+	+/−	Data not available	Data not available

[a] LPS, lipopolysaccharide; IL, interleukin; TNF, tumor necrosis factor. IL-8 expression was constitutive in culture.
++/+++, increased mRNA expression as documented by QPCR (quantitative polymerase chain reaction) compared with control.

programmed cell death cascade of events in fetal membranes are all promoters of PROM.

DISTINCT INFLAMMATORY AND MOLECULAR PATHWAYS IN PRETERM DELIVERY AND PRETERM PREMATURE RUPTURE OF THE MEMBRANES

The etiological factors associated with PTD and pPROM are identical. Both conditions are associated with infection, smoking, socioeconomic factors, racial differences, nutritional status, multiple gestation, and polyhydramnios. The maternal and fetal inflammatory response increases production and release of the inflammatory cytokines (IL-1, IL-6, IL-8, TNF-α) that induce prostaglandin production, leading to cervical ripening and prostaglandin-mediated contractility. These factors are common to both PTD and pPROM and are elevated in the AF even in the absence of microbial invasion of intra-amniotic cavity (MIAC) and IAI, when compared with term labor.[77-81] However, some women experience pPROM, whereas some experience PTD without ROM. Based on our findings it appears that certain molecular factors involved in women with pPROM are absent or minimally present in women with preterm labor without ROM.

In an attempt to delineate the pathways that differentiate PTL from PROM, we have identified three major pathways that are definitive. They are inflammatory cytokines, increased MMP activity, and apoptosis. MMP activity and apoptosis are most strongly associated with PROM, whereas inflammatory cytokines are increased in both of these conditions. As discussed earlier in this chapter, most of these cytokines induce prostaglandin production from placental tissues, resulting in contractions. This suggests that one or more of these cytokines may act as a switch between the pathways that promote PROM vs PTL. Cytokines may increase MMP activity or accelerate apoptosis, each of which is associated with PROM.

In an attempt to identify the factors that determine which pathway is followed (i.e. PTL vs

PROM), the effect of individual cytokine stimulation on activation of the MMP and apoptosis pathways was examined. The results are summarized in Tables 7.6 and 7.7. In a dose-dependent manner, TNF can activate MMPs, whereas both IL-1β and TNF can activate apoptosis, both of which are associated with PROM. Conversely, IL-6 is neither an activator of MMPs nor an inducer of apoptosis. We propose that during intra-amniotic infection, the outcome will be determined based on the concentration of the individual cytokines in the amniotic fluid. IL-6 seems to have a higher concentration (in the microgram range) than the other two (picogram range). Additionally, as a prostaglandin stimulant, IL-6 may lead to preterm labor and directly promote PROM.[82] Conversely, IL-1β and TNF may direct the events that promote PROM over PTL.

Table 7.6 Inflammatory cytokine induction of matrix metalloproteinase (MMP) expression and activity from cultured human fetal membranes

Gene expression	IL-1	IL-6	TNF	Control
MMP2	+	+	+	+
MMP9	+	+	+	−
MMP2 specific activity[a]	+	+	+	+
MMP9 specific activity[a]	−	−	+	−

IL, interleukin; TNF, tumor necrosis factor.
[a] Documented by zymogram analysis using gelatin substrate.

Table 7.7 Matrix metalloproteinase (MMP) and caspase activity in inflammatory cytokine-stimulated amniochorion compared with unstimulated controls

Activity assay	IL-1β	IL-6	TNF
MMP2	NC[a]	NC	NC
MMP9	NC	NC	↑[b]
Caspase 2	↑	NC	↑
Caspase 3	↑	NC	↑
Caspase 8	↑	NC	↑
Caspase 9	↑	NC	↑
TUNEL-positive cells[c]	55%	25%	80%

IL, interleukin; TNF, tumor necrosis factor.
[a] NC, no change.
[b] ↑, increase.
[c] Unstimulated control membranes showed ~15% TUNEL-positive cells.

GENETIC PREDISPOSITION IN PRETERM PREMATURE RUPTURE OF THE MEMBRANES

Although the etiologies associated with PTL and pPROM are the same, the disparities observed in the phenotype (PTL vs pPROM) in different individuals are the results of divergent molecular pathways. This difference among individuals in clinical presentations may be attributable to genetically determined predispositions in key genes involved in multiple pathways that lead to the outcome. The single nucleotide polymorphisms (SNPs) in various genes and their interaction with environmental factors such as infection (IAI, bacterial vaginosis), nutrition, smoking, and other epidemiological factors can result in different phenotypic expression based on the type of gene–gene interaction and gene–environment interaction. Studies are currently underway examining the association of SNPs with MMP, cytokine, and other genes involved in the pathways that lead to pPROM. Strauss and colleagues[83–86] have reported SNP association studies performed to document ethnic disparity in the pPROM rate between African-Americans and Caucasians. Some of the recent findings are listed in Table 7.8. Many case–control studies are currently underway looking at genotypic and allelic frequency differences in the inflammatory and other pathway genes involved in preterm labor, pPROM, and PTD. Identification of polymorphisms and their association with the disease process will aid early identification of women at risk for pPROM and potentially lead to interventions based on these findings.

REFERENCES

1. Mercer BM. Preterm premature rupture of the membranes. Obstet Gynecol 2003; 101:178–193.
2. Mossman HW. Vertebrate Fetal Membranes. New Jersey: Rutgers University Press; 1987.
3. Hay ED. Extracellular matrix. J Cell Biol 1981; 9:205s–223s.
4. Behzad F, Dickinson MR, Charlton A, Aplin JD. Brief communication: sliding displacement of amnion and chorion following controlled laser wounding suggests a mechanism for short-term sealing of ruptured membranes. Placenta 1994; 15:775–778.
5. Bourne GL. The microscopic anatomy of human amnion and chorion. Am J Obstet Gynecol 1960; 79:1070–1073.
6. Malak TM, Ockleford CD, Bell SC et al. Confocal immunofluorescence localization of collagen types I, III, IV, V and VI and their ultrastructural organization in term human fetal membranes. Placenta 1993; 14:385–406.
7. Aplin JD, Campbell S, Allen TD. The extracellular matrix of human amniotic epithelium: ultrastructure, composition and deposition. J Cell Sci 1985; 79:119–136.
8. Bryant-Greenwood GD. The extracellular matrix of the human fetal membranes: structure and function. Placenta 1998; 19:1–11.
9. French JI, McGregor JA. The pathobiology of premature rupture of membranes. Semin Perinatol 1996; 20:344–368.
10. Aplin JD, Campbell S. An immunofluorescence study of extracellular matrix associated with cytotrophoblast of the chorion laeve. Placenta 1985; 6:469–479.
11. Skinner SJ, Campos GA, Liggins GC. Collagen content of human amniotic membranes: effect of gestation length and premature rupture. Obstet Gynecol 1981; 57:487–489.
12. Vadillo-Ortega F, Gonzalez-Avila G, Karchmer S et al. Collagen metabolism in premature rupture of amniotic membranes. Obstet Gynecol 1990; 75:84–88.
13. Kanayama N, Terao T, Kawashima Y, Horiuchi K, Fujimoto D. Collagen types in normal and prematurely ruptured amniotic membranes. Am J Obstet Gynecol 1985; 153:899–903

Table 7.8 Recently published reports on gene polymorphisms and their association with preterm premature rupture of the membrane (pPROM)

Gene	SNP	Significance	Reference
MMP9	14 CA-repeat (MMP9 promoter region)	High risk of pPROM in African-Americans	83
MMP8	+17 (G) and −381 (G)	The minor alleles in complete linkage dysequilibrium. High risk of having pPROM	84
TNF-α	−308	High risk of pPROM in African-Americans	85
CARD15	2936 insC	No significant association documented in pPROM	86
TLR4	896 A>G	No significant association documented in pPROM	86

SNP, single nucleotide polymorphism; MMP8, MMP9, matrix metalloproteinases; TNF-α, tumor necrosis factor-α; TLR4, toll-like receptor 4.

14. Meirowitz NB, Smulian JC, Hahn RA et al. Collagen messenger RNA expression in the human amniochorion in premature rupture of membranes. Am J Obstet Gynecol 2002; 187:1679–1685.

15. Malak TM, Bell SC. Structural characteristics of term human fetal membranes: a novel zone of extreme morphological alteration within the rupture site. Br J Obstet Gynaecol 1994; 101:375–386.

16. McLaren J, Malak TM, Bell SC. Structural characteristics of term human fetal membranes prior to labour: identification of an area of altered morphology overlying the cervix. Hum Reprod 1999; 14:237–241.

17. Malak T, Mullholland G, Bell S. Structural and morphometric characteristics of the fetal membranes in preterm birth. J Reprod Fertil 1993; 12:48.

18. Malak T, Mullholland G, Bell S. Morphometric characteristics of the decidua, cytotrophoblast and connective tissue of the prelabour ruptured fetal membrane. Ann NY Acad Sci 1994; 734:430–433.

19. French JI, McGregor JA. The pathobiology of premature rupture of membranes. Semin Perinatol 1996; 20:344–368.

20. Gibbs RS, Blanco JD. Premature rupture of the membranes. Obstet Gynecol 1982; 60:671–679.

21. Mercer BM, Lewis R. Preterm labor and preterm premature rupture of the membranes. Diagnosis and management. Infect Dis Clin North Am 1997; 1:177–201.

22. Naeye RL, Peters EC. Causes and consequences of premature rupture of fetal membranes. Lancet 1980; 1:192–194.

23. Gugino LJ, Buerger PT, Wactawski-Wende J, Fisher J. Chorioamnionitis: the association between clinical and histological diagnosis. Prim Care Update Ob Gyns 1998; 5:148.

24. Quinn PA, Butany J, Taylor J, Hannah W. Chorioamnionitis: its association with pregnancy outcome and microbial infection. Am J Obstet Gynecol 1987; 156:379–387.

25. McGregor JA, Lawellin D, Franco-Buff A, Todd JK, Makowski EL. Protease production by microorganisms associated with reproductive tract infection. Am J Obstet Gynecol 1986; 154:109–114.

26. Schoonmaker JN, Lawellin DW, Lunt B, McGregor JA. Bacteria and inflammatory cells reduce chorioamniotic membrane integrity and tensile strength. Obstet Gynecol 1989; 74:590–596.

27. MacGregor JA, Lawellin D, Franco-Buff A, Todd JK, Makowski EL. Protease production by microorganisms associated with reproductive tract infection. Am J Obstet Gynecol 1986; 154:109–114.

28. Sbarra AJ, Thomas GB, Cetrulo CL et al. Effect of bacterial growth on the bursting pressure of fetal membranes in vitro. Obstet Gynecol 1987; 70:107–110.

29. McGregor JA, Schoonmaker J, Lunt BD, Lawellin DW. Antibiotic inhibition of bacterially induced fetal membrane weakening. Obstet Gynecol 1990; 76:124–128.

30. Roemro R, Mazor M. Infection and preterm labor. Clin Obstet Gynecol 1988; 31:553–584.

31. Gomez R, Ghezzi F, Romero R et al. Premature labor and intra-amniotic infection. Clinical aspects and role of the cytokines in diagnosis and pathophysiology. Clin Perinatol 1995; 22:281–342.

32. Skinner SJ, Campos GA, Liggins GC. Collagen content of human amniotic membranes: effect of gestation length and premature rupture. Obstet Gynecol 1981; 57:487–489.

33. Bryant-Greenwood GD, Yamamoto SY. Control of peripartal collagenolysis in the human chorion-decidua. Am J Obstet Gynecol 1995; 172:63–70.

34. Woesner FJ. Matrix metalloproteinases and their inhibitors in connective tissue remodeling. FASEB J 1991; 5:2145–2154.

35. Draper D, McGregor J, Hall J et al. Elevated protease activities in human amnion and chorion correlate with preterm premature rupture of membranes. Am J Obstet Gynecol 1995; 173:1506–1512.

36. Hampson V, Liu D, Billett E, Kirk S. Amniotic membrane collagen content and type distribution in women with preterm premature rupture of the membranes in pregnancy. Br J Obstet Gynaecol 1997; 104:1087–1091.

37. Vadillo-Ortega F, Gonzalez-Avila G, Furth EE et al. 92-kd type IV collagenase (matrix metalloproteinase-9) activity in human amniochorion increases with labor. Am J Pathol 1995; 146: 148–156.

38. So T. The role of matrix metalloproteinases for premature rupture of the membranes. Nippon Sanka Fujinka Gakkai Zasshi 1993; 45:227–233.

39. Vadillo-Ortega F, Hernandez A, Gonzalez-Avila G et al. Increased matrix metalloproteinase activity and reduced tissue inhibitor of metalloproteinases-1 levels in amniotic fluids from pregnancies complicated by premature rupture of membranes. Am J Obstet Gynecol. 1996; 174:1371–1376.

40. Fortunato SJ, Menon R, Lombardi SJ. Collagenolytic enzymes (gelatinases) and their inhibitors in human amniochorionic membranes. Am J Obstet Gynecol 1997; 77:731–741.

41. Fortunato SJ, Menon R, Lombardi SJ. Presence of four tissue inhibitors of matrix metalloproteinases (TIMP 1, 2, 3 and 4) in human fetal membranes. Am J Reprod Immunol 1998; 40:395–400.

42. Fortunato SJ, Menon R, Lombardi SJ. MMP/TIMP imbalance in amniotic fluid during PROM: an indirect support for endogenous pathway to membrane rupture. J Perinat Med 1999; 27:362–368.

43. Fortunato SJ, Menon R, Lombardi SJ. Amniochorion gelatinase–gelatinase inhibitor imbalance in vitro: a possible infectious pathway to rupture. Obstet Gynecol 2000; 95:240–244.

44. Athayde N, Edwin SS, Romero R, Gomez R et al. A role for matrix metalloproteinase-9 in spontaneous rupture of the fetal membranes. Am J Obstet Gynecol 1998; 179:1248–1253.

45. McLaren J, Taylor DJ, Bell SC. Increased concentration of pro-matrix metalloproteinase 9 in term fetal membranes overlying the cervix before labor: implications for membrane remodeling and rupture. Am J Obstet Gynecol 2000; 182:409–416.

46. Uchide K, Ueno H, Inoue M et al. Matrix metalloproteinase-9 and tensile strength of fetal membranes in uncomplicated labor. Obstet Gynecol 2000; 95:851–855.

47. Fortunato SJ, LaFleur B, Menon R. Amniotic fluid concentrations of collagenase-1 and collagenase-3 are increased in polyhydramnios. Am J Reprod Immunol 2003; 49:120–125.

48. Lawen A. Apoptosis – an introduction. Bioessays 2003; 25:888–896.

49. Kerr JF, Wyllie AH, Currie AR. Apoptosis: a basic biological phenomenon with wide-ranging implications in tissue kinetics. Br J Cancer 1972; 26:239–257.

50. Ko LJ, Prives C. p53: puzzle and paradigm. Genes Dev 1996; 10:1054–1072.

51. Cryns VL, Yuan J. The cutting edge: caspases in apoptosis and disease. In: Lockshin RA, Zakeri Z, Tilly JL, eds. When Cells Die. New York: Wiley-Liss; 1998: 177–210.

52. Nicholson DW. ICE/CED3-like proteases as therapeutic targets for the control of inappropriate apoptosis. Nat Biotechnol 1996; 14: 297–301.

53. Watanabe D, Suda T, Nagata S. Expression of Fas in B cells of the mouse germinal center and Fas-dependent killing of activated B cells. Int Immunol 1995; 7:1949–1956.

54. Hsu H, Huang J, Shu HB, Baichwal V, Goeddel DV. TNF-dependent recruitment of the protein kinase RIP to the TNF receptor-1 signaling complex. Immunity 1996; 4:387–396.

55. Muzio M, Chinnaiyan AM, Kischkel FC et al. FLICE, a novel FADD-homologous ICE/CED-3-like protease, is recruited to the CD95 (Fas/APO-1) death-inducing signaling complex. Cell 1996; 85:817–827.

56. Vincenz C, Dixit VM. Fas-associated death domain protein interleukin-1beta-converting enzyme 2 (FLICE2), an ICE/Ced-3 homologue, is proximally involved in CD95- and p55-mediated death signaling. J Biol Chem 1997; 272:6578–6583.

57. Hsu H, Huang J, Shu HB, Baichwal V, Goeddel DV. TNF-dependent recruitment of the protein kinase RIP to the TNF receptor-1 signaling complex. Immunity 1996; 4:387–396.

58. Duan H, Dixit VM. RAIDD is a new 'death' adaptor molecule. Nature 1997; 385:86–89.

59. Wallach D, Varfolomeev EE, Malinin NL et al. Tumor necrosis factor receptor and Fas signaling mechanisms Annu Rev Immunol 1999; 17:331–367.

60. Varfolomeev EE, Schuchmann M, Luria V et al. Targeted disruption of the mouse Caspase 8 gene ablates cell death induction by the TNF receptors, Fas/Apo1, and DR3 and is lethal prenatally. Immunity 1998; 9:267–276.

61. Srinivasula SM, Ahmad M, Fernandes-Alnemri T, Litwack G, Alnemri ES. Molecular ordering of the Fas-apoptotic pathway: the Fas/APO-1 protease Mch5 is a CrmA-inhibitable protease that activates multiple Ced-3/ICE-like cysteine proteases. Proc Natl Acad Sci USA 1996; 93:14486–14491.

62. Pan G, O'Rourke K, Dixit VM. Caspase-9, Bcl-XL, and Apaf-1 form a ternary complex. J Biol Chem 1998; 273:5841–5845.

63. Lei H, Furth EE, Kalluri R, Chiou T et al. A program of cell death and extracellular matrix degradation is activated in the amnion before the onset of labor. J Clin Invest 1996; 98:1971–1978.

64. Oltvai ZN, Milliman CL, Korsmeyer SJ. Bcl-2 heterodimerizes in vivo with a conserved homolog, Bax, that accelerates programmed cell death. Cell 1993; 74:609–619.

65. Reed JC. Bcl-2 and the regulation of programmed cell death. J Cell Biol 1994; 124:1–6.

66. Fortunato SJ, Menon R, Bryant C, Lombardi SJ. Programmed cell death (apoptosis) as a possible pathway to metalloproteinase activation and fetal membrane degradation in premature rupture of membranes. Am J Obstet Gynecol 2000; 182:1468–1476.

67. Tryggvason K, Huhtala P, Tuuttila A et al. Structure and expression of type IV collagenase genes. Cell Differ Dev 1990; 32:307–312.

68. Fortunato SJ, Menon R, Lombardi SJ. Support for an infection-induced apoptotic pathway in human fetal membranes. Am J Obstet Gynecol 2001; 184:1392–1397.

69. Fortunato SJ, Menon R, Swan KF, Lyden TW. Organ culture of amniochorionic membrane in vitro. Am J Reprod Immunol 1994; 32:184–187.

70. Menon R, Swan KF, Lyden TW, Rote NS, Fortunato SJ. Expression of inflammatory cytokines (IL-1 beta and IL-6) in amniochorion. Am J Obstet Gynecol 1995; 172:493–500.

71. Fortunato SJ, Menon R, Swan KF. Expression of TNF-alpha and TNFR p55 in cultured amniochorion. Am J Reprod Immunol 1994; 32:188–195.

72. Fortunato SJ, Menon R, Swan KF. Amniochorion: a source of interleukin-8. Am J Reprod Immunol 1995; 34:156–162.

73. Fortunato SJ, Menon R, Lombardi SJ. IL-15, a novel cytokine produced by human fetal membranes increases during preterm labor. Am J Reprod Immunol 1998; 39:16–23.

74. Fortunato SJ, Menon RP, Swan KF, Menon R. Release of inflammatory cytokines (IL-1, IL-6, IL-8 and TNF-α) from human fetal membranes in response to endotoxic lipopolysaccharide mimics amniotic fluid concentrations. Am J Obstet Gynecol 1996; 174:1855–1862.

75. Fortunato SJ, Lombardi SJ, Menon R. Immunoreactivity of human fetal membranes to peptidoglycan polysaccharide (PGPS): cytokine response. J Perinat Med 1998; 26:442–447.

76. Kent ASH, Sullivan MHF, Elder MG. Transfer of cytokines through human fetal membranes. J Reprod Fertil 1994; 100:81–84.

77. Mercer BM, Lewis R. Preterm labor and preterm premature rupture of the membranes. Diagnosis and management. Infect Dis Clin North Am 1997; 11(1):177–201.

78. McGregor JA, French JI. Preterm birth: the role of infection and inflammation. Medscape Womens Health 1997; 2:1.

79. Gomez R, Romero R, Edwin SS, David C. Pathogenesis of preterm labor and preterm premature rupture of membranes associated with intraamniotic infection. Infect Dis Clin North Am 1997; 11:135–176.

80. Keelan JA, Coleman M, Mitchell MD. The molecular mechanisms of term and preterm labor: recent progress and clinical implications. Clin Obstet Gynecol 1997; 40:460–478.

81. Mazor M, Chaim W, Horowitz S, Romero R, Glezerman M. The biomolecular mechanisms of preterm labor in women with intrauterine infection. Isr J Med Sci 1994; 30:317–322.

82. Dudley DJ, Hunter C, Mitchell MD, Varner MW. Clinical value of amniotic fluid interleukin-6 determinations in the management of preterm labour. Br J Obstet Gynaecol 1994; 101:592–597.

83. Ferrand PE, Parry S, Sammel M et al. A polymorphism in the matrix metalloproteinase-9 promoter is associated with increased risk of preterm premature rupture of membranes in African Americans. Mol Hum Reprod 2002; 8:494–501.

84. Wang H, Parry S, Macones G et al. Functionally significant SNP MMP8 promoter haplotypes and preterm premature rupture of membranes (PPROM). Hum Mol Genet 2004; 13:2659–2669.

85. Roberts AK, Monzon-Bordonaba F, Van Deerlin PG et al. Association of polymorphism within the promoter of the tumor necrosis factor alpha gene with increased risk of preterm premature rupture of the fetal membranes. Am J Obstet Gynecol 1999; 180:1297–1302.

86. Ferrand PE, Fujimoto T, Chennathukuzhi V et al. The CARD15 2936insC mutation and TLR4 896 A>G polymorphism in African Americans and risk of preterm premature rupture of membranes (PPROM). Mol Hum Reprod 2002; 8:1031–1034.

8. Maternal inflammatory conditions and pregnancy

Mandish K Dhanjal and Catherine Nelson-Piercy

INTRODUCTION

Pregnancy induces changes in the maternal immune system in order to protect the fetus from immunological attack by the mother. This occurs with a shift from a prevailing Th1 response (cell-mediated immunity) to a Th2 response (humoral immunity). These changes revert postpartum.

Pre-existing maternal disease may be modulated in pregnancy by the effects of the altered immunological status according to the underlying pathophysiology of the disease in question. Immune-mediated diseases are those most likely to be affected. In rheumatoid arthritis (RA), a Th1-type immune response is predominant, which may be ameliorated; in idiopathic thrombocytopenic purpura (ITP) a Th2-type prevails, which can be exacerbated. The fetus may be integral as an antigenic stimulus with the passage of fetal cells through the placenta and into the maternal circulation (microchimerism). Alternatively, the fetus can itself be affected by autoantibodies involved in maternal disease, as in neonatal lupus erythematosus and neonatal thrombocytopenia in ITP.

Management of these inflammatory disorders is now extending to the use of drugs aimed at specifically altering the immune response, such as anti-tumor necrosis factor (anti-TNF) and intravenous immunoglobulin (IVIG). The use of such drugs in pregnancy will be discussed.

RHEUMATOID ARTHRITIS

Rheumatoid arthritis is a chronic systemic inflammatory disorder producing a deforming symmetrical polyarthritis with synovitis of joint and tendon sheaths, articular cartilage loss, and erosion of juxta-articular bone. This leads to progressive joint damage that causes severe disability. Extra-articular involvement can occur, usually after the onset of joint disease. This includes anemia, vasculitis (may affect the neurons), pulmonary effusions and fibrosis, pericarditis, amyloidosis, and a secondary Sjögren's syndrome (exocrine salivary and lacrimal glands' inflammation causing dry eyes and dry mouth). Nodules may occur in subcutaneous, pulmonary, and scleral tissues. In general, RA improves in pregnancy and flares postpartum.

INCIDENCE

The prevalence is 0.5–1% in most populations. There is a high prevalence in Pima Indians (5.3%) and Chippewa Indians (6.8%), supporting a genetic role in increased risk.[1] RA is three times more common in women than men, and approximately 1 in every 1000–2000 pregnancies is affected.

GENETICS

The main genetic risk factor is human leukocyte antigen (HLA) DRB1 alleles, with the strongest susceptibility being HLA-DRB1*0404 and DRB1*0401 alleles. TNF alleles are also linked with RA.[1]

INFLAMMATORY PATHOLOGY

RA is initiated by CD4+ T cells, which are activated in response to an as-yet unknown endogenous or exogenous antigen (Figure 8.1). Candidate auto-antigens recently identified are citrullinated protein, proteins derived from cartilage, heavy-chain binding protein, and peptides derived from HLA class II molecules.[2]

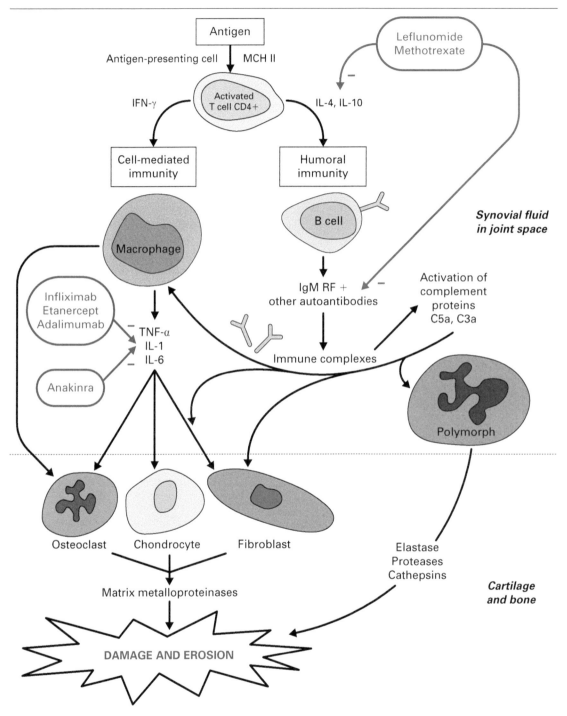

Figure 8.1 Inflammatory pathway in rheumatoid arthritis and drug actions.

The activated CD4+ T cells stimulate:

1. Monocytes, macrophages, and synovial fibroblasts to produce TNF-α, and the interleukins IL-1 and IL-6, which are the key cytokines that drive inflammation in RA. Large amounts of TNF-α and IL-1 are found in synovial fluid. These cells will also secrete matrix metalloproteinases (MMPs) as well as stimulating angiogenesis. The synovium becomes inflamed and proliferates.
2. B cells to produce antibodies, including rheumatoid factor. The precise pathogenic role of rheumatoid factor is not known, but may involve activation of complement through the formation of immune complexes which are present in synovial fluid. This results in recruitment of polymorphs which secrete elastase and proteases, and further monocytes, macrophages, and synovial fibroblasts.
3. Osteoclastogenesis directly and via TNF-α, IL-1, and IL-6.

This cascade of cytokine and enzyme production results in the irreversible destruction of cartilage and damage to bones.[3,4]

RA has previously been considered to be a predominately cell-mediated autoimmune disease (Th1). One theory supporting its amelioration in pregnancy is the shift away from a Th1 response. However, recent findings of highly disease-specific autoantibodies against citrullinated peptide in the serum of patients with RA have underscored the importance of humoral immunity (Th2) in the disease.[2] Very recent clinical trials using B-cell depletion support the concept that humoral immunity plays a significant role in the course of the disease.[5] This may explain why over 25% of women with RA experience worsening of symptoms in pregnancy.[6]

EFFECT OF PREGNANCY ON RHEUMATOID ARTHRITIS

RA symptoms improve during pregnancy and deteriorate postpartum.

Older retrospective and prospective studies based on personal recall of events have shown a 66–80% degree of improvement.[7–9] However, a widespread variability in disease response was found in a large prospective study of 140 pregnant women with RA, which used standardized assessment of joint symptoms, examination of inflamed joints, and the Health Assessment Questionnaire.[6] The study confirmed that two-thirds of the women reported an improvement in joint swelling and pain by the third trimester of pregnancy, but only 16% went into complete remission. Significantly, 27% had substantial disability during pregnancy, of whom one-third recalled little disability prior to pregnancy. Disease response in a previous pregnancy was predictive of response in the index pregnancy.

There have been various theories for the improvement of RA in pregnancy. Hormonal changes, with raised cortisol and estrogen in pregnancy, have been suspected, but cortisol levels do not correlate with symptoms[10] and estrogen levels are similar in RA cases and controls.[1] However, the combined oral contraceptive pill, with its supraphysiological estrogen dose, is protective.[1] Placental clearance of immune complexes, pregnancy-associated plasma protein A, and pregnancy-specific proteins such as α_2-glycoprotein (PAG) have been implicated, and in experimental models α_2-glycoprotein improves arthritis.[9]

Maternal–fetal (paternal) HLA incompatibility has recently been found to be protective in RA.[8] It was found that 76% of women whose RA went into remission during pregnancy had maternal–fetal disparities in the HLA-DRB1, -DQA, and -DQB alleles compared with 25% in whom the disease remained active.[8] It is thought that maternal HLA class II antigens (probably DR or DQ) form complexes with self-peptides, causing activation of maternal T lymphocytes that results in tissue damage. Fetal class II antigens can pass to the mother through cell trafficking. One theory is that when maternal and paternally inherited fetal class II antigens are disparate, maternal HLA will combine with fetal antigens, hence reducing the number of maternal HLA–self-peptide complexes. This would result in improvement of the disease in pregnancy.

Alternatively, genetic defects in the HLA-DR and -DQ region or major histocompatibility complex (MHC) passenger genes could give rise to the primary antigen in RA. Sharing of HLA antigens could then result in disease activity. Disparate genes and their peptide products would result in amelioration.[11]

Postpartum, particularly after the first pregnancy, there may be deterioration in RA or new-onset disease. However, the UK study showed no consistent pattern, although most women reported worsening in pain and swelling, with an increase in the mean number of inflamed joints, but this could not be predicted from previous postpartum relapse.[6] Lack of treatment was not the reason for postpartum flares. It may be that a reversal of the pregnancy-associated factors alluded to above could result in flare. Studies have noted that breast-feeding explains most of the increased risk post-partum, which occurs within 3–4 months.[1,12] This may be due to the proinflammatory hormone pro-lactin, which exhibits Th1-type cytokine effects.[1] Bromocriptine, which inhibits prolactin release, has a modest protective effect on postpartum flare.[6]

Miscarriage before disease onset but not fecundity (length of time of unprotected intercourse before first pregnancy) has recently been shown to be associated with the progression of joint damage in women with RA over a 2-year follow-up.[13]

DIAGNOSING A FLARE

Patients experience a worsening of joint pain and/or extra-articular involvement associated with anemia, leukocytosis, and thrombocytosis. A raised ESR (erythrocyte sedimentation rate) is unhelpful, as this occurs in normal pregnancy. RA can be monitored during and after pregnancy by the swollen joint count and RA disease activity index (RADAI), without major interference from pregnancy-related symptoms.[12]

EFFECT OF RHEUMATOID ARTHRITIS ON PREGNANCY

RA is not associated with infertility[14,15] or spontaneous miscarriage.[13] However, low-titer antiphospholipid antibody occasionally occurs with RA. Unexpectedly, an increased risk of pre-eclampsia in those with inflammatory arthritides was shown in a population-based Norwegian study spanning over 12 years, which has not previously been reported in smaller uncontrolled studies.[16] This could be linked to the association of HLA-DR4 with both RA and pre-eclampsia, or possibly a treatment effect related to steroid use.

There is a higher rate of induction of labor and cesarean section in women with RA.[16] Rheumatoid joints are generally unstable or fixed. Immobility in hip and knee joints may not permit vaginal delivery. Very rarely, bacteremia occurring during labor, results in septic arthritis of an affected or surgically corrected joint. Atlantoaxial subluxation, when the neck is extended during general anesthetic for cesarean section, is rare but potentially very serious as it can lead to spinal cord compression.

Fetal concerns relate to the few cases of congenital heart block that can occur in the minority of mothers with RA who have anti-Ro antibodies: see systemic lupus erythematosus (SLE) section. The main concerns relate to the safety of medications used during pregnancy and lactation.

TREATMENT OF RHEUMATOID ARTHRITIS (AND OTHER RHEUMATIC DISORDERS) IN PREGNANCY

The aim of treatment in RA is to relieve the symptoms and signs of disease, maintain physical function, and retard progression of joint damage and disability. This is achievable using analgesics, anti-inflammatory drugs, and disease-modifying agents. The safety of such medications is relevant in the pregnant and breast-feeding woman.

Paracetamol (acetaminophen) is safe in pregnancy and is the first-line analgesic.

Non-steroidal anti-inflammatory drugs (NSAIDs) are cyclo-oxygenase (COX) inhibitors that are non-selective against the two isoenzymes COX-1 and COX-2. They are generally avoided due to premature closure of the fetal ductus arteriosus via their inhibition of prostaglandin E_2 production, which would ordinarily relax the pulmonary vessels.[17] However, ductal flow impairment is rare before 27 weeks and resolves within 24 hours of NSAID discontinuation, and indomethacin (used in the short term at later gestations for the arrest of preterm labor) appears to be safe. NSAIDs also affect the fetal kidney, causing reversible oligohydramnios.[17] NSAIDs can be used before 28–32 weeks in some circumstances: for example, if steroids are being avoided due to the presence of osteopenia or osteoporosis.[10]

There have been recent concerns over the use of aspirin and NSAIDs pre-pregnancy and in the first trimester. Although they were initially not considered teratogenic, some data are emerging of an association between NSAIDs, cardiac defects, and orofacial clefts.[18] Analgesic doses of NSAIDs have been associated with miscarriage.[19] They have also been implicated as a cause of reversible female infertility due to the luteinized unruptured follicle (LUF) syndrome via their COX-2 inhibitory effects.[20] COX-2 is thought to be necessary for follicular rupture, and hence ovum release at ovulation. Salicylates (in analgesic doses) and NSAIDs may increase the risk of neonatal hemorrhage via inhibition of platelet function.[17]

The recently introduced COX-2 inhibitors, although currently contraindicated in pregnancy, have been reported to show only minor renal and no ductal effects on the fetus when used to prevent premature labor. Their effects on LUF syndrome are as yet unknown: some drugs have been withdrawn due to cardiovascular risk.[21]

Corticosteroids are preferable to NSAIDs for symptom control. Their dose may be limited by the maternal side effects of hypertension, gestational diabetes, and osteoporosis. They have been shown to increase the incidence of preterm rupture of membranes when used throughout pregnancy.[10] Only 10% of the dose of prednisolone crosses to the fetus. An association between very large doses of steroids and cleft lip and/or cleft palate has been found in animal studies. However, the association between oral cleft in the newborn and maternal corticosteroid use in human pregnancy is controversial. Some studies in humans suggest an increased risk of cleft lip and/or cleft palate following first-trimester exposure, but other studies have shown no increased risk of abortion, stillbirth, congenital malformations, adverse fetal effects, or neonatal death attributable to maternal steroid therapy.[10,17,22–25] Fetal adrenal suppression is a rare occurrence.[17] Hydrocortisone is used to cover the stress of labor in women who have been on >7.5 mg of prednisolone daily for more than 2 weeks. Prednisolone is safe in breast-feeding mothers since only 10% of active drug is secreted into breast milk.[17]

Disease-modifying antirheumatoid drugs (DMARDs) are second-line agents in the treatment of RA (Table 8.1). In non-pregnant populations with early and established RA, they are better than placebo in controlling symptoms and signs in patients previously treated with only NSAIDs. Progression of structural damage is slowed by sulfasalazine, methotrexate, and leflunomide, although the latter two drugs are contraindicated in pregnancy. DMARDs produce remission in only 20% of patients.[17]

The mechanism of action of these drugs in RA is complex and remains incompletely understood. Inhibitory effects on inflammatory pathways, immune responses, and cell activation have been described in experimental systems and clinical studies. Table 8.1 shows the effects of these drugs. Figure 8.2 shows the balance between efficacy and toxicity of these drugs.

Hydroxychloroquine, at doses up to 200 mg twice daily, can be continued or initiated in pregnancy for symptom control in a patient not responding to

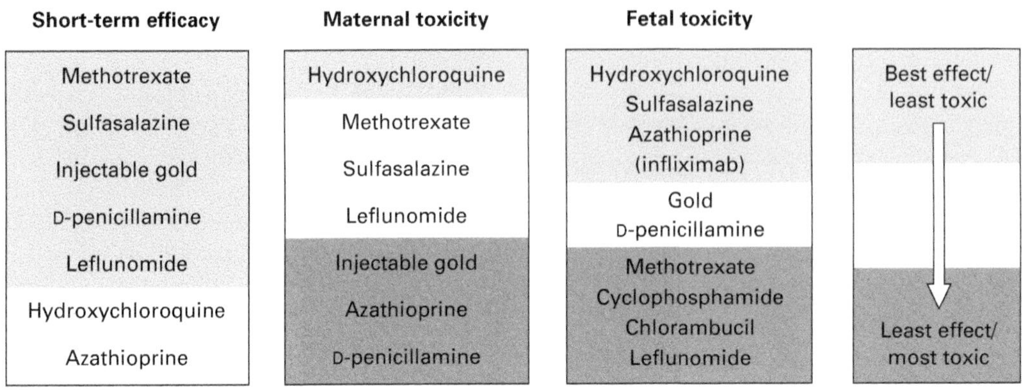

Short-term efficacy	Maternal toxicity	Fetal toxicity	
Methotrexate Sulfasalazine Injectable gold D-penicillamine Leflunomide Hydroxychloroquine Azathioprine	Hydroxychloroquine Methotrexate Sulfasalazine Leflunomide Injectable gold Azathioprine D-penicillamine	Hydroxychloroquine Sulfasalazine Azathioprine (infliximab) Gold D-penicillamine Methotrexate Cyclophosphamide Chlorambucil Leflunomide	Best effect/ least toxic ↓ Least effect/ most toxic

Figure 8.2 DMARDs efficacy–toxicity balance.

Table 8.1 Disease-modifying drugs in rheumatoid arthritis (DMARDs)

Drug	Main action	Route	$t_{1/2}$	Side effects	Fetal effects
Hydroxychloroquine	Antimalarial	po	1–2 months	GI upset, retinopathy, epilepsy	Only reported with chloroquinine
Sulfasalazine		po	Sulfapyridine 18 hours, mesalazine 6 hours	Rashes, GI upset, BM suppression	
Penicillamine	Chelating agent	po	Long	BM suppression, drug-induced autoimmune diseases: immune complex nephritis, SLE, MG, polymyositis	Congenital collagen defect in 5%
Gold	Chelating agent	po/im		Blood disorders, diarrhea, immune complex nephritis	Teratogenic in animals
Methotrexate	Folic acid antagonist	po	Long	BM suppression, pulmonary fibrosis	Teratogenic, fetotoxic
Cyclophosphamide	Alkylating agent	po/iv			
Chlorambucil	Alkylating agent		1.8 hours		
Azathioprine	Cytotoxic	po	4–6 hours	BM suppression, hepatotoxic, GI upset, herpes zoster	Infertility in exposed female fetus
Cyclosporine		po	6 hours	Nephrotoxic	IUGR
Leflunomide	Inhibits de-novo pyrimidine synthesis	po	15–18 days[a]	Hepatotoxic: ↑ transaminases in 2–4%, hepatocellular necrosis 0.02–0.04% Weight loss, diarrhea, hypertension	Teratogenic, fetotoxic
Infliximab	Chimeric anti-TNF-α Ab	iv	9 days	Infections, especially opportunistic and TB, lymphoma,[b] serious anaphylaxis 0.4%, drug-induced autoimmune SLE, demyelinating disease, haematological abnormalities	No increase in fetal birth defects/fetal loss in 96 women
Entanercept	Binds TNF-α and TNF-β	sc	4 days	Skin irritation 50–80% (dose-dependent)	Unknown
Adalimumab	Human anti-TNF-α Ab	sc	2 weeks		Unknown
Anakinra	Human IL-1 receptor antagonist	sc	6 hours	Infections mainly bacterial ↑ 5-fold	Unknown

po, oral; im, intramuscular; iv, intravenous; sc, subcutaneous; TB, tuberculosis; BM, bone marrow; GI, gastrointestinal; SLE, systemic lupus erythematosus; MG, myasthenia gravis; IUGR, intrauterine growth restriction; TNF, tumor necrosis factor; IL-1, interleukin-1.
[a]Can remain in circulation for 2 years
[b]Lymphoma also increased in those with severe rheumatoid arthritis; therefore, drug effect uncertain.

acetaminophen and steroids, despite the knowledge that the drug passes freely to the fetus. Concerns regarding fetal retinopathy and ototoxicity relate to chloroquine only.[26] No increase in the perinatal mortality rate (PNMR) or congenital malformations have been found with hydroxychloroquine use when compared with controls, or when compared with the background population.[17,26]

Sulfasalazine has been used extensively in the treatment of inflammatory bowel disease in pregnancy and appears to be safe. It may be continued throughout pregnancy, although concomitant high-dose folate supplementation (5 mg) is recommended.[17]

Use of drugs in renal transplant patients has provided much of the safety data on drugs such as azathioprine, which is the most common cytotoxic drug used in RA and SLE. It seems safe; however, an increase in intrauterine growth restriction (IUGR) in transplant patients is noted and neonatal immunosuppression is a theoretical risk.[17] Traditional advice to avoid breast-feeding while receiving azathioprine is based on a single study of only two patients, where metabolites of azathioprine were detected in the breast milk. No resulting neonatal toxicity or adverse effects were reported.[27] It is preferred to cyclosporine. Methotrexate is highly teratogenic and should be discontinued at least 3 months prior to conception, with folic acid supplementation given preconceptually.[17] D-penicillamine is generally stopped before conception because of the small risk of congenital collagen defects.[17] However, as it is particularly useful in the management of the extra-articular features of RA, it is sometimes used later in pregnancy.[10] Gold salts can be continued during pregnancy if they are controlling disease, although most would avoid initiation of treatment during pregnancy.[10,17]

NEWER DMARDS: LEFLUNOMIDE AND TNF ANTAGONISTS (INFLIXIMAB, ETANERCEPT, ADALIMUMAB)

Leflunomide must be stopped preconceptionally, but due to its extensive enterohepatic recirculation, it can persist in blood for up to 2 years. It is there-fore recommended that an elimination protocol is followed using cholestyramine to bind the drug, both in men and women wishing to conceive.[3]

TNF-α regulates production of IL-1, and together these two cytokines orchestrate rheumatoid inflammation and damage (see Figure 8.1). TNF antagonists are amongst the most effective treatments in RA. They demonstrate a rapid response, usually within a few weeks. They are used in the treatment of moderate to severe RA with persistent disease activity despite best available, but also potentially toxic and immunosuppressive, standard therapy.[3] They are not licensed for use in pregnancy; however, women do conceive while using drugs for which little pregnancy data are available. By collating the pregnancy outcomes and neonatal data of such cases, useful information is gleaned (see Table 8.1).

TNF antagonists are associated with an increase in infections, although RA itself is associated with a twofold increase in serious infection. The 40-fold increase in tuberculosis with adalimumab is 10 times greater than with infliximab and is due to reactivation of latent disease. Anti-TNF therapy is therefore contraindicated in the presence of active serious infections and latent untreated tuberculosis. It is not advisable in moderate or severe congestive cardiac failure and in demyelinating syndromes. The efficacy of these agents outside pregnancy is improved by combining them with methotrexate, probably because methotrexate limits the production of antibodies against the TNF antagonists.[3]

Infliximab neutralizes the biological activity of TNF-α by binding to both the soluble and membrane-bound protein. In Europe, infliximab is approved for the treatment of Crohn's disease, RA, and ankylosing spondylitis. It has been shown to be more effective than methotrexate in RA.[3] In a study of 96 women taking infliximab within 3 months of conception and/or during the first trimester of pregnancy,[28] the rate of live births, miscarriages, and therapeutic terminations observed was similar to those expected in a healthy population. One baby was delivered at 24 weeks, but died shortly after birth with intracranial and intrapulmonary bleeding. The mother was on other drugs, including azathioprine. One baby had tetralogy of Fallot, another had intestinal malrotation, but was also exposed to leflunomide, a known teratogen in animals.

Etanercept has an efficacy equivalent to methotrexate, but high doses have a more rapid response in the first 2 weeks of use.[3]

SYSTEMIC LUPUS ERYTHEMATOSUS

SLE is a multisystem autoimmune rheumatic disorder. Table 8.2 outlines the common clinical features and Table 8.3 shows the clinical and serological features required for diagnosis of this condition.

Pregnancy runs a variable course and is dependent on various factors, including disease activity at conception; associated anti-Ro, anti-La, or antiphospholipid antibodies; associated hypertension; and renal disease.

INCIDENCE

SLE is a disease of mainly young women, being 10–20 times more common in women than in men. It is becoming of increasing relevance to obstetricians as the incidence continues to rise, although

Table 8.2 Clinical features of systemic lupus erythematosus

System	Clinical features
General	Fever, anorexia
Joints	Arthralgia, arthritis
Skin	Photosensitivity, butterfly rash, Raynaud's phenomenon, livedo reticularis, vasculitis, purpura, urticaria, alopecia
Blood	Anemia (normocytic or hemolytic), leukopenia, thrombocytopenia
CNS	Asceptic meningitis, stroke, demyelination, headache, fits, chorea, mono- and polyneuropathy, cranial nerve lesions, autonomic disorder
Psychiatric	Anxiety, depression, psychosis, cognitive dysfunction
Renal	Glomerulonephritis
Chest	Pleurisy, pleural effusion, restrictive lung disease, pulmonary hypertension
Cardiovascular	Pericarditis, endocarditis, valve lesions, cardiomyopathy

Table 8.3 Summary of American Rheumatism Association classification criteria for systemic lupus erythematosus

System	Four features required simultaneously or following each other
Mucocutaneous	Facial butterfly rash Discoid lupus Photosensitivity skin rash Oral/nasopharyngeal ulceration
Joints	Non-erosive arthritis involving ≥2 peripheral joints
CVS/respiratory	Pleurisy/pericarditis
Renal	Proteinuria >0.5 g/day
CNS	Psychosis/fits
Hematological	1 of: • Hemolytic anaemia • Leukopenia: >4 on ≥2 occasions • Lymphopenia: <1.5 on ≥2 occasions • Thrombocytopenia: <100
Immunological	1 of: • Antibody to native DNA in abnormal titer • Antibody to smooth muscle nuclear antigen • Positive finding of antiphospholipid antibodies (including IgG or IgM anticardiolipin antibodies and lupus anticoagulant)

From Hochberg.[29]

this could be a reflection of diagnosing milder cases. In the UK the overall incidence is 4 cases/ 100 000/year.[30] The ethnic variation in prevalence of SLE is shown in Table 8.4.

INFLAMMATORY PATHOLOGY

SLE is predominately a Th2 disease (humoral immunity) and is characterized by the presence of numerous autoantibodies, as shown in Table 8.5.

Antibodies to double-stranded DNA (anti-dsDNA) are the most specific antibodies found in

Table 8.4 Ethnic variation in systemic lupus erythematosus (SLE) prevalence in the UK

Ethnic group in UK	Prevalence of SLE/100 000 women
Afro-Caribbean	206
Asian	91
Caucasian	36
Overall pregnant women	~100

From Johnson et al.[30]

Table 8.5 Common autoantibodies in systemic lupus erythematosus

	Antigen against which autoantibody produced	Prevalence (%)
Intracellular	dsDNA (ssDNA)	40–90
	Histones	30–80
	Sm	10–30
	RNP	20–30
	Ro/SSA	10–15
	La/SSB	10–15
	hsp	30
Cell membrane	Cardiolipin (phospholipids)	20–40
	Lupus anticoagulant	15–20
	Neuronal antigen	70–90% with CNS involvement; 10% without
	Lymphocyte	45–75
	Red cell	10
	Platelet	10
Extracellular	Rheumatoid factor	25
	C1q	20–45

From Rahman and Isenberg.[31]

SLE. They are raised in active disease and hence can be used in monitoring disease activity. They are specific to SLE, and deposits have been found in the glomeruli of patients with lupus nephritis. The most damaging is the IgG isotype.[31]

> The immunopathological pathway is still unknown, but it is considered that B cells producing autoantibodies, T cells, the complement system, and apoptosis are involved, as shown in the postulated mechanism in Figure 8.3. The underlying antigenic stimulus in SLE is unknown, but contenders include DNA and histone in complex, or perhaps viral DNA-binding proteins.

Apoptosis or programmed cell death may be central to exposing the suspected antigen (DNA/histone complex) within cell blebs on the surface of the dying cell. Prevailing B cells continuously exposed to this self-antigen (or viral antigen with molecular mimicry) undergo antigen-driven somatic mutation whereby mutations accumulate in the expressed immunoglobulin gene sequences until the antibody released acts specifically against this antigen. This process is assisted by T helper cells, which preferentially support a Th2 response. Th2 cells produce an abundance of IL-10, which inhibits the Th1 cell-mediated response, and hence macrophage and natural killer cell cytotoxicity. There is also a reduction in T-suppressor cells; hence, production of autoantibody continues unchecked.[31]

Antibody–antigen immune complexes are not cleared effectively by monocytes as complement activation is deficient; hence, autoantibody persists and reaches the target organ, e.g. kidney. It is no longer suspected that immune complexes are deposited here. The favored hypothesis is that antibody binds to nucleosome–histone complexes, and the positively charged histone binds to the negatively charged heparan sulfate on the basement membrane in the glomerulus. This is damaging to the glomerulus.[31]

Generation of antiphospholipid antibody is suspected to occur against phospholipids combined to the plasma protein β_2-glycoprotein 1, which occurs on the outer surface of the blebs of the apoptotic cells.[31]

Other autoantibodies may be generated by epitope spreading: this occurs when previously unexposed cryptic epitopes are exposed to self during an immune response. These epitopes are considered foreign, and antibodies are generated against them.

LUPUS FLARES

Flares of SLE in pregnancy most often affect the joints and skin.[32] It can be difficult to diagnose a flare in pregnancy, as many features such as facial erythema, musculoskeletal pain, fatigue, hair loss, edema, anemia, and raised ESR also occur in normal pregnancy. Additionally, there may be difficulty in distinguishing active lupus nephritis from preeclampsia, particularly beyond 20 weeks, as both can present with proteinuria, hypertension, deteriorating renal function, and thrombocytopenia. Immunological testing plays a key role in diagnosis and this and other useful distinguishing features are shown in Table 8.6.

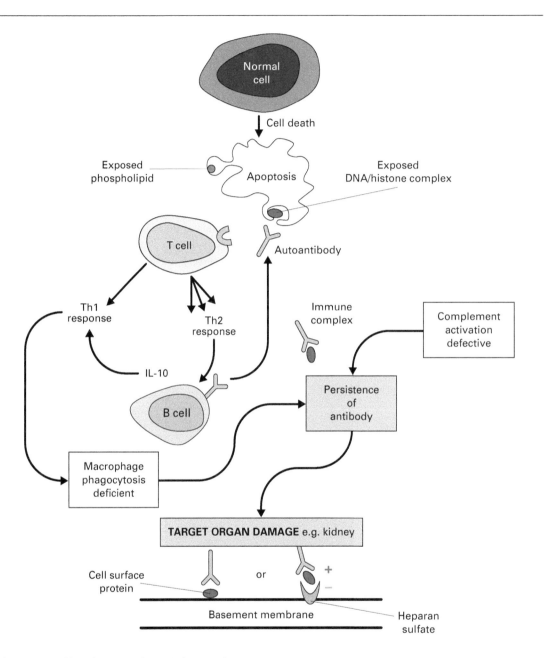

Figure 8.3 Possible pathogenesis of systemic lupus erythematosus.

Table 8.6 Useful distinguishing features between lupus nephritis and pre-eclampsia

	Feature	Active lupus nephritis	Pre-eclampsia
Clinical	Onset/remission	Remission not related to delivery	Usually acute onset and remits postnatally
	Joint and skin symptoms	Present	Absent
Immunology	ANA	Positive	Usually negative
	dsDNA Ab	Rising titer	Absent
	C3, C4, CH50: classical complement pathway	Low	Normal (but can be low)
	Ba, Bb: alternative complement pathway	High	Normal
	CH50/Ba	Low	High
	WCC/lymphocytes	Low	Normal
Urine	Hematuria	Present	Absent
	Casts	Present	Absent
Histopathology	Renal biopsy[a]	Glomerulonephritis	Acute atherosis

WCC, white cell count.
[a]Rarely performed in pregnancy.

EFFECT OF PREGNANCY ON SLE

The impact of pregnancy on SLE remains controversial. Despite numerous retrospective and prospective studies, including some with matched non-pregnant controls, there is no clear agreement as to the exact influence pregnancy has on the course of SLE, with reports of lupus flare varying from 13 to 75%.[32–34] Study comparisons have been limited by differences in study entry criteria and design, variability of disease activity at conception, criteria used for lupus flare, routine steroid administration, and variations in the continuation of stabilizing drug treatment.

> In studies with carefully matched non-pregnant controls, no excessive rate of lupus flares was noted in pregnancy. However, when patients are used as their own controls, an excessive rate of flare is noted.[35]

Relapse is more likely in women with active disease at conception (10–30% flare with inactive disease vs 60% with active disease), lupus nephritis, and hypertension.[32,33] Variability exists regarding timing of flares, with reported postpartum flares ranging from 6 to 51%.[32,34,36–38] Flares increase in those women who stop treatment with antimalarials,[26] but are not prevented by the prophylactic use of steroids.[32]

SLE is a predominately Th2 disease that would be expected to be exaggerated in the Th2-positive milieu of pregnancy. Persistently high levels of the Th2-response cytokine IL-10 have been found in pregnant patients with SLE compared with healthy pregnant controls.[39] Significantly higher levels of IL-10 and soluble tumor necrosis factor receptors (sTNFR I) occur in those women with active disease during pregnancy and postpartum, which may help explain postnatal flares.

Pregnancy does not appear to affect the long-term prognosis of SLE.[40] Unusual symptoms in SLE such as chorea can be made worse by pregnancy specifically.[40]

LUPUS NEPHRITIS

Numerous studies yield conflicting results regarding the effect of pregnancy on lupus nephritis. Quiescent disease at conception is associated with less deterioration during pregnancy in several series, with flare rates ranging from 7.4 to 32%.[35] Active disease at conception has reported flare rates of 48–62% in pregnancy.[35] In the only prospective case–control study of lupus nephritis in pregnancy to date, 78 pregnancies (in 56 patients) were age- and time-matched with 78 non-pregnant controls, all of whom had SLE nephritis at diagnosis.[35] In this well-conducted single-center study, no differences in exacerbation of renal disease activity (44.6% vs 41.9%) or deterioration in renal function (17.3% vs 24%) were noted between cases and controls, respectively. There were no differences in the amount of steroids taken. Controls were on more immunosuppressive and antimalarial agents.

EFFECT OF SLE ON PREGNANCY

> SLE is associated with increased risks of spontaneous miscarriage, fetal death, preterm delivery, IUGR, and pre-eclampsia. Fertility is unaffected, although cyclophosphamide treatment may induce infertility due to ovarian failure.

The increase in spontaneous miscarriage in women with SLE is directly related to the presence of antiphospholipid antibodies, which occur in 32.6% (13.5–51.7%) of SLE pregnancies.[41] Recurrent pregnancy loss may be treated with aspirin or with aspirin and low-molecular-weight heparins (LMWH). The role of antiphospholipid syndrome (APS) in miscarriage is discussed fully in Chapter 5. Late fetal losses are related to secondary APS, active disease, hypertension, and renal impairment.[32,36] These are declining in incidence, reflecting the improvements in obstetric and neonatal management of these high-risk pregnancies as well as improved ascertainment and hence inclusion in recent data series of milder cases of SLE.

Recent studies have shown stillbirth rates of up to 3.2% and total fetal loss rates (spontaneous miscarriage and stillbirths) of 5–26%.[32,34,36–38,42] In a case–control prospective study, the Toronto group confirmed that active disease results in poorer fetal outcome[36] (Table 8.7). One series, in which 55% of women were antiphospholipid positive, had high stillbirth rates of 12% and fetal loss rates of 26%. They demonstrated a doubling of risk of early and late fetal loss in the women with lupus nephritis.[32] Recent series of pregnant women with lupus nephritis have shown stillbirth rates of 4–9% and total fetal loss rates of 22–38%.[35,43–45]

> Women with APS are at risk of arterial and venous thromboses. If they have previously had a thrombosis, the recurrence risk is 70%. Such patients will be on long-term anticoagulation with aspirin or warfarin. They require high-dose LMWH, e.g. enoxaparin 40 mg twice daily, and aspirin throughout pregnancy.[10,46]

SLE is associated with an increase in IUGR and preterm delivery. In 638 lupus pregnancies, a median of 9.4% (range 2–39.5%) had IUGR; 33.4% (7.8–63.2%) resulted in preterm delivery, with 7.5% (5.6–37.9%) having preterm rupture of membranes (pPROM).[32,34,37,38,41,42] Researchers disagree as to whether[33,42,47] or not[34,36,41] disease activity or lupus nephritis is associated with preterm delivery.

The Toronto group found that of the 38.4% preterm deliveries in their study of lupus pregnancies, 61% were due to spontaneous onset of preterm labor. The rest were iatrogenic deliveries for maternal or fetal complications, mainly maternal hypertensive disease and fetal syndrome. Although no significant correlation was found with lupus disease activity, those with preterm delivery were on larger amounts of prednisolone, which the group speculates may be associated independently with preterm delivery.[41] Inactive disease rather than controlled disease may be the determining factor in extending SLE pregnancies to full term.

Pre-eclampsia has been shown to be increased in those women with active lupus at conception (28.5% compared with 6.4% with quiescent disease

Table 8.7 Fetal loss with systemic lupus erythematosus (SLE)

	Pregnant patients with SLE			Healthy pregnant women
	Overall	Inactive disease	Active disease	
Stillbirth rate (%)	1.7	0	12.5	1.7
Total fetal loss (%)	16.9	13.7	37.5	5.1

From Georgiou et al.[36]

at conception). Hypertension and pre-eclampsia are increased in those women with any renal disease, including lupus nephritis in remission.[33] Pre-eclampsia rates as high as 66% have been reported in those women with lupus nephritis, compared with 14% in those without renal involvement.[48] These high rates may reflect the difficulty in distinguishing pre-eclampsia from renal flare in pregnancy.

Severe SLE can result in maternal death, which is usually the result of lung, renal, or cardiac involvement, or of catastrophic APS.

NEONATAL LUPUS ERYTHEMATOSUS

These conditions occur due to transplacental transfer of pathological maternal IgG autoantibodies directed against the intracellular ribonucleoproteins Ro, La, and occasionally U_1 (U_1RNP). In the neonate they result in immunologically mediated damage to the skin, heart, blood, and liver.[49]

These autoantibodies are present mainly in those with SLE, but can be found in other connective tissue diseases as well as in currently asymptomatic individuals who may go on to develop a connective tissue disease in the future. It is the presence of anti-Ro with or without anti-La antibodies rather than the type of associated autoimmune disease that is a risk factor for neonatal lupus erythematosus (NLE). More than 90% of mothers of affected offspring have anti-Ro antibodies and 50–70% have anti-La antibodies. About 30% of patients with SLE are anti-Ro positive. Mothers of babies with neonatal lupus have a higher frequency of HLA-DR3, often with A1 and B8.[10]

A recent large prospective study of 128 infants born to anti-Ro-positive women with or without anti-La or anti-U_1 antibodies has shown that 52% of the infants will have NLE if their mother has an autoimmune disease, or if she had a previously affected child.[49]

Congenital heart block (CHB) is the most serious abnormality and affects 1.6–2% of children born to mothers with the antibodies.[49,50]

CHB is due to damage to the atrioventricular node. The incidence increases to 10.5% if a previous child is affected,[49] and has been reported as high as 50% when two previous children are affected.[10] It can be detected from 16–24 weeks' gestation and may be fatal. Dexamethasone may prevent progression from incomplete to complete fetal heart block.[10] Recently, IVIG in combination with prednisolone has been shown to prevent recurrence of CHB.[51] If complete heart block occurs, the neonate may require a cardiac pacemaker. Plasmapheresis treatment has been used with varied effects.[10]

Sinus bradycardia occurs in 9–16.7% of cases, suggesting that the sinoatrial node may also be damaged. A prolonged QT interval occurs in 37.5–41% of cases, which is important as this can result in sudden infant death.[49,50] Endomyocardial fibrosis and pericarditis have also been described.[40]

The mechanism of cardiac damage is unclear. It may be due to a humoral response, with anti-Ro or anti-La antibodies directly damaging the conduction system in the fetal heart, but the mother's heart is not affected. A cell-mediated mechanism has been proposed, with transplacental transfer of maternal cells to the fetus, which leads to maternal microchimerism and tissue damage (see Systemic sclerosis section). Myocyte-specific phenotype maternal cells have been found in all sections taken from the hearts of four children who died from NLE, equating to up to 2.2% of myocytes being of maternal origin. This compared with a negligible 0–0.1% of cells being of maternal origin in 25% of the heart sections taken from four controls.[52] It is not clear whether these maternal cells are contributing to the pathogenesis or secondary process of repair of cardiac injury in NLE.

Cutaneous NLE manifests as annular inflammatory lesions similar to those of adult subacute cutaneous lupus, usually on the face and scalp, which appear after sun or UV light exposure in the first 2 weeks of life. It occurs in 16% of cases, but the incidence is greater in those with anti-Ro and anti-La antibodies rather than anti-Ro alone.[49] Some skin lesions are associated with antibodies against U_1RNP, a protein that is found in normal human skin cells. The rash disappears spontaneously within 6 months, suggesting a direct antibody-mediated mechanism. Residual hypopigmentation or telangiectasia may persist for up to 2 years, but scarring is unusual. Sunlight and phototherapy should be avoided.[10]

It was found that 27% of neonates with anti Ro/La will be neutropenic, anemic, or thrombocytopenic.[49] This resolves by the age of 1 and infants are usually asymptomatic. A protein similar to Ro occurs on the membrane of neutrophils, and Ro antigen is present on the surface of red blood cells (RBCs). These are thought to be attacked by the autoantibodies.

Abnormal liver function tests, usually either elevated transaminases or γGT (γ-glutamyl transpeptidase), occur in 25% of cases and resolve in 1 year and tend not to be associated with jaundice.[49]

TREATMENT OF SLE IN PREGNANCY

(See Table 8.1 and refer to treatment sub-section under Rheumatoid arthritis section for more details on individual drugs.)

Preconception counseling in a multidisciplinary setting will allow assessment of disease activity, hypertension, renal lupus, and antibody status. Recommendations can be made on timing of pregnancy, ideally when in remission, and explanation of risks. Adjustments in teratogenic treatments can be made, such as the discontinuation of methotrexate, cyclophosphamide, ACE (angiotensin-converting enzyme) inhibitors, and angiotensin-II receptor antagonists, if this is clinically feasible.

Patients with antiphospholipid antibodies should be advised to start low-dose aspirin, 75 mg daily, preconception or from when the pregnancy test is positive. They should commence prophylactic doses of LMWH if they have had a previous arterial/venous thrombosis or recurrent miscarriage or adverse pregnancy outcome (IUGR, severe preeclampsia, or abruption). The dose may need to be increased if there are combination thrombophilias.

> Disease flares must be actively managed and corticosteroids are the drug of choice.

Hydroxychloroquine should be continued in pregnancy, as stopping it has been shown to double the incidence of flare in patients with SLE in the next 6 months in non-pregnant patients.[26] It also has a very long half-life, so discontinuation will not prevent fetal exposure. Azathioprine is also usually continued, as this acts as a 'steroid-sparing' agent. Differentiation of active renal lupus from pre-eclampsia is notoriously difficult and the two conditions may be superimposed. Distinguishing features are shown in Table 8.6. Hypertension should be controlled with methyldopa. Nifedipine, labetalol, or hydralazine can be used as second-line agents.

SYSTEMIC SCLEROSIS (SCLERODERMA)

Systemic sclerosis (SSc) is an autoimmune connective tissue disease causing a small vessel vasculitis, and cutaneous and visceral fibrosis. Table 8.8 shows the different clinical forms of systemic sclerosis. Of these, diffuse cutaneous systemic sclerosis is the most severe and is associated with significant morbidity and mortality. The median survival time is approximately 11 years.[53]

INCIDENCE

The UK incidence is 300 cases per year, with a prevalence of 1 in 10 000. SSc affects women approximately four times as often as men, with this ratio increasing during the childbearing years to 10:1. The mean age of onset is the early 40s.[54]

INFLAMMATORY PATHOLOGY

A stimulating antigen in a susceptible individual leads to a complex interplay between immunological and vascular factors that results in connective tissue abnormalities in different organs, causing different subsets of the disease. Some of the mechanisms implicated in pathogenesis of SSc are indicated in Figure 8.4.

Table 8.8 Clinical forms of systemic sclerosis

	Raynaud's phenomenon	Skin changes	Visceral involvement	Autoantibodies against antigen
Prescleroderma	✓ (+ nailfold capillary changes)		✗	Topoisomerase I (Scl-70) nucleolar centromere
Limited cutaneous systemic sclerosis (formerly CREST syndrome)	✓	✓ or ✗ Acral: hands (sclerodactyly), face, feet	10–15 years later: Pulmonary hypertension (+/− interstitial lung disease) Calcinosis Telangiectasia GI disease	Centromere (70–80%)
Diffuse cutaneous systemic sclerosis	✓ (+ nailfold capillary dilatation, and drop out)	Truncal and acral skin Tendon friction rubs	Early: Interstitial lung disease, renal, GI and cardiac involvement	Topoisomerase I (30%)
Scleroderma sine scleroderma	✓ or ✗	✗	Presentation: Pulmonary fibrosis, renal crisis, cardiac or GI disease	Topoisomerase I centromere RNA-polymerase I

GI, gastrointestinal.

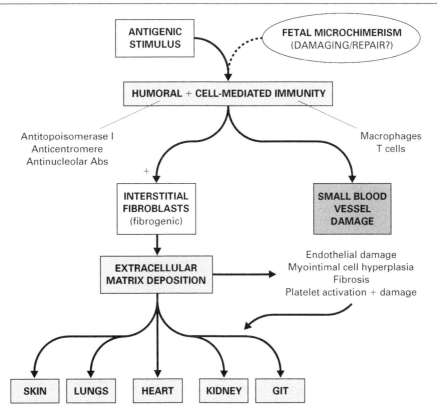

Figure 8.4 Pathogenesis of systemic sclerosis.

MICROCHIMERISM IN SYSTEMIC SCLEROSIS

> Microchimerism is the coexistence of two distinct cell populations, originating from different individuals, in a single person. Fetal cells transfer into the maternal circulation from 4 to 6 weeks' gestation and continue until delivery such that at 36 weeks all pregnant women have detectable fetal cells in their blood.[55]

Fetal cells can be detected in maternal blood 27 years on.[56] This cellular trafficking is bidirectional, and maternal cells can also transfer into the fetus. Maternal cells have been found more frequently in those with juvenile idiopathic inflammatory myopathies compared with controls,[57] as well as being found in the myocardium of babies with NLE affected by heart block.[52]

SSc was the first disease to be associated with microchimerism when Nelson et al found affected women to have a significantly greater number of microchimeric cells in their circulation than healthy controls.[58] Male cells are detected in affected tissues from skin and different organs.[59] Male T cells with a CD4+ phenotype that can react against maternal histocompatibility antigens resulting in damage have been found in lesional skin.[60]

The alternative hypothesis is that, rather than instigating damage, these fetal cells are actually involved in tissue repair and have a long-term protective effect on course of the disease. Evidence for this comes from women with SSc who have never been pregnant (nulliparous) and hence not been exposed to fetal cell trafficking. They have an earlier onset of the disease and have more pulmonary involvement and death than parous women.[61] Additionally, nulliparous women have been found to have an increased risk of developing SSc than parous women.[62]

RENAL CRISIS

It is essential, but difficult, to differentiate a renal crisis from pre-eclampsia in SSc (Table 8.9). High-dose steroids can precipitate a renal crisis, especially in early diffuse disease.[63] Anti-RNA polymerase is associated with renal SSc. Delay in treatment may be fatal.

EFFECT OF PREGNANCY ON SYSTEMIC SCLEROSIS

> SSc symptoms tend to be unaffected by pregnancy.

A retrospective study in Washington, DC, found no change in symptoms in 88%, improvement in 5%, and deterioration in 7% of cases.[64] They found that the figures in a prospective study were 61%, 20%, and 19%, respectively.[65] The same group, in a recent large prospective case-controlled study of 91 pregnancies in 59 women with SSc, found that Raynaud's phenomenon improved during pregnancy and deteriorated postpartum.[54] This may be due to the peripheral vasodilatation that occurs in pregnant women. Also, 27% of patients with diffuse disease noted a temporary increase in skin thickening, which was not apparent postpartum. Esophageal reflux deteriorated as a result of the physiological relaxation of the esophageal sphincter in pregnancy. There is a danger that this can lead to aspiration pneumonia, and, if this occurs on the background of severe pulmonary fibrosis, it can be fatal.

There is no evidence that pregnancy worsens the already poor outcome of those women with cardiac or respiratory disease, although those with severe pulmonary fibrosis and pulmonary hypertension are at extremely high risk of postpartum deterioration, as with pulmonary hypertension from any cause.[65] Pulmonary hypertension occurs in 15% of those with limited cutaneous SSc who are ACA positive, and in 25% of those with diffuse cutaneous SSc who are U_3RNP positive. Lung fibrosis occurs in the majority of those with antitopoisomerase I, irrespective of SSc subset, and 15% of them will develop secondary pulmonary hypertension.

Renal flares are thought not to increase in pregnancy, although it is difficult with the few series available to come to any firm conclusion. Renal crises are more common in the first 4–5 years of diagnosis of diffuse systemic sclerosis, and hence women who happen to fall pregnant during this time may be affected. Certainly, both the women with renal crises in the Washington study had early diffuse systemic sclerosis (<4 years), a finding echoed in retrospective studies.[64,65]

In general, women with limited SSc without organ involvement do better than those with diffuse disease. The extent of diffuse disease and systemic involvement (particularly lung, cardiac, and renal) influences prognosis, but there are no absolute rules.

> Those women with early disease (less than 4 years), diffuse disease, or antitopoisomerase (anti-ScL-70) antibodies are at greater risk of having more active aggressive disease than those with long-standing disease and anticentromere antibodies. Women with renal involvement often have associated hypertension, and rapid deterioration is possible.

The Washington group found maternal death rates of 1.9%.[65] Ten-year survival of women with SSc is unchanged by pregnancy.[10]

EFFECT OF SYSTEMIC SCLEROSIS ON PREGNANCY

SSc does not affect fertility.[15] Case–control studies have found no increase in miscarriage in women with SSc (limited cutaneous or diffuse) compared to women with RA or to normal controls.[15,54,64] However, 42% of women with late diffuse disease miscarried compared to only 13% in the rest of the SSc patients.[54] The presence of antiphospholipid antibodies was not revealed.

There is an increased risk of premature delivery,[54,64] with 22% occurring in those with limited disease, 28% in diffuse disease, and 5% in controls. Women with early diffuse SSc (< 4 years) had the highest rates of preterm birth of 65% compared with 24% in the rest of the patients combined. The true incidence of preterm birth will be slightly less, as these figures include infants born at 37 weeks.[54] Half of the cases were a result of preterm labor and pPROM, and the others were caused by iatrogenic preterm delivery for maternal or fetal compromise.

There is no increased risk of pre-eclampsia in the absence of hypertension or renal involvement.

TREATMENT

(See Table 8.1 and refer to treatment section under rheumatoid arthritis for more details on individual drugs.)

Preconception counseling allows assessment of the extent of organ involvement.

> Pregnancy is not recommended in those women with renal impairment, severe cardiomyopathy, severe restrictive lung disease, or pulmonary hypertension.

Those women with early diffuse disease should delay pregnancy until the disease stabilizes to decrease the risk of renal crises.[65] This is usually 3–5 years from the onset of symptoms. Disease-remitting drugs such as D-penicillamine and cyclosporin A (cyclosporine) should preferably be discontinued before conception if the disease is stable, although inadvertent first trimester exposure should not cause undue concern.

A multidisciplinary team approach with frequent joint obstetric and medical care is appropriate. Blood pressure monitoring is essential, as hypertension may indicate a renal crisis. Urgent attempts should be made to differentiate this from pre-eclampsia, as delay in treatment of a renal crisis with an ACE inhibitor can be fatal (see Table 8.9). These drugs have revolutionized the management and survival in renal systemic sclerosis and should not be withheld in pregnancy. They are usually contraindicated, but in SSc the benefit outweighs the risk of fetal renal toxicity. If doubt remains, then ACE inhibitors should be commenced and delivery performed. Delivery will not reverse a renal crisis but will result in improvement in pre-eclampsia.

Table 8.9 Differentiating between renal crisis and pre-eclampsia in systemic sclerosis

	Renal crisis	Pre-eclampsia
Hypertension	Acute onset; severe, often malignant	Usually acute onset; may be severe
Proteinuria	+/−	Present
Thrombocytopenia	+/−	+/−
Abnormal liver function tests	−	+/−
Creatinine	Daily increases	+/− increase, but slower
Treatment	ACE inhibitors	Delivery

ACE, angiotensin-converting enzyme.

Management of SSc during pregnancy is largely symptomatic. Raynaud's phenomenon usually improves, but, if not, calcium antagonists may be used. Ranitidine or proton-pump inhibitors can be used for reflux but NSAIDs are best avoided, as previously discussed. Corticosteroids (more than 15 mg prednisolone per day and betamethasone for fetal lung maturity) must be avoided in early diffuse SSc, since they can precipitate a renal crisis.[63] Azathioprine would be more appropriate in this instance. It is best to avoid β-adrenergic agonists for preterm labor, since SSc patients may have silent myocardial damage, which makes them more vulnerable to ischemia and pulmonary edema. Atosiban or nifedipine would be preferable for tocolysis.

Thickened tight skin and blood vessel involvement can make venepuncture, venous access, blood pressure measurement, and regional anesthesia difficult. However, epidural anesthesia and analgesia is encouraged, as vasodilation improves skin perfusion of the extremities. Other measures to reduce problems related to Raynaud's phenomenon include warming of the delivery room and any intravenous fluids as well as wearing of socks and gloves. General anesthesia may be complicated by difficult endotracheal intubation. Cesarean sections are performed for obstetric reasons and heal well if care is taken with skin closure.

Postnatal vigilance is essential, especially in those women with cardiac, pulmonary, or renal involvement. The most recent data, although derived from a retrospective postal questionnaire, suggest that outcomes are not significantly worse than controls, provided pregnancy is well-timed and carefully monitored.[10] Clinicians are therefore becoming more optimistic in counseling women with systemic sclerosis considering pregnancy.

IDIOPATHIC THROMBOCYTOPENIC PURPURA

Idiopathic thrombocytopenic purpura (ITP) is an autoimmune condition with antibodies binding to platelets, resulting in their premature destruction by the reticuloendothelial system (RES). It is char-

acterized by a persistent thrombocytopenia, with a peripheral platelet count of $<150 \times 10^9$/L. In pregnancy, these antibodies can cross the placenta and affect the fetus or neonate, causing thrombocytopenia, which occasionally results in intracranial hemorrhage.

INCIDENCE

ITP is a rare condition, which occurs in 5.8–6.6 per 100 000 people in the UK.[66] There is a female preponderance of the disease (female:male ratio = 3:1), affecting mainly women of childbearing age. Hence, the incidence in pregnancy is increased to 1–2 per 1000 pregnancies.

INFLAMMATORY PATHOLOGY

ITP was initially suspected to be an autoimmune disease when babies born to affected mothers developed a transient neonatal thrombocytopenia. Plasma taken from those patients with ITP and transfused into healthy patients also resulted in a transient thrombocytopenia in the recipients.[67]

It is now known that in ITP there are immunoglobulin G (IgG) autoantibodies against multiple platelet surface antigens. These platelet-associated IgG (PAIgG) are a heterogeneous group of antibodies against various glycoprotein complexes, including glycoprotein IIb/IIIa, Ib/IX, Ia/IIa, IV, and V complexes, as well as antibodies against other platelet determinants.[67] Although it is not known what initiates the production of these autoantibodies in ITP, there is a generation of new autoantibodies against other platelet antigens by epitope spread, such that by the time the disease manifests itself clinically, most patients will have antibodies against several platelet surface antigens.

Increased numbers of HLA-DR+ T cells, soluble interleukin-2 receptors, and a cytokine profile suggesting the activation of precursor T-helper cells and type 1 T-helper cells have been found in adults with ITP. In these patients, T cells exposed to fragments of glycoprotein IIb/IIIa (but not native proteins) will stimulate antibody synthesis.[67]

Platelets coated with IgG autoantibodies are cleared by tissue macrophages, mainly in the spleen and liver (RES). Normally, there is a compensatory increase in platelet production, but in ITP platelet production may be impaired by the further destruction of intramedullary antibody-coated platelets. The result is a worsening thrombocytopenia.

DIAGNOSIS

ITP may have been previously diagnosed, but one-third of cases are diagnosed for the first time in pregnancy with routine testing of the blood count for anemia.[68]

The platelet count normally falls in pregnancy due to a hemodilutional effect and platelet consumption in the placenta. By delivery, 5.4–8.3% of healthy women are thrombocytopenic, based on ranges in non-pregnant populations, with counts of $<150 \times 10^9$/L. Gestational thrombocytopenia (GT) accounts for 75% of these cases, with only 3% due to ITP. Only 5% have platelet counts of $<100 \times 10^9$/L. Ranges of $109–341 \times 10^9$/L and $123–359 \times 10^9$/L have now been established for pregnancy in two different centers.[69,70]

The diagnosis of ITP is one of exclusion, as there is no reliable confirmatory test. Hence, when a low platelet count is incidentally discovered in pregnancy, other causes of thrombocytopenia must be excluded (Table 8.10). A blood film will pick up platelet clumps due to ethylenediaminetetraacetic acid (EDTA)-induced platelet aggregation, which occurs in 0.1% of adults. This spurious thrombocytopenia is confirmed by the finding of a normal platelet count when a repeat sample is taken in citrate.[71]

Differentiating ITP from GT in this context can be difficult. GT is a benign disorder where the platelet count falls as gestation advances, rarely falling to $<80 \times 10^9$/L. However, counts as low as 50×10^9/L have been reported. GT is common, has a favorable outcome, and has no association with maternal hemorrhage or fetal or neonatal thrombocytopenia.[72,73] Recognition may prevent unnecessary intervention. In GT, the platelet count is normal pre-pregnancy and normalizes again within

Table 8.10 Causes of thrombocytopenia in pregnancy

Primary causes	Secondary causes
Spurious: EDTA-induced platelet aggregation	Other autoimmune disorders: SLE, antiphospholipid syndrome (APS)
Gestational thrombocytopenia (GT)	Immunodeficiency states – IgA deficiency, common variable hypogammaglobulinemia
Pre-eclampsia and HELLP syndrome	Infection: HIV, hepatitis C, sepsis, malaria
Autoimmune: idiopathic (ITP)	Drugs, e.g. heparin, quinine, teicoplanin
Disseminated intravascular coagulation (DIC)	Lymphoproliferative disorders: acute/chronic leukemia, lymphoma
Folate deficiency	
Microangiopathic hemolytic processes: HUS/TTP	
Congenital platelet disorders: May–Hegglin anomaly	
Hypersplenism, e.g. malaria	
Myelodysplasia	

EDTA, ethylenediaminetetraacetic acid; ITP, idiopathic thrombocytopenic purpura; HUS/TTP, hemolytic-uremic syndrome/thrombotic thrombocytopenic purpura; SLE, systemic lupus erythematosus; IgA, immunoglobulin A; HIV, human immunodeficiency virus.

2–3 months of delivery. In ITP, the platelet count may be low pre-pregnancy. Also, an acute fall in platelets is unlikely to be GT. Testing for platelet autoantibodies is unhelpful. Increased levels of PAIgG can be detected in most patients with ITP but are not sufficiently sensitive or specific (estimated sensitivity 49–66%, estimated specificity 78–92%, estimated positive predictive value 80–83%) for diagnosis.[67] Additionally, these antibodies do not predict the likelihood of neonatal thrombocytopenia.

Assays for antibodies to specific platelet membrane glycoproteins IIb/IIIa and Ib/IX are less sensitive (50–65%), but more specific (90%) in ITP. These may be useful in women with a combination of bone marrow failure associated with ITP, ITP refractory to first- and second-line treatment, drug-dependent immune thrombocytopenia, and rare disorders such as monoclonal gammopathies and acquired autoantibody-mediated thrombasthenia.[66]

Bone marrow examination is not recommended in pregnancy unless lympho- or myeloproliferative disease is suspected.[73]

Occasionally, ITP presents for the first time in pregnancy with a severe thrombocytopenia. Symptomatic patients complain of mucocutaneous bleeding (bruising, petechiae, purpura, epistaxis, conjunctival hemorrhage, or bleeding gums) or of more severe bleeding (gastrointestinal, hematuria, or deep tissue bleeding). Table 8.11 shows the clinical findings related to the degree of thrombocytopenia.

EFFECTS OF PREGNANCY ON ITP

ITP in pregnancy results from adult chronic disease in 70% of women.[68] Such women can get an exacerbation in pregnancy, which may be due to the Th2 milieu. The greatest rate of decline and lowest platelet count occurs in the third trimester.[69] As explained above, ITP may occur de novo in pregnancy.

EFFECTS OF ITP ON PREGNANCY

In an 11-year retrospective study of 119 pregnancies in 92 women, Webert et al found that, in general, pregnancy was safe for both mother and fetus, although about one-third of the women required treatment for thrombocytopenia or bleeding.[68] Two-thirds of women had no symptoms, and only 3.4% had severe hemorrhage, including gastrointestinal bleeding, hematuria, and hematoma formation. Their platelet counts ranged from 3 to 117×10^9/L.

Delivery is the time of maximum concern for both the mother and thrombocytopenic fetus. The maternal risk revolves around postpartum hemorrhage and epidural use, and the fetal concern around intracranial hemorrhage secondary to a traumatic delivery. No antenatal measures reliably predict neonatal status, and maternal response to intervention does not guarantee a favorable neonatal outcome.[68,70,74,75] This may be because of different autoantibody specificities, as occurs in myasthenia gravis (see below). Only previous neonatal outcome provides a useful predictor of the neonatal platelet count in the subsequent pregnancy.[67,68] Identifying the fetus at risk of thrombocytopenia by fetal blood sampling, either antenatally with cordocentesis, or fetal scalp blood analysis during labor, is not recommended.[66,70] The risk of fetal death with cordocentesis, even in fetuses at low risk of bleeding, is 1–2%. This outweighs the risk of intracranial hemorrhage. Fetal scalp blood sampling (FBS) produces artificially low results as a result of clotting of blood with exposure of vernix or amniotic fluid, and can cause significant hemorrhage in an affected fetus. The positive predictive value of FBS to determine severe neonatal thrombocytopenia is only 50%.[75]

Recent studies have shown that the risk of maternal and fetal hemorrhage is not reduced with cesarean section compared with an uncomplicated vaginal delivery.[68,70,75] It is therefore recommended that cesarean section is only performed for obstetric reasons. Ventouse delivery should be avoided, but the use of outlet forceps should be considered if there is delay in the second stage.

With active management of the third stage using Syntocinon (oxytocin), there is seldom excessive bleeding from the placental bed. However, there is a real risk of bleeding from surgical incisions, soft-tissue injuries, or tears. An umbilical cord platelet count should be taken.

NEONATE

As a result of investigative and publication bias, it was initially considered that neonatal thrombocytopenia occurred in 52% of neonates, with significant morbidity in 12%. However, more recent studies show that 9% of neonates of mothers with presumed ITP have platelet counts of $<50 \times 10^9$/L and 4% have counts $<20 \times 10^9$/L.[76] In 710 neonates born to mothers with presumed ITP, the risk of

Table 8.11 Clinical consequences of thrombocytopenia

Platelet count ($\times 10^9$/L)	Clinical findings
<10	Internal bleeding
10–30	Spontaneous development of ecchymoses or petechiae
30–50	Excessive bruising with minor trauma
>50	Incidentally discovered

intracranial hemorrhage or other major bleeding complication is 1.1% (0–1.5%), which, although low, is higher than among infants of healthy mothers.[68,75] This risk will be enhanced if alloantibodies are present. There are no studies showing that this risk is reduced by cesarean section.[67]

The neonatal platelet count tends to worsen in the first few days of life, with the nadir on days 2–5 when the splenic circulation becomes established. This is when most hemorrhagic events occur in the neonate.

TREATMENT

Treatment is required in ITP if a patient is symptomatic or has an unacceptably low platelet count near delivery which would put her at risk of maternal hemorrhage (Table 8.12). The aim is to keep the platelets $>30 \times 10^9$/L throughout pregnancy and $>50 \times 10^9$/L near term. Treatment is unlikely to cause elevation of the fetal platelet count in an affected fetus.

Therapy for pregnant women with ITP is similar to that for non-pregnant patients, with the mainstay of treatment being either steroids or high-dose intravenous human IgG (IVIG), although there have been no randomized controlled trials comparing the two. Both are considered to be equally effective in improving the platelet count in patients with ITP. Anti-D has recently been used for treatment and has yielded promising results.

Table 8.12 Guide to treatment and delivery options with degree of thrombocytopenia

Platelet count $\times 10^9$/L	Action
<20	Treat
>20	Treat if symptomatic[73]
30	Possibly safe for vaginal delivery[77]
>50	Safe for vaginal delivery and cesarean section[73]
>80[a]	Considered safe for epidural

[a]Use of thrombelastography may help in future.

CORTICOSTEROIDS

Prednisolone is commenced at 1 mg/kg (prepregnancy weight) and reduced to the minimum dose, which maintains a platelet count $>50 \times 10^9$/L, or $>80 \times 10^9$/L if aiming to use a regional anesthetic.[69,73] Response rates are 50–75%, depending on the intensity and duration of treatment. Most responses occur within the first 3 weeks. The incidence of continuous remission varies from <5% to >30%.[67]

Alternatively, a low dose of prednisolone (e.g. 10 mg) could be commenced and increased gradually if necessary to achieve the desired platelet count. The advantages of this are that the total dose of steroid used will be less, although the time taken to achieve an acceptable count may be delayed. This option could be considered in a patient with a count between 20 and 50×10^9/L, with several weeks before delivery.

INTRAVENOUS MONOMERIC POLYVALENT HUMAN IMMUNOGLOBULIN

IVIG acts by blocking the Fc receptors of platelet autoantibodies.[78] The onset of action is quicker than with steroids and anti-D, with a satisfactory response occurring in 3 days of treatment. The response rate is 80% for 2–3 weeks. Hence, IVIG can be used if there are only a few days until delivery or if a high maintenance dose of steroids is required to achieve an acceptable platelet count.

Traditionally, 0.4 g/kg/day is administered for 5 days, although 1 g/kg over 8 hours, repeated after 2 days if there has been an inadequate response, has been used successfully and may be more convenient.[69] Also, 1 g/kg for 2–3 days has been used to treat internal bleeding when platelets are $<15 \times 10^9$/L despite treatment for several days with steroids or when progressive or extensive purpura present.

There is an infective risk with IVIG because of the use of pooled sera. Sustained remission is infrequent; therefore, repeated infusions may be required to maintain the platelet count.[67] Exogenous IgG may not cross the placenta, and hence will not have an effect on fetal platelets. The cost is considerably greater than with steroids. Renal failure and pulmonary insufficiency may occur, as may anaphylaxis in recipients who have congenital IgA deficiency. IVIG should be used discriminately and not in mild cases of ITP where the benefit is unproven.

ANTI-D IMMUNOGLOBULIN

Anti-D is a polyclonal antibody mainly of IgG subclasses I and III which binds to the D antigen on the surface of RBCs in rhesus-positive patients. Antibody-coated RBCs and platelets are cleared by the RES, but RBCs are preferentially destroyed compared with platelets.[78] The result is an increase in platelet numbers, as they have been spared destruction, and a mild hemolysis. Rhesus-negative patients do not respond, and splenectomized patients respond less well.

Anti-D is increasingly used for the treatment of ITP outside pregnancy in rhesus-positive patients. It is as effective as steroids in the treatment of ITP, and is less toxic, but more expensive. It is cheaper than IVIG and is derived from a smaller donor pool.[67] Conveniently, a single infusion of 75 µg/kg administered over 2–5 minutes resulted in a mean platelet increase of 46×10^9/L in 52 HIV-negative adults, which was higher when the hemoglobin concentration (Hb) was >12 g/dl. The effect lasts for more than 3 weeks in 50% of responders, with no difference in duration of response when comparing IVIG and anti-D.[78] In a smaller study of 13 HIV-negative patients, the median platelet increase was 43×10^9/L after 24 hours and 153×10^9/L after 1 week.[79] The dose of anti-D used is 10 times higher than used for prophylaxis against rhesus disease. These high doses lead to post-transfusion reactions in 3.2% (fever, chills, and headaches) and some degree of hemolysis.[78] Side effects can be limited by first administering acetaminophen and 20 mg prednisolone.[79] The mean Hb decrease from hemolysis is 0.8 g/dl.

The use of anti-D for treatment of ITP in pregnancy is limited by the fear of fetal or neonatal hemolysis. However, there was no fetal or neonatal hemolysis in a recent small study of 8 rhesus-positive pregnant women with ITP treated with anti-D during second and third trimesters.[80] The platelet response rate was 75% by 7 days post-transfusion, similar to 72% outside of pregnancy.[78] The median platelet increase was 54×10^9/L. However, two-thirds of responders required additional treatment (steroids/IVIG) to attain a platelet count adequate for delivery or epidural. Mild side effects occurred in 50% of patients and the Hb fell >2 g/dl in one patient.

SEVERE SYMPTOMATIC REFRACTORY ITP

When oral steroids or IVIG have not helped increase the platelet count, high-dose IV methylprednisolone (1 g) can be used in combination with IVIG. Azathioprine has also been used. Danazol, cyclophosphamide, and vinca alkaloids, which have been used outwith pregnancy, are teratogenic and hence avoided.

Splenectomy is now hardly ever indicated in the pregnant patient with ITP, but remains an option if all other attempts to increase the platelet count to safe levels fail. It is best carried out in the second trimester, because surgery is best tolerated then and the size of the uterus does not make the operation technically difficult.

Platelets should be available for transfusion at delivery if the patient still has severe thrombocytopenia, but should not be given prophylactically, as they will simply be destroyed.

MYASTHENIA GRAVIS

Myasthenia gravis (MG) is an autoimmune neuromuscular disorder that affects neuromuscular transmission, causing fatigable weakness of the skeletal muscles following repetitive activity. It results in ptosis, diplopia, difficulty speaking, and occasionally respiratory distress due to fatigue of the intercostal muscles.

INCIDENCE

MG is a rare condition that occurs twice as commonly in women as in men. Its onset is usually at less than 40 years of age, and hence it occurs during the childbearing age. The prevalence is 6.4 per 100 000 deliveries.[81]

INFLAMMATORY PATHOLOGY

Disease-specific serum IgG autoantibodies against the nicotinic acetylcholine receptors (anti-AChR Ab) at the motor endplate of striated muscle occur in 85% of MG patients.[82] These antibodies act by antibody-induced reduction of AChR numbers, complement-mediated damage to the postsynaptic membrane, and antibody blocking of AChRs.[82] The neuromuscular transmission of the action potential will therefore be disrupted, as the effect of acetylcholine released from the presynaptic membrane is blocked (Figure 8.5).

In the 15% of patients with clinical MG and no detectable antibody (seronegative MG), antibody directed to other neuromuscular junction targets is implicated, including the recently identified antibodies against MuSK (muscle-specific protein kinase), which is involved with anchoring and clustering of AChRs at the postsynaptic membrane.[82]

Antibodies can cross the placenta and cause neonatal myasthenia gravis (NMG). It is considered that NMG is due to the production of antifetal AChR Ab, which acts against one of the two different isoforms of the AChR, which are each made up of 5 subunits. The adult form is present in innervated muscle and has two α and one β, δ, and ε

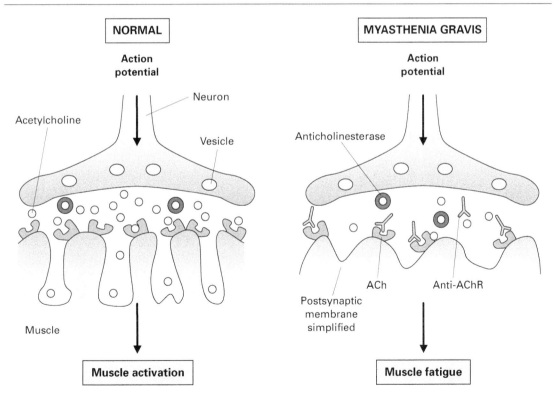

Figure 8.5 Schematic diagram of pathogenesis of myasthenia gravis.

subunits. In the fetal form present in immature or denervated muscle and in thymic myoid cells, the ε subunit is replaced by the γ subunit.[83,84] Patients form antibodies to both isoforms, but one may be more prevalent. Women with subclinical disease can have Ab fetal AChR, and hence have affected neonates.

The thymus gland is likely to be involved in the pathogenesis of MG.[82] It is abnormal in 75% of patients with MG: thymic hyperplasia in 85% and thymic tumors in 15% of the women. The thymus contains muscle-like myoid cells that express AChR. In MG, these are surrounded by activated T cells and germinal centers which are sites of B-cell memory generation. The thymic cells in myasthenics secrete anti-AChR antibodies.

The trigger for MG could be an alteration of the AChR autoantigen in the thymus, molecular mimicry with an immune response to an infectious agent that resembles the AChR, or fetal cell trafficking with the finding that fetal AChR antibodies are significantly more common in women presenting with MG after pregnancy compared with women presenting before pregnancy.[85]

Many patients respond to thymectomy, and 25% do not require further treatment. Previous thymectomy decreases the risk of pregnancy-associated complications.[86]

EFFECT OF PREGNANCY ON MG

> The course of myasthenia gravis during pregnancy is variable, unpredictable, and can change in subsequent pregnancies.

Exacerbations do not correlate with preconception disease activity.[86] There are only a few case series reported in the literature, none of which are controlled. In a total of 152 pregnancies in women with MG from four different case series, 50% were unchanged, 20% improved, and 30% were worse.[86–89] Exacerbations are not trimester-specific. Postpartum flares occur, with a rate of 28% in one recent study.[86]

Of those who are asymptomatic and not on treatment preconception, 17% relapse mildly in preg-

nancy, which is controlled with anticholinesterase (AChE) alone. Severe respiratory crisis can occur with relapse, requiring corticosteroids, azathioprine, plasmapharesis, IVIG, and sometimes intubation, which have all helped to reduce mortality. Puerperal infections can result in a severe deterioration and should be treated promptly.[87] The long-term outcome of MG is not worsened by pregnancy.[86]

EFFECT OF MG ON PREGNANCY

Analysis of a large patient cohort database in Norway with 127 pregnant myasthenics and 1.9 million controls has shown no increase in the rate of assisted vaginal delivery or postpartum hemorrhage in affected patients.[81] This is not surprising, as MG does not affect the smooth muscle of myometrium, and therefore contractions and uterine involution are not impaired. Interestingly, an increased cesarean section rate was observed, but these were mainly elective cesareans. Those women with preclinical MG or those in complete clinical remission of MG are more likely to have labor induced. This may explain why they have slower progress and protracted labors compared with controls. However, there is no increase in their assisted vaginal birth or cesarean section rate.[90]

There is an increased incidence of preterm rupture of membranes in myasthenics (5.5% vs 1.7%), but no increase in IUGR or preterm delivery.[81,86] The perinatal mortality rate (PNMR) is unaffected, but the death rate due to severe fetal anomalies is increased.[81,86] There is an increase in adverse perinatal outcome in those women with asymptomatic preclinical MG or those women in remission,[90] implicating the role of antifetal AChR antibody.

> Neonatal myasthenia gravis occurs in 6–30% of patients and is considered to be due to the passive transplacental transfer of fetal AChR antibodies.[86,87,89]

Studies are conflicting as to whether there is a correlation between the different types of anti-AChR Ab titer and disease. There is no association between maternal symptom severity and NMG.[90] There are two clinical forms of NMG:

1. *Typical transient NMG (TNMG)* (71%) presents with poor sucking and generalized hypotonia by 4 days of life. Respiratory distress is usually mild, but may be severe and life-threatening, requiring ventilation.[89] It usually lasts for 3 weeks, but occasionally persists for 4 months. It responds well to oral or parenteral AChE (see below). Alpha-fetoprotein (AFP) from the placenta has been shown to inhibit antibody binding to the fetal AChR, which may be why the fetus is unaffected and moves normally.[86] The occurrence of TNMG is not affected by the outcome of any previous pregnancy,[89] but in a woman in her first pregnancy it can be predicted by a high antifetal:antiadult AChR Ab ratio.[84]

2. *Atypical NMG: arthrogryposis multiplex congenital (AMC)* (29%) results from lack of fetal movement in utero and results in multiple congenital joint contractures and polyhydramnios. In MG it is thought that AMC is due to selective antibody-mediated inhibition of particular functional epitopes on the fetal AChR – different from those in TNMG – which when blocked can cause fetal paralysis.[83] Fetal and neonatal death is common. This form of NMG is associated with pulmonary hypoplasia and other fetal anomalies that can be severe and involve different organs; this may be due to antibody reacting with other fetal antigens, causing systemic anomalies unrelated to lack of fetal movement. Mothers may be symptomatic or asymptomatic (preclinical or in remission).[81,90] There is a high recurrence risk (up to 100%) of fetal deformities. It is potentially treatable with extensive plasma exchange.[83]

Breast-feeding should be avoided in mothers with babies who have NMG, as the harmful anti-AChR antibodies are present in breast milk.

TREATMENT

Anticholinesterase inhibitor drugs such as pyridostigmine prevent the breakdown of acetylcholine and can be safely continued in pregnancy. Higher doses may be required as the pregnancy advances.

Parenteral administration is best during labor. Rather than administering large doses, which can cause gastrointestinal upset in breast-fed newborns, shorter dose intervals should be used.[86]

Second-line drugs include corticosteroids, azathioprine, and sometimes cyclosporin A (cyclosporine) (see Table 8.1). Cyclosporin A (cyclosporine) is used in transplant patients from whom most of the safety data are derived. It may be associated with spontaneous abortion, prematurity, and IUGR. Withdrawal of these agents may lead to a life-threatening exacerbation. Serial plasmapheresis, which results in removal of autoantibodies, and high-dose IVIG have been successfully used for myasthenic crises in pregnancy and to prevent neonatal death.[86]

Magnesium sulfate for seizure prophylaxis or treatment in pre-eclampsia is contraindicated, as it can precipitate a myasthenic crisis. Narcotics should be used with caution, as they can reduce respiratory drive. Regional analgesia is safe.

REFERENCES

1. Silman AJ, Pearson JE. Epidemiology and genetics of rheumatoid arthritis. Arthritis Res 2002; 4 (suppl 3):S265–S272.
2. Bläß S, Engel JM, Burmester GR. The immunologic homunculus in rheumatoid arthritis. Arthritis Rheum 1999; 42:2499–2506.
3. Wood AJ. New drugs for rheumatoid arthritis. N Engl J Med 2004; 350:2167–2179
4. Choy EH, Panayi GS. Cytokine pathways and joint inflammation in rheumatoid arthritis. N Engl J Med 2001; 344:907–916.
5. Dorner T, Egerer K, Feist E, Burmester GR. Rheumatoid factor revisited. Curr Opin Rheumatol 2004; 16:246–253.
6. Barrett JH, Brennan P, Fiddler M et al. Does rheumatoid arthritis remit during pregnancy and relapse postpartum? Results from a nationwide study in the United Kingdom performed prospectively from late pregnancy. Arthritis Rheum 1999; 42:1219–1227.
7. Hench AB. The ameliorating effect of pregnancy on chronic atrophic (infectious rheumatoid) arthritis; fibrositis and intermittent hydrothosis. Proc Mayo Clinic 1938; 13:161.
8. Nelson JL, Hughes KA, Smith AG et al. Maternal–fetal disparity in HLA class II alloantigens and the pregnancy-induced amelioration of rheumatoid arthritis. N Engl J Med 1993; 329:466–471.
9. Unger A, Kay A, Griffin AJ, Panayi G. Disease activity and pregnancy associated alpha 2-glycoprotein in rheumatoid arthritis during pregnancy. Br Med J (Clin Res Ed) 1983; 286:750–752.
10. Nelson-Piercy C, Khamashta MA. Autoimmune rheumatic disorders and vasculitis in pregnancy. In: Warrell DA, Cox TM, Firth JD, Benz EJ, eds. Oxford Textbook of Medicine, 4th edn. Oxford: Oxford University Press; 2003.
11. Gill TJ. Maternal–fetal interactions and disease. N Engl J Med 1993; 329:500–501.

12. Østensen M, Fuhrer L, Mathieu R et al. A prospective study of pregnant patients with rheumatoid arthritis and ankylosing spondylitis using validated clinical instruments. Ann Rheum Dis 2004; 63: 1212–1217.

13. Van Dunne FM, Lard LR, Rook D et al. Miscarriage but not fecundity is associated with progression of joint destruction in rheumatoid arthritis. Ann Rheum Dis 2004; 63:956–960.

14. Pope JE, Bellamy N, Stevens A. The lack of associations between rheumatoid arthritis and both nulliparity and infertility. Semin Arthritis Rheum 1999; 28:342–350.

15. Steen VD, Medsger TA. Fertility and pregnancy outcome in women with systemic sclerosis. Arthritis Rheum 1999; 42:763–768.

16. Skomsvoll JF, Østensen M, Irgens LM et al. Pregnancy complications and delivery practice in women with connective tissue disease and inflammatory rheumatic disease in Norway. Acta Obstet Gynecol Scand 2000; 79:490–495.

17. Janssen NM, Genta MS. The effects of immunosuppressive and anti-inflammatory medications on fertility, pregnancy and lactation. Arch Intern Med 2000; 160:610–619.

18. Ericson A, Källén BAJ. Nonsteroidal anti-inflammatory drugs in early pregnancy. Reprod Toxicol 2001; 15:371–375.

19. Nielsen GL, Sørensen HT, Larsen H, Pedersen L. Risk of adverse birth outcome and miscarriage in pregnant users of non-steroidal anti-inflammatory drugs: population-based observational study and case-control study. BMJ 2001; 322:266–270.

20. Stone S, Khamashta MA, Nelson-Piercy C. Nonsteroidal anti-inflammatory drugs and reversible female infertility: is there a link? Drug Safety 2002; 25:545–551.

21. Anon. Taking stock of coxibs. Drug Ther Bull 2005; 43: 1–6.

22. Fraser FC, Sajoo A. Teratogenic potential of corticosteroids in humans. Teratology 1995; 51:45–46.

23. Park-Wyllie L, Mazzotta P, Pastuszak A et al. Birth defects after maternal exposure to corticosteroids: prospective cohort study and meta-analysis of epidemiological studies. Teratology 2000; 62:385–392.

24. Gur C, Diav-Citrin O, Shechtman S et al. Pregnancy outcome after first trimester exposure to corticosteroids: a prospective controlled study. Reprod Toxicol 2004; 18:93–101.

25. Pradat P, Robert-Gnansia E, Di Tanna GL et al. First trimester exposure to corticosteroids and oral clefts. Birth Defects Res A Clin Mol Teratol 2003; 67:968–970.

26. Costedoat-Chalumeau N, Amoura Z, Duhaut P et al. Safety of hydroxychloroquine in pregnant patients with connective tissue diseases. Arthritis Rheum 2003; 48:3207–3211.

27. Coulam CB, Zincke H, Strioff S. Pregnancy after renal transplantation: estrogen secretion. Transplantation 1982; 33:556–558.

28. Katz JA, Antoni C, Keenan GF et al. Outcome of pregnancy in women receiving infliximab for the treatment of Crohn's disease and rheumatoid arthritis. Am J Gastroenterol 2004; 99:2385–2392.

29. Hochberg MC. Updating the American College of Rheumatology revised criteria for the classification of systemic lupus erythematosus. Arthritis Rheum 1997; 40:1725.

30. Johnson AE, Gordon C, Palmer RG, Bacon PA. The prevalence and incidence of systemic lupus erythematosus in Birmingham, England. Relationship to ethnicity and country of birth. Arthritis Rheum 1995; 38:551–558.

31. Rahman A, Isenberg D. Systemic lupus erythematosus and related disorders. In: Warrell DA, Cox TM, Firth JD, Benz EJ, eds. Oxford Textbook of Medicine, 4th edn. Oxford: Oxford University Press; 2003.

32. Cortés-Hernández J, Ordi-Ros J, Paredes F et al. Clinical predictors of fetal and maternal outcome in systemic lupus erythematosus: a prospective study of 103 pregnancies. Rheumatology 2002; 41: 643–650.

33. Cervera R, Font J, Carmona F et al. Pregnancy outcome in systemic lupus erythematosus: good news for the new millennium. Autoimmun Rev 2002; 1:354–359.

34. Lima F, Buchanan NMM, Khamashta MA et al. Obstetric outcome in systemic lupus erythematosus. Semin Arthritis Rheum 1995; 25:184–192.

35. Tandon A, Ibañez D, Gladman DD et al. The effect of pregnancy on lupus nephritis. Arthritis Rheum 2004; 50:3941–3946.

36. Georgiou PE, Politi EN, Sakka V et al. Outcome of lupus pregnancy: a controlled study. Rheumatology 2000; 39:1014–1019.

37. Lê Thi Huong DL, Wechsler B, Vauthier-Brouzes D et al. Outcome of planned pregnancies in systemic lupus erythematosus: a prospective study on 62 pregnancies. Br J Rheumatol 1997; 36:772–777.

38. Carmona F, Font J, Cervera R et al. Obstetrical outcome of pregnancy in patients with systemic lupus erythematosus. A study of 60 cases. Eur J Obstet Gynecol Reprod Biol 1999; 83:137–142.

39. Doria A, Ghirardello A, Iaccarino L et al. Pregnancy, cytokines, and disease activity in systemic lupus erythematosus. Arthritis Rheum 2004; 51:989–995.

40. de Swiet M. Antiphospholipid syndrome, systemic lupus erythematosus and other connective tissue diseases. In: de Swiet M, eds. Medical Disorders in Obstetric Practice 4th edn. Oxford: Blackwell Science; 2002: 267–281.

41. Clark CA, Spitzer KA, Nadler JN et al. Preterm deliveries in women with systemic lupus erythematosus. J Rheumatol 2003; 30:2127–2132.

42. Mok MY, Leung PY, Lao TH et al. Clinical predictors of fetal and maternal outcome in Chinese patients with systemic lupus erythematosus. Ann Rheum Dis 2004; 63:1705–1706.

43. Rahman FZ, Rahman J, Al-Suleiman SA, Rahman MS. Pregnancy outcome in lupus nephropathy. Arch Gynecol Obstet 2005; 271: 222–226.

44. Le Thi Huong D, Wechsler B, Vauthier-Brouzes D et al. Pregnancy in past or present lupus nephritis: a study of 32 pregnancies from a single centre. Ann Rheum Dis 2001; 60:599–604.

45. Moroni G, Quaglini S, Caloni M et al. Pregnancy in lupus nephritis. Am J Kidney Dis 2002; 40:713–720.

46. Lockshin MD, Erkan D. Treatment of the antiphospholipid syndrome. N Engl J Med 2003; 349:1177–1179.

47. Petri M. Hopkins Lupus Pregnancy Center: 1987 to 1996. Rheum Dis Clin North Am 1997; 23:1–13.

48. Lockshin MD, Sammaritano LR. Rheumatic disease. In: Barron WM, Lindheimer MD, eds. Medical Disorders During Pregnancy, 3rd edn. St Louis: Mosby; 2000: 355–391.

49. Cimaz R, Spence DL, Hornberger L, Silverman ED. Incidence and spectrum of neonatal lupus erythematosus: a prospective study of infants born to mothers with anti-Ro antibodies. J Pediatr 2003; 142:678–683.

50. Brucato A, Frassi M, Franceschini F et al. Risk of congenital complete heart block in newborns of mothers with anti-Ro/SSA antibodies detected by counterimmunoelectrophoresis: a prospective study of 100 women. Arthritis Rheum 2001; 44:1832–1835.

51. Kaaja R, Julkunen H. Prevention of recurrence of congenital heart block with intravenous immunoglobulin and corticosteroid therapy: comment on the editorial by Buyon et al. Arthritis Rheum 2003; 48:280–281.

52. Stevens AM, Hermes HM, Rutledge JC et al. Myocardial-tissue-specific phenotype of maternal microchimerism in neonatal lupus congenital heart block. Lancet 2003; 362:1617–1623.

53. Lambe M, Björnådal L, Neregård P et al. Childbearing and the risk of scleroderma: a population-based study in Sweden. Am J Epidemiol 2004; 159:162–166.

54. Steen VD. Pregnancy in women with systemic sclerosis. Obstet Gynecol 1999; 94:15–20.

55. Ariga H, Ohto H, Busch MP et al. Kinetics of fetal cellular and cell-free DNA in the maternal circulation during and after pregnancy: implications for noninvasive prenatal diagnosis. Transfusion 2001; 41:1524–1530.

56. Bianchi DW, Zickwolf GK, Weil GJ et al. Male progenitor cells persist in maternal blood for as long as 27 years postpartum. Proc Natl Acad Sci USA 1996; 93:705–708.

57. Artlett CM, Miller FW, Rider LG. Persistent maternally derived peripheral microchimerism is associated with the juvenile idiopathic inflammatory myopathies. Rheumatology (Oxford) 2001; 40:1279–1284.

58. Nelson JL, Furst DE, Maloney S et al. Microchimerism and HLA-compatible relationships of pregnancy in scleroderma. Lancet 1998; 351:559–562.

59. Artlett CM, Smith JB, Jimenez SA. Identification of fetal DNA and cells in skin lesions from women with systemic sclerosis. N Engl J Med 1998; 338:1186–1191.

60. Scaletti C, Vultaggio A, Bonifacio S et al. Th2-orientated profile of male offspring T cells present in women with systemic sclerosis and reactive with maternal major histocompatibility complex antigens. Arthritis Rheum 2002; 46:445–450.

61. Artlett CM, Rasheed M, Russo-Stieglitz KE et al. Influence of prior pregnancies on disease course and cause of death in systemic sclerosis. Ann Rheum Dis 2002; 61:346–350.

62. Pisa FE, Bovenzi M, Romeo L et al. Reproductive factors and the risk of scleroderma: an Italian case–control study. Arthritis Rheum 2002; 46:451–456.

63. Steen VD, Medsger TA. Case–control study of corticosteroids and other drugs that either precipitate or protect from the development of scleroderma renal crisis. Arthritis Rheum 1998; 41: 1613–1619.

64. Steen VD, Conte C, Day N et al. Pregnancy in women with systemic sclerosis. Arthritis Rheum 1989; 32:151–157.

65. Steen VD. Pregnancy in systemic sclerosis. Scand J Rheumatol 1998; 27 (Suppl 107): 72–75.

66. British Committee for Standards in Haematology, General Haematology Task Force. Guidelines for the investigation and management of idiopathic thrombocytopenic purpura in adults, children and in pregnancy. Br J Haematol 2003; 120:574–596.

67. Cines DB, Blanchette VS. Immune thrombocytopenic purpura. N Engl J Med 2002; 346:995–1008.

68. Webert KE, Mittal R, Sigouin C et al. A retrospective 11-year analysis of obstetric patients with idiopathic thrombocytopenic purpura. Blood 2003; 102:4306–4311.

69. Burrows RF, Kelton JG. Incidentally detected thrombocytopenia in healthy mothers and their infants. N Engl J Med 1988; 319: 142–145.

70. Sainio S, Kekomäki R, Riikonen S, Teramo K. Maternal thrombocytopenia at term: a population-based study. Acta Obstet Gynecol Scand 2000; 79:744–749.

71. Pegels JG, Bruynes EC, von Engelfriet CP, dem Borne AE. Pseudothrombocytopenia: an immunologic study on platelet antibodies dependent on ethylene diamine tetra-acetate. Blood 1982; 59:157–161.

72. Aster RH. Gestational thrombocytopenia: a plea for conservative management. N Engl J Med 1990; 323:264–266.

73. Letsky EA, Greaves M. Guidelines on the investigation and management of thrombocytopenia in pregnancy and neonatal alloimmune thrombocytopenia. Br J Haematol 1996; 95:21–26.

74. Fujimura K, Harada Y, Fujimoto T et al. Nationwide study of idiopathic thrombocytopenic purpura in pregnant women and the clinical influence on neonates. Int J Hematol 2002; 75:426–433.

75. Payne SD, Resnik R, Moore TR et al. Maternal characteristics and risk of severe neonatal thrombocytopenia and intracranial hemorrhage in pregnancies complicated by autoimmune thrombocytopenia. Am J Obstet Gynecol 1997; 177:149–155.

76. Gill KK, Kelton JG. Management of idiopathic thrombocytopenic purpura in pregnancy. Semin Hematol 2000; 37:275–289.

77. Lichtin A. The ITP practice guideline: what, why, and for whom? Blood 1996; 88:1–2.

78. Scaradavou A, Woo B, Woloski BMR et al. Intravenous anti-D treatment of immune thrombocytopenic purpura: experience in 272 patients. Blood 1997; 89:2689–2700.

79. Newman GC, Novoa MV, Fodero EM et al. A dose of 75 µg/kg/d of i.v. anti-D increases the platelet count more rapidly and for a longer period of time than 50 µg/kg/d in adults with immune thrombocytopenic purpura. Br J Haematol 2001; 112:1076–1078.

80. Michel M, Novoa MV, Bussel JB. Intravenous anti-D as a treatment for immune thrombocytopenic purpura (ITP) during pregnancy. Br J Haematol 2003; 123:142–146.

81. Hoff JM, Daltveit AK, Gilhus NE. Myasthenia gravis: consequences for pregnancy, delivery, and the newborn. Neurology 2003; 61: 1362–1366.

82. Thanvi BR, Lo TCN. Update on myasthenia gravis. Postgrad Med J 2004; 80:690–700.

83. Polizzi A, Huson SM, Vincent A. Teratogen update: maternal myasthenia gravis as a cause of congenital arthrogryphosis. Teratology 2000; 62:332–341.

84. Gardnerova M, Eymard B, Morel E et al. The fetal/adult acetylcholine receptor antibody ratio in mothers with myasthenia gravis as a marker for transfer of the disease to the newborn. Neurology 1997; 48:50–54.

85. Matthews I, Sims G, Ledwidge S et al. Antibodies to acetylcholine receptor in parous women with myasthenia: evidence for immunization by fetal antigen. Lab Invest 2002; 82:1407–1417.

86. Batocchi AP, Majolini L, Evoli A et al. Course and treatment of myasthenia gravis during pregnancy. Neurology 1999; 52:447–452.

87. Djelmis J, Sostarko M, Mayer D, Ivanisevic M. Myasthenia gravis in pregnancy: report on 69 cases. Eur J Obstet Gynecol Reprod Biol 2002; 104:21–25.

88. Mitchell PJ, Bebbington M. Myasthenia gravis in pregnancy. Obstet Gynecol 1992; 80:178–181.

89. Téllez-Zenteno JF, Hernández-Ronquillo L, Salinas V, Estanol B, da Silva O. Myasthenia gravis and pregnancy: clinical implications and neonatal outcome. BMC Musculoskelet Disord 2004; 5:42.

90. Hoff JM, Daltveit AK, Gilhus NE. Asymptomatic myasthenis gravis influences pregnancy and birth. Eur J Neurol 2004; 11:559–562.

9. Pre-eclampsia and the systemic inflammatory response

Chris WG Redman and Ian L Sargent

PRE-ECLAMPSIA IS A TWO-STAGE DISORDER WITH MATERNAL AND FETAL COMPONENTS

Pre-eclampsia is a potentially dangerous and highly variable complication of the second half of pregnancy, labor, or the early puerperium. It causes many signs that reflect pansystemic disturbances but few symptoms, which are suffered late in its evolution. It is neither predictable nor preventable and, to date, its precise cause or causes are unknown. The simple signs that are used for clinical screening are new hypertension and proteinuria, both regressing after delivery. These signs are components of all current definitions but derive from consensus not an understanding of the pathogenesis of pre-eclampsia. There is no specific diagnostic feature that on its own allows unequivocal recognition. The disorder is a syndrome, a cluster of signs, all of which, in isolation, could have other causes.

It has been known for nearly 100 years that pre-eclampsia originates in the placenta. The presence of a placenta is both necessary and sufficient to cause the disorder.[1] A fetus is not required, as pre-eclampsia can occur with hydatidiform mole, a complication of pregnancy characterized by dysregulated trophoblast proliferation without a fetus. A uterus is probably not required, because pre-eclampsia may develop with abdominal pregnancy where the placenta implants in the peritoneum.[2] Delivery removes the causative organ, namely the placenta, and cures the condition.

Although pre-eclampsia is a placental disorder, the placenta does not have to be abnormal for a pregnant woman to suffer pre-eclampsia. The disease constitutes a spectrum of what is called maternal and placental pre-eclampsia:[3] with placental pre-eclampsia, there is an abnormal placenta in a normal woman; with maternal pre-eclampsia, there is a normal placenta within an abnormal woman, suffering some sort of long-term problem. In practice, many presentations are a mixture of both types in varying degrees.

The placental problem is hypoxia secondary to a poor uteroplacental supply. This fails because of events in the first half of pregnancy, which in essence comprise poor growth and development of the early placenta. This is called poor placentation. The maternal problem comprises the sequelae of a systemic inflammatory response, involving the entire inflammatory network of the circulation, including the endothelium. Whereas the first stage is difficult or impossible to detect clinically, the second stage is the clinical sydrome. The sequence of events has been highlighted by the two-stage hypothesis for pre-eclampsia.[1]

INNATE AND ADAPTIVE IMMUNITY

Inflammatory responses evolved before the adaptive immune responses. The latter is present only in vertebrates and is an evolutionary and functional elaboration of the former. The more primitive innate (inflammatory) system responds quickly and is relatively non-specific. The adaptive immune system develops slowly but has a precise action that delivers antigen-specific responses with immunological 'memory'. The innate and adaptive systems are asymmetrically interdependent. The innate system does not need the adaptive system to function, whereas the adaptive system cannot function without signals from the innate system. This is important in relation to this chapter. A systemic inflammatory response is not necessarily generated by antigen-specific stimulation. In relation to normal and abnormal pregnancy it may not result, indeed almost certainly does not result, from antigenic stimulation by the genetically foreign fetus.

The adaptive immune system distinguishes self from non-self antigens and responds to the latter. The innate immune system reacts, more widely, to 'danger'[4] using a range of 'pattern recognition receptors' that have evolved to respond in a broad but stereotyped way. The danger signal may be external (from pathogens) or internal (from products of trauma, ischemia, necrosis, or oxidative stress that reflect damage). When inflammatory cells are activated they release signals such as cytokines or chemokines that, in turn, attract and 'instruct' adaptive immune cells (T or B lymphocytes) to generate antigen-specific responses from antibodies or cytotoxic cells. Hence the two systems, innate and adaptive, operate together and in sequence.

In this chapter the inflammatory system is considered to be the sum of events involving innate rather than adaptive immune changes. The two stages of pre-eclampsia involve the innate immune system in different ways: in the first stage, there is an important element localized to the placental bed; in the second stage, a diffuse systemic response predominates.

During placentation, natural killer (NK) cells play an important role in the decidua, where they are a prominent part of a decidual inflammatory response (although they are lymphocytes, they belong to the innate immune system). Decidual NK cells are a specialized subset of NK cells already present preconceptually in the endometrium of the luteal phase. They are considered to facilitate placentation by secreting cytokines that promote infiltration of the spiral arteries by invasive trophoblast. The nature of these interactions and their genetic control are described elsewhere in this book. In this chapter only systemic inflammatory responses will be described.

SYSTEMIC INFLAMMATORY RESPONSES

A systemic inflammatory response (SIR) differs markedly from local inflammatory responses, which are confined to one position in tissues. The response is diffuse, involving all cells and protein systems within blood and, by secondary extension, affects inflammatory networks outside the circulation in target organs.

The primary inflammatory cells are the phagocytes (granulocytes, monocytes) and NK cells, but an SIR also involves endothelial cells, which become diffusely activated. Such cells can produce a range of proinflammatory cytokines, can stimulate, as well as be stimulated by, inflammatory leukocytes, and can present antigen to T cells after appropriate stimulation. Platelets and a variety of humoral components also participate (Table 9.1). Other cells in tissues, such as hepatocytes and adipocytes, which are not normally considered to be inflammatory, have central roles (see below). The SIR is therefore not simple. It contains complex cross-regulating and synergistic pathways that are incompletely understood. This inflammatory network has a wider range than may be appreciated, and many two-way interactions between its components. For example, blood coagulation is not only activated by inflammatory processes but also thrombin, the final trigger to coagulation, also stimulates inflammation via specific receptors.

Table 9.1 Components of the inflammatory or innate immune system

Inflammatory leukocytes:

- Granulocytes
- Monocytes
- Natural killer lymphocytes
- Certain B cells producing 'natural antibodies'

Endothelium
Platelets
Coagulation cascade
Complement system
Cytokines and chemokines
Adipocytes
Hepatocytes

SYSTEMIC INFLAMMATION AND OXIDATIVE STRESS

Oxidative stress is a dysequilibrium between anti-oxidant defenses and production of reactive oxygen species in favor of the latter. Reactive oxygen species are toxic because they trigger chain reactions with several cell components – including lipids, DNA, and proteins – that lead to a loss of cell integrity, enzyme function, and genomic stability. Natural antioxidant mechanisms have evolved to limit oxidative damage. The process is discussed in extended detail elsewhere in this book.

The key feature, which is central to this chapter, is that oxidative stress and chronic inflammation are related, perhaps inseparable, phenomena.[5] An inflammatory response generates oxidative stress – e.g. the respiratory burst of activated immune phagocytes – that releases reactive oxygen intermediates into the microenvironment. In a converse fashion, oxidative stress from other causes stimulates an inflammatory response. The products of oxidative stress, such as lipid peroxides, are intrinsically proinflammatory.

METABOLISM AND THE SYSTEMIC INFLAMMATORY RESPONSE

Systemic inflammation has complex effects on metabolism, of which many are stimulated by components of the acute phase response. Inflammatory responses, stimulated by endotoxin, tumor necrosis factor-α (TNF-α), or other proinflammatory factors, cause insulin resistance and hyperlipidemia. The hyperlipidemia of sepsis has been known for many years (see review[6]). The inflammatory cytokine TNF-α is an important mediator of these changes because it induces insulin resistance and inhibits lipogenesis while increasing lipolysis.[7] It inhibits proximal steps of insulin signaling in varying ways, depending on cell type. Increased release of free fatty acids (FFAs) contributes also to insulin resistance peripherally (see review[8]).

Obesity is associated with an SIR. A cluster of clinical features, including obesity, is variously called the metabolic syndrome, syndrome X, or the insulin resistance syndrome (see review[9]). Components of the syndrome include insulin resistance, impaired glucose tolerance or overt diabetes, dyslipidemia, and hypertension. The syndrome arises because adipose tissue is not merely an energy store but a source of proinflammatory cytokines and other metabolic mediators, including TNF-α, interleukin-6 (IL-6), leptin, a hormone that regulates appetite and energy expenditure, and plasminogen activator-1 (PAI-1). Thus, body mass index (BMI) is significantly correlated with circulating leptin, TNF-α, and IL-6 in humans.[10] Leptin has proinflammatory actions[11] as does TNF-α. The net effect is that obesity is a state of chronic systemic inflammation. IL-6 induces the acute phase response,[12] so that elevated C-reactive protein (CRP) is a typical feature of the metabolic syndrome, but other acute phase reactants such as plasma fibrinogen are similarly increased.

Systemic inflammation is accompanied by an increase in triglyceride-rich lipoproteins, a reduction in high-density lipoprotein (HDL) cholesterol, and impairment of cholesterol transport. These metabolic alterations, which promote atherosclerosis, may explain an epidemiological link between chronic inflammation and cardiovascular disease.[13]

SYSTEMIC INFLAMMATION AND THE ACUTE PHASE RESPONSE

The complete range of events stimulated by systemic inflammation is termed the acute phase response. The term is misleading because it also includes chronic changes. The response is not identical under all situations. It comprises alterations in circulating plasma protein proteins as well as fever, anemia, leukocytosis, and metabolic adaptations, especially involving the liver and adipose tissue (summarized elsewhere[14]). Proteins linked to the acute phase response, known as acute phase proteins, are typically synthesized in the liver: they are classified as positive if they increase with systemic inflammation (CRP is the best known) or negative if they decrease with systemic inflammation (e.g. albumin).

CRP is the classical acute phase reactant. Circulating concentrations can increase within hours by several orders of magnitude in response to inflammatory stimuli. Human CRP binds with highest affinity to phosphocholine residues, but also to a variety of other intrinsic and extrinsic ligands, including damaged cell membranes. Extrinsic factors that bind to CRP include constituents of microorganisms. It functions as a typical component of the innate immune system, acting as a scavenger protein and responding to a range of 'dangerous' molecules.[15] Some acute phase proteins are listed in Table 9.2.

SYSTEMIC INFLAMMATORY RESPONSE AND PREGNANCY

Even normal pregnancy is characterized by a mild SIR, which is apparent before implantation in the luteal phase of the menstrual cycle, as shown in several papers, e.g. Sacks et al.[16] Its activity increases as pregnancy advances. In pre-eclampsia the response is more intense but, in general, does not differ in type but only in degree.[17]

In normal pregnancy the mild changes do not indicate that pregnant women are ill. Many features of pregnancy that are considered to be physiological are indicators of the associated acute phase response, and include reduced plasma albumin,[18] and increases in plasma fibrinogen,[19] PAI-1,[20] ceruloplasmin,[21] and many other compounds. The intensity of such features increases modestly as normal gestation advances. CRP, the classical acute phase reactant, has not been studied in detail during pregnancy. What little evidence there is points to a significant but small increase in the circulation, which begins in the first trimester.[16]

Leukocytosis is already evident in the first trimester[22] (see Table 9.3), and increases as pregnancy advances and the cells appear to be activated.[23] Phagocytosis[24] and the chemiluminescent responses of polymorphonuclear leukocytes (PMNs) after stimulation with serum-opsonized zymosan are increased.[25] Circulating soluble neutrophil elastase concentrations are an indirect index

Table 9.2 Changes in concentrations of plasma proteins in the acute phase response

Type of protein	Example
Proteins whose plasma concentrations increase – positive acute phase reactants	
Proteinase inhibitors	α_1-Antitrypsin
	α_1-Antichymotrypsin
Coagulation proteins	Fibrinogen
	Prothrombin
	Factor VIII
	Plasminogen
	Plasminogen activator inhibitor-1
Complement proteins	Complement 1s
	Complement 2
	Factor B
	Complement 3, 4, 5
	Mannose-binding lectin
Transport proteins	Haptoglobin
	Hemopexin
	Ceruloplasmin
Participants in inflammatory responses	Soluble phospholipase A_2
	Interleukin-1 receptor antagonist
	Lipopolysaccharide-binding protein
Miscellaneous	C-reactive protein
	Serum amyloid A
	Fibronectin
	Ferritin
	α1-Acid glycoprotein
Proteins whose plasma concentrations decrease – negative acute phase reactants	
Miscellaneous	Albumin
	Transferrin
	Insulin-like growth factor 1
	Transthyretin
	High-density lipoproteins
	Low-density lipoproteins

of neutrophil activation and are significantly higher in normal pregnancy than in non-pregnant women.[26] However, not all investigators agree that granulocytes are activated, with contrary findings in normal pregnancy, as reported by Beilin et al[27] and others. The reasons for these discrepancies are not clear.

Monocytes also show evidence of activation in terms of a monocytosis,[22] activation of phagocytic activity,[28] and priming[29] (Figure 9.1). Hence, the

Table 9.3 The systemic inflammatory network is stimulated in pre-eclampsia relative to normal pregnancy

Part of network affected	Reference
Leukocytosis[a]	Terrone et al[58]
Increased leukocyte activation[a]	Sacks et al[29]
(Complement activation[a,b]	Haeger et al[59]
Activation of the clotting system[a]	Perry and Martin[60]
Activation of platelets[a]	Konijnenborg et al[61]
Markers of endothelial activation[a]	Taylor et al[62]
Markers of oxidative stress[a]	Gratacos et al[63]
Hypertriglyceridemia[a]	Hubel[55]
Increased circulating proinflammatory cytokines:	
Tumour necrosis factor-α[a]	Vince et al[64]
Interleukin-6[a]	Greer et al[5]
Interleukin-8[a,b]	Stallmach et al[66]

[a] Significant change(s) relative to normal non-pregnant women.
[b] Not all authors agree, see text.
There are usually multiple references to justify each change.

weight of evidence is overwhelmingly in favor of systemic leukocyte priming or activation during normal pregnancy.

As pregnancy advances, the SIR strengthens and peaks during the third trimester. But it was not until the late 1990s that the concept of systemic activation was formally consolidated using flow cytometric examination of fresh unstimulated leukocytes.[17,30]

Measurements of more comprehensive inflammatory markers of circulating leukocytes showed that activation during pregnancy extends to lymphocytes and monocytes, as well as granulocytes.[30] Other evidence for a pregnancy-induced SIR comes from measuring circulating inflammatory cytokines. Because TNF-α, a classical inflammatory cytokine, has a short half-life in the circulation, levels of its circulating soluble receptors are sometimes used as surrogate markers of higher average circulating levels.[31] By this indirect measure,[32] or by direct assay, circulating TNF-α is increased in normal pregnancy.[33] Plasma IL-6 is similarly increased.[34] In sum, normal pregnancy can be viewed as a state of mild systemic inflammation complete with evidence for an acute phase reaction and activation of multiple components of the inflammatory network.

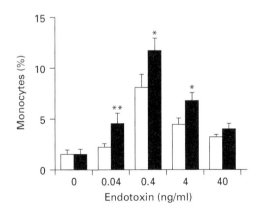
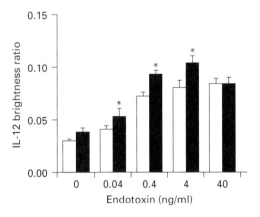

Figure 9.1 Monocytes are primed to respond to an inflammatory stimulus in pregnancy compared with non-pregnancy. The responses in terms of intracellular production of interleukin-12 (IL-12) have been measured by flow cytometry in two ways: first, by the proportion of positively labeled monocytes (left); secondly, by the intensity of the labeling (right). Samples from healthy pregnant women in the third trimester ($n = 12$, black columns) were compared with samples from non-pregnant women of childbearing age ($n = 12$, open columns). (Reproduced with permission from Sacks et al.[29])

METABOLIC CHANGES AND THE INFLAMMATORY RESPONSE IN NORMAL PREGNANCY

The metabolic adaptations of systemic inflammation – namely an acute phase response (as discussed above), oxidative stress, hyperlipidaemia, and increased insulin resistance – also occur during normal pregnancy.

Circulating markers of oxidative stress are increased at least in the third trimester.[35] In normal pregnancy, insulin resistance develops early and persists until delivery. The major change is between 16 and 26 weeks of gestation.[36] Hypertriglyceridemia, as occurs in systemic inflammation also, becomes detectable in the second trimester.[37] The cause of the insulin resistance is undecided. There are potential secreted placental factors, such as human placental growth hormone[38] and the adipokine resistin,[39] which cause insulin resistance. The fact that inflammatory responses themselves can engender insulin resistance raises the possibility that they contribute to the insulin resistance and ensuing metabolic changes of pregnancy.

DOES THE SYSTEMIC INFLAMMATORY RESPONSE IN NORMAL PREGNANCY ARISE FROM SPECIFIC MATERNAL T-CELL IMMUNITY TO THE ALLOGENEIC FETUS?

From the previously stated relation between innate and adaptive immunity, it should be clear that inflammatory responses, in general, do not imply that there is some form of antigen-specific response and, in the context of pregnancy, of alloimmune recognition of the genetically foreign fetus.

The major interface between mother and fetus, the large syncytiotrophoblast layer in contact with maternal blood, expresses no polymorphic human leukocyte antigens (HLA), which are the main drivers of immune rejection. Immune rejection is executed by cytotoxic T cells that bind these antigens. But, the placental hemochorial surface is formed from a huge syncytium, which by its nature

could not be susceptible to cytolytic attack from single T cells. Nevertheless, the concept of maternal immune rejection of the 'foreign' fetus continues to be developed. Although in mouse pregnancy this may be appropriate, there is so far little direct evidence that such processes occur in human pregnancy. The concepts are centered on what is called the Th1/Th2 phenomenon.

SYSTEMIC INFLAMMATORY RESPONSE AND THE Th1/Th2 PHENOMENON

The Th1/Th2 classification was first developed in relation to the functions of T helper (Th) cells, which differentiate into two subtypes depending on the nature of the adaptive response that they induce. Th1 cells characteristically secrete interferon-gamma (IFN-γ) and promote antigen-specific cell-mediated immunity (cytotoxicity), whereas Th2 cells are distinguished by interleukin-4 (IL-4) production and stimulate the development of humoral immunity (antibodies). Graft rejection is a type 1 phenomenon. The hypothesis, first proposed by Wegmann and colleagues,[40] is that Th1 responses are suppressed in normal pregnancy to avoid immune rejection of the fetus. There is evidence of such regulation in human pregnancy in that Th1 activity is partially suppressed.[29,41] In the apparent absence of a placental target for maternal T cells, it is not possible at the moment to understand the consequences of this concept. Moreover, the Th1/Th2 paradigm is now considered to be oversimplified and needs to be adapted to take account of the rapidly expanding knowledge of the complexity of the interactions between the innate and adaptive immune systems.[42]

The bias of immune responses to type 1 or type 2 depends on the activity of the innate immune system. The bias is not limited to T cells and their responses, but includes cells of the innate immune system such as NK[43] or NKT cells,[44] of which the latter are characterized by a fixed repertoire of T-cell receptors as well as having clear NK cell attributes. There is evidence that the bias that Th cells adopt depends on the cytokine milieu created by

NKT cells, which appear to play a dominant role in immunoregulation.[45] Rather than discussing a Th1 or Th2 bias, which implies a key role for T helper cells, it is better to refer to the type 1 or type 2 bias to include the innate as well as adaptive immune responses which acknowledges the potential role of NK or NKT cells.

It is not yet known how normal pregnancy provokes a mild maternal systemic response: that it arises from the placenta is self-evident, but yet, as already mentioned, it appears to be heralded in the luteal phase of the menstrual cycle before the placenta exists. It is further enhanced during the first trimester before the uteroplacental circulation develops. At this stage it might originate with endocrine factors or simply be a distant echo of more profound local inflammation associated with menstruation, implantation, and placentation. Studies of women with pre-eclampsia have revealed some insights.

PRE-ECLAMPSIA IS ASSOCIATED WITH A MORE EXTREME SYSTEMIC INFLAMMATORY RESPONSE THAN OCCURS IN NORMAL PREGNANCY

The syndrome of pre-eclampsia is astonishingly diverse because it arises from the sum of the circulatory disturbances caused by systemic maternal endothelial cell dysfunction or activation.[46] Subsequent work of many investigators has strengthened the concept. Pathological alterations in the endothelium can be seen in the kidney, for example, as glomerular endotheliosis,[47] the specific renal lesion of pre-eclampsia.

Since endothelium is an integral part of the inflammatory network, activated endothelium activates leukocytes and vice versa.[48,49] Therefore, as expected, the systemic endothelial dysfunction is combined with an SIR such that, on average, all the markers of inflammation that are already changed in normal pregnancy (see above) are more severely affected in pre-eclampsia, affecting not only endothelial cells and leukocytes but also other components to varying degrees (see Table

9.3). But which is the primary change in pregnancy or pre-eclampsia – leukocytic or endothelial – is not clear.

Only recently has it been appreciated that what has been considered to be the pathology of pre-eclampsia evolves from processes that are an intrinsic part of normal pregnancy, albeit in a less intense form. We have proposed that pre-eclampsia develops when the systemic inflammatory process, common to all women in the second half of their pregnancies, causes one or other maternal system to decompensate.[17] This implies that the syndrome is not a separate condition but the extreme end of a continuum of maternal SIRs caused by pregnancy itself, which explains why pre-eclampsia is impossible to distinguish clearly – in terms of any definition, diagnos-tic test, or pathological lesion – from normal pregnancy.

Previously, inflammation was equated with systemic sepsis, which causes hypotension and shock. This seems incompatible with the concepts that are presented here. In fact, the endothelium (which is part of the inflammatory system) controls the microcirculation and is a potential source of potent vasoconstrictors such as endothelin-1 or thromboxane A_2. Several authors have shown how proinflammatory stimuli can impair endothelial-dependent relaxation: see, for example, Hingorani et al.[50] The hypotension of sepsis represents end-stage decompensation of vascular homeostasis. Animal experiments support the concept. A rat model of preeclampsia depends on using a classical proinflammatory stimulus: namely, a single administration of endotoxin to pregnant rats at 14 days of pregnancy. This causes new hypertension and proteinuria, which persist until the end of pregnancy. The same dose has no effect on non-pregnant animals.[51] Infusion of the proinflammatory cytokine TNF-α provokes systemic hypertension, but only in pregnant and not in non-pregnant rats.[52] These experiments show how systemic inflammation can cause hypertension and the features of pre-eclampsia. Sepsis is associated with fever, which is not considered to be a feature of pre-eclampsia. However, fever does occur significantly more often in pre-eclamptic women during labor, even after adjustment for confounding factors.[53] In terms of adaptive immunity, type 1 responses are not suppressed to the same degree in pre-eclampsia as they are in normal pregnancy.[41] This observation has been confirmed by other investigators (e.g. Sakai et al[54]) and interpreted to indicate that there is activation of a partial maternal alloimmune rejection of the fetus. But, as discussed already, there is little direct evidence to support this hypothesis and no evidence for allospecific immune rejection mechanisms.

PRE-ECLAMPSIA, OXIDATIVE STRESS, AND OTHER METABOLIC CHANGES

Metabolic markers of systemic inflammation are associated with, and intensified in, pre-eclampsia (see Table 9.3). It has already been mentioned that inflammation and oxidative stress are closely related. The oxidative stress of pre-eclampsia, which is not localized to the placenta but disseminated in the maternal circulation,[55] is an expected component of the systemic inflammatory response. Consistent with the continuum of inflammatory responses in pregnancy, it is intensified relative to normal pregnancy.[55,56] Of great clinical relevance is the fact that antioxidants, including the antioxidant vitamins that have a potential use in preventing pre-eclampsia,[57] also have anti-inflammatory actions.[5]

Whether the other metabolic changes that have been associated with systemic inflammation also occur in pre-eclampsia is not agreed. There is evidence for a more intense acute phase response, which – with respect to some markers, e.g. ceruloplasmin,[67] complement proteins C3 and Factor B,[68] or serum albumin[18] – is more marked than in normal pregnancy. Serum CRP may be elevated[69] but there is difficulty in separating the changes due to pre-eclampsia from the chronic changes associated with risk features such as obesity. Some investigators can find evidence of insulin resistance in pre-eclampsia,[70] whereas others cannot.[71] As with measures of serum CRP, it is a concern whether the changes are specific to the woman or to the pregnancy.

THE ROLE OF THE PLACENTA

The basic role of the placenta in pre-eclampsia has already been described, as has its contribution to both maternal and placental pre-eclampsia.

But how does a placental problem become a generalized maternal problem? One or several undefined placental factors must circulate to cause the maternal disorder. The factor would presumably be released during all pregnancies to account for the SIR encountered in normal pregnant women, and be atypically increased when the placenta is oxidatively stressed. There are three interrelated possibilities:

- dissemination of growth factors, their soluble regulators, or inflammatory cytokines released by syncytiotrophoblast
- placental oxidative stress
- placental debris.

A strong candidate is the soluble receptor for vascular endothelial growth factor (VEGFR-1), also known as sFlt-1 (soluble fms-like tyrosine kinase-1). It binds to vascular endothelial and placental growth factors and neutralizes their angiogenic activities.[72] VEGF is an important survival factor for endothelium, so systemic inhibition would be expected to cause generalized endothelial dysfunction. This has been confirmed in human and animal studies. For example, neutralizing monoclonal antibody to VEGF mimics the antiangiogenic actions of sFlt-1. In clinical trials of its use for the treatment of certain cancers, hypertension and proteinuria – the principal signs of pre-eclampsia – are the commonest side effects.[73] Likewise, the infusion of sFlt-1 into rats[74] causes these signs to appear and glomerular lesions that are the same as those seen specifically in pre-eclampsia, namely glomerular endotheliosis.[47]

Serum Flt-1 is increased in pre-eclampsia.[74] Because it is complexed to VEGF, its high levels in pre-eclampsia can explain the variable reports of changes of plasma VEGF in this condition: if total VEGF is measured it is increased, whereas if only free VEGF is assayed it is reduced. In non-pregnant individuals, sFlt-1 is synthesized and released by endothelial cells[75] and peripheral blood monocytes.[76] But during pregnancy the circulating sFlt-1 seems also to originate from the placenta.[74] Hence, its blood plasma concentrations decline rapidly after delivery.[74] It is also produced by trophoblast cells in culture,[77] in greater amounts under conditions of oxidative stress. If sFlt-1 were the main cause of pre-eclampsia, this could explain the paradoxical protective effect of cigarette smoking on the occurrence of pre-eclampsia, which was first noted 40 years ago[78] and has been repeatedly confirmed. Non-pregnant cigarette smokers have lower levels of circulating sFlt-1 than controls who do not smoke.[79]

It should be remembered that sFlt-1 is also released by endothelium and monocytes,[75,76] which are activated in pre-eclampsia. These inflammatory cells may also be a source of this factor in pre-eclampsia, both in the mother and the placenta. But, in non-pregnant individuals, with chronic medical conditions that are associated with mild systemic inflammatory responses, circulating sFLt-1 is, in general, decreased.[80,81]

It is possible that syncytiotrophoblasts could synthesize and release the excessive amounts of pro-inflammatory cytokines that cause the systemic responses considered in this chapter. But an analysis of production from chorionic villous explants failed to show the expected increases in protein or mRNA for TNF-α, IL-6, IL-α, and IL-1β[82] when tissues from pre-eclamptic and normal pregnancies were compared. Moreover, although peripheral and uterine vein blood concentrations of TNF-α were increased relative to control, there was no gradient between the two sources.[82] Thus, there is no convincing evidence that the pre-eclamptic placenta disseminates inflammatory cytokines into the maternal circulation.

Dissemination may also involve oxidative stress, and the disseminators may be inflammatory leukocytes themselves exposed to oxidatively altered trophoblast in the intervillous space. Thus, leukocytes in the uterine vein are significantly activated relative to those in the peripheral circulation in pre-eclampsia. Whereas the local mechanisms of activa-tion are not known, transient hypoxia in the inter-villous space could account for at least some of the observed changes.[83]

Cellular, subcellular, and molecular debris from the syncytial surface of the placenta is shed into the maternal circulation. We have proposed that its clearance constitutes the systemic inflammatory stimulus in normal and pre-eclamptic pregnancies. Debris is detected in the plasma of normal pregnant women but in significantly increased amounts in pre-eclampsia and is probably the product of syncytial apoptosis and necrosis (Figure 9.2), which is reviewed in greater detail elsewhere.[84]

The debris includes syncytiotrophoblast microparticles,[85] which are the hallmark of apoptosis and are thought to be the result of turnover and renewal of the syncytial surface of chorionic villi.[86] Such apoptosis of normal human syncytiotrophoblast can be visualized by electron microscopy.[87] Apoptosis rates are significantly increased in the syncytiotrophoblast in pre-eclampsia.[88] In addition, in-vitro hypoxia induces apoptosis of cultured human cytotrophoblasts.[89] Hence, if syncytiotrophoblast microparticles were derived from apoptotic processes, then the observation that more circulates in pre-eclampsia may be related to the degree of apoptosis in, and shedding from, the syncytiotrophoblast. In pre-eclampsia, other circulating markers of syncytial debris, including cytokeratin[90] and soluble fetal DNA,[91] are also increased. At the other end of the spectrum is the evidence for increased shedding of multinucleate syncytial fragments,[92] a process that was once called trophoblast deportation.

Increasing placental size would be expected to increase the amount of syncytial debris, which would explain why pre-eclampsia is predominantly a disorder of the third trimester, when the placenta is fully grown. It is also larger with multiple pregnancies, which also amplifies the likelihood of pre-eclampsia. In a second context, shedding would be associated with placental oxidative stress, as with the most severe pre-eclampsia, typically of early onset, and associated with intense fetal growth retardation. The placentas are usually abnormally small. Here, it must be presumed that there is an

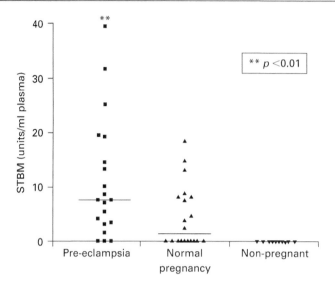

Figure 9.2 Measurements of syncytiotrophoblast microparticles (STBM) measure in plasma samples taken from non-pregnant women of childbearing age and women with pre-eclampsia matched for maternal and gestational age and for parity. (Reproduced with permission from Knight et al.[85])

alteration in the quality of the inflammatory stimulus generated by the placenta: e.g. by its content of peroxidized lipids.[93]

The current evidence is that circulating placental debris is likely to be a part of the systemic inflammatory stimulus associated with both normal and pre-eclamptic pregnancies. We have shown that syncytial microparticles are directly damaging to endothelium,[94] which is thereby stimulated to release proinflammatory substances.[95] They can also activate neutrophils in vitro,[96] and our preliminary evidence is that they are directly proinflammatory (Redman and Sargent, unpublished work). It is possible that this circulating debris comprises a danger signal in pregnancy to which the inflammatory system responds appropriately.

MATERNAL PREDISPOSING FACTORS

The metabolic, endothelial, vascular, and inflammatory changes of pre-eclampsia are similar to those of the metabolic syndrome or syndrome X.[97] The components of this syndrome predispose to pre-eclampsia and include obesity (many authors, e.g. Ros et al[98]), diabetes,[99] and chronic hypertension.[100] Low-grade systemic inflammation is a feature of all these conditions in men or non-pregnant women. It also is evident in chronic arterial disease such as ischemic heart disease.[101] Arterial disease and chronic hypertension are closely associated and the latter is also associated with an SIR.

Knowledge of the role of systemic inflammation in normal pregnancy, pre-eclampsia, and these medical conditions allows some insights. The established systemic inflammation of women with the medical conditions creates a higher baseline upon which the changes of pregnancy and pre-eclampsia are superimposed. Hence, the change of even a normal pregnancy may be enough to tip the scales in favor of pre-eclamptic features. Because there is a diffuse scale of intensities, the model also explains the overlap between normality and pre-eclampsia, which makes clinical recognition imprecise under the best circumstances (Figure 9.3).

Constitutions that contribute to these medical conditions not only predispose to pre-eclampsia but also affect the long-term prognosis of women

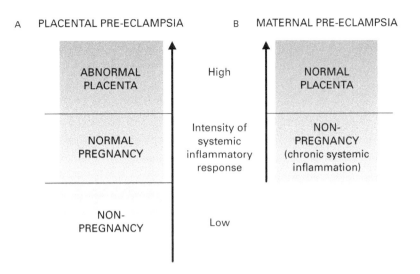

Figure 9.3 Placental and maternal pre-eclampsia. A hypothetical gray scale of increasing systemic inflammation is shown. In a completely normal woman, although normal pregnancy stimulates a systemic inflammatory response (SIR), it is not intense enough to generate the signs of pre-eclampsia. To do that requires the abnormal stimulus from an oxidatively stressed placenta. (A) In a woman with a chronic SIR associated with conditions such as chronic hypertension, diabetes, or obesity that predispose to pre-eclampsia, the starting point is abnormal enough such that even a normal placenta can stimulate a systemic response on an intensity to give the signs of pre-eclampsia. (B) In clinical practice there are many mixed presentations with both maternal constitution and placental ischemia contributing to the presentation.

who suffer pre-eclampsia. These women are, for example, several times more likely to develop cardiovascular diseases, making pregnancy an important way of screening for individual susceptibility for these conditions.[97] It has been proposed that pregnancy is a cardiovascular and metabolic stress test[102] that reveals consitutional tendencies, which become manifest in later life (Figure 9.4).

CONCLUSIONS

Pregnancy is a systemic inflammatory stress for women, especially the second half of pregnancy. The stress is probably generated by both endocrine and placental factors. That there is systemic inflammation does not necessarily mean that the maternal immune system is reacting to fetal (paternal) antigens. The placental stimulus may consist of sFlt-1

or syncytial debris, or both, released into the maternal circulation from the syncytiotrophoblast surface of the placenta, which signals danger to the maternal innate immune system, especially if the placenta is hypoxic. When the threshold for sustaining homeostasis is reached and there is excessive involvement of maternal endothelial integrity, pre-eclampsia ensues. These clinically apparent features constitute the second stage of pre-eclampsia. Many, but not all, cases of pre-eclampsia are associated with poor placentation. This constitutes the first stage, which would appear to have a different origin involving decidual immune responses. Second-stage responses, which we propose are all secondary to the SIR, could explain why women bearing pregnancies with unusually large placentas (an excessively large inflammatory stimulus) are susceptible to pre-eclampsia. Chronic systemic inflammation in women who are obese, chronically hypertensive,

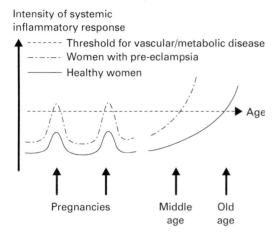

Figure 9.4 Pregnancy is a stress test revealing a propensity to medical conditions that will occur in later life. Each pregnancy generates an inflammatory response that – in those with underlying medical conditions – may cause maternal responses to cross the thresholds for overt disease, which otherwise becomes apparent in later life. (Adapted from Sattar and Greer.[102])

or diabetic contributes to pre-eclampsia superimposed on the added stimulus from even a normal pregnancy. This explains why these women are particularly susceptible to pre-eclampsia. Many of the metabolic features of normal and pre-eclamptic pregnancy such as insulin resistance, hyperlipidemia, increased blood coagulability, or hypoalbuminemia, previously seen in isolation as hormonally induced, could instead be different consequences of the one process of a systemic inflammatory response.

REFERENCES

1. Redman CWG. Current topic. Pre-eclampsia and the placenta. Placenta 1991; 12:301–308.
2. Piering WF, Garancis JG, Becker CG, Beres JA, Lemann J Jr. Preeclampsia related to a functioning extrauterine placenta: report of a case and 25-year follow-up. Am J Kidney Dis 1993; 21:310–313.
3. Ness RB, Roberts JM. Heterogeneous causes constituting the single syndrome of preeclampsia: a hypothesis and its implications. Am J Obstet Gynecol 1996; 175:1365–1370.
4. Matzinger P. The danger model: a renewed sense of self. Science 2002; 296:301–305.
5. Hensley K, Robinson KA, Gabbita SP, Salsman S, Floyd RA. Reactive oxygen species, cell signaling, and cell injury. Free Radic Biol Med 200; 28:1456–1462.
6. Harris HW, Gosnell JE, Kumwenda ZL. The lipemia of sepsis: triglyceride-rich lipoproteins as agents of innate immunity. J Endotoxin Res 2000; 6:421–430.
7. Sethi JK, Hotamisligil GS. The role of TNF alpha in adipocyte metabolism. Semin Cell Dev Biol 1999; 10:19–29.
8. Hirosumi J, Tuncman G, Chang L et al. A central role for JNK in obesity and insulin resistance. Nature 2002; 420:333–336.
9. Isomaa B. A major health hazard: the metabolic syndrome. Life Sci 2003; 73:2395–2411.
10. Mantzoros CS, Moschos S, Avramopoulos I et al. Leptin concentrations in relation to body mass index and the tumor necrosis factor-alpha system in humans. J Clin Endocrinol Metab 1997; 82:3408–3413.
11. Zarkesh-Esfahani H, Pockley G, Metcalfe RA et al. High-dose leptin activates human leukocytes via receptor expression on monocytes. J Immunol 2001; 167:4593–4599.
12. Yudkin JS, Stehouwer CD, Emeis JJ et al. C-reactive protein in healthy subjects: associations with obesity, insulin resistance, and endothelial dysfunction: a potential role for cytokines originating from adipose tissue? Arterioscler Thromb Vasc Biol 1999; 19:972–978.
13. Hansson GK, Libby P, Schönbeck U et al. Innate and adaptive immunity in the pathogenesis of atherosclerosis. Circ Res 2002; 91:281–291.
14. Gabay C, Kushner I. Acute-phase proteins and other systemic responses to inflammation. N Engl J Med 1999; 340:448–454.
15. Pepys MB, Hirschfield GM. C-reactive protein: a critical update. J Clin Invest 2003; 111:1805–1812.
16. Sacks GP, Seyani L, Lavery S et al. Maternal C-reactive protein levels are raised at 4 weeks gestation. Hum Reprod 2004; 19:1025–1030.
17. Redman CWG, Sacks GP. Sargent IL. Preeclampsia, an excessive maternal inflammatory response to pregnancy. Am J Obstet Gynecol 1999; 180:499–506.
18. Studd JW, Blainey JD, Bailey DE. Serum protein changes in the preeclampsia–eclampsia syndrome. J Obstet Gynaecol Br Commonw 1970; 77:796–801.
19. Gatti L, Tenconi PM, Guarneri D et al. Hemostatic parameters and platelet activation by flow-cytometry in normal pregnancy: a longitudinal study. Int J Clin Lab Res 1994; 24:217–219.
20. Halligan A, Bonnar J, Sheppard B et al. Haemostatic, fibrinolytic and endothelial variables in normal pregnancies and pre-eclampsia. Br J Obstet Gynaecol 1994; 101:488–492.
21. Haram K, Augensen K, Elsayed S. Serum protein pattern in normal pregnancy with special reference to acute-phase reactants. Br J Obstet Gynaecol 1983; 90:139–145.
22. Smarason AK, Gunnarsson A, Alfredsson JH et al. Monocytosis and monocytic infiltration of decidua in early pregnancy. J Clin Lab Immunol 1986; 21:1–5.
23. Rebelo I, Carvalho Guerra F, Pereira Leite L et al. Lactoferrin as a sensitive blood marker of neutrophil activation in normal pregnancies. Eur J Obstet Gynecol Reprod Biol 1995; 62:189–194.
24. Barriga C, Rodriguez AB, Ortega E. Increased phagocytic activity of polymorphonuclear leukocytes during pregnancy. Eur J Obstet Gynecol Reprod Biol 1994; 57: 43–46.
25. Kuroiwa A, Miyamoto K, Okabe N et al. Re-evaluation of the phagocytic respiratory burst in the physiological or inflammatory state and in ageing. J Clin Lab Immunol 1989; 29:189–191.
26. Greer IA, Haddad NG, Dawes J et al. Neutrophil activation in pregnancy-induced hypertension. Br J Obstet Gynaecol 1989; 96:978–982.

27. Beilin LJ, Croft KD, Michael CA et al. Neutrophil platelet-activating factor in normal and hypertensive pregnancy and in pregnancy-induced hypertension. Clin Sci (Lond) 1993; 85:63–70.

28. Koumandakis E, Koumandaki I, Kaklamani et al. Enhanced phagocytosis of mononuclear phagocytes in pregnancy. Br J Obstet Gynaecol 1986; 93:1150–1154.

29. Sacks GP, Redman CW, Sargent IL. Monocytes are primed to produce the Th1 type cytokine IL-12 in normal human pregnancy: an intracellular flow cytometric analysis of peripheral blood mononuclear cells. Clin Exp Immunol 2003; 131:490–497.

30. Sacks GP, Studena K, Sargent IL et al. Normal pregnancy and preeclampsia both produce inflammatory changes in peripheral blood leukocytes akin to those of sepsis. Am J Obstet Gynecol 1998; 179:80–86.

31. Vince GS, Starkey PM, Austgulen R et al. Interleukin-6, tumour necrosis factor and soluble tumour necrosis factor receptors in women with pre-eclampsia. Br J Obstet Gynaecol 1995; 102:20–25.

32. Arntzen KJ, Liabakk NB, Jacobsen G et al. Soluble tumor necrosis factor receptor in serum and urine throughout normal pregnancy and at delivery. Am J Reprod Immunol 1995; 34:163–169.

33. Melczer Z, Banhidy F, Csomor S et al. Influence of leptin and the TNF system on insulin resistance in pregnancy and their effect on anthropometric parameters of newborns. Acta Obstet Gynecol Scand 2003; 82:432–438.

34. Austgulen R, Lien E, Liabakk NB et al. Increased levels of cytokines and cytokine activity modifiers in normal pregnancy. Eur J Obstet Gynecol Reprod Biol 1994; 57:149–155.

35. Morris JM, Gopaul NK, Endresen MJ et al. Circulating markers of oxidative stress are raised in normal pregnancy and pre-eclampsia. Br J Obstet Gynaecol 1998; 105:1195–1199.

36. Stanley K, Fraser R, Bruce C. Physiological changes in insulin resistance in human pregnancy: longitudinal study with the hyperinsulinaemic euglycaemic clamp technique. Br J Obstet Gynaecol 1998; 105:756–759.

37. Martin U, Davies C, Hayavi S, Hartland A, Dunne F. Is normal pregnancy atherogenic? Clin Sci (Lond) 1999; 96:421–425.

38. Barbour LA, Shao J, Qiao L et al. Human placental growth hormone causes severe insulin resistance in transgenic mice. Am J Obstet Gynecol 2002; 186:512–517.

39. Yura S, Sagawa N, Itoh H et al. Resistin is expressed in the human placenta. J Clin Endocrinol Metab 2003; 88:1394–1397.

40. Wegmann TG, Lin H, Guilbert L et al. Bidirectional cytokine interactions in the materal–fetal relationship: is successful pregnancy a Th2 phenomenon? Immunol Today 1993; 14:353–356.

41. Saito S, Sakai M, Sasaki Y et al. Quantitative analysis of peripheral blood Th0, Th1, Th2 and the Th1:Th2 cell ratio during normal human pregnancy and preeclampsia. Clin Exp Immunol 1999; 117:550–555.

42. Chaouat G. Innately moving away from the Th1/Th2 paradigm in pregnancy. Clin Exp Immunol 2003; 131:393–395.

43. Loza MJ, Perussia B. Final steps of natural killer cell maturation: a model for type 1–type 2 differentiation? Nat Immunol 2001; 2:917–924.

44. Lee PT, Benlagha K, Teyton L et al. Distinct functional lineages of human V(alpha)24 natural killer T cells. J Exp Med 2002; 195:637–641.

45. Oki S, Chiba A, Yamamura T et al. The clinical implication and molecular mechanism of preferential IL-4 production by modified glycolipid-stimulated NKT cells. J Clin Invest 2004; 113:1631–1640

46. Roberts JM, Taylor RN, Musci TJ et al. Preeclampsia, an endothelial cell disorder. Am J Obstet Gynecol 1989; 161:1200–1204.

47. Gaber LW, Spargo BH, Lindheimer MD. Renal pathology in pre-eclampsia. Ballière's Clin Obstet Gynaecol 1994; 8:443–468.

48. Zimmerman GA, Prescott SM, McIntyre TM. Endothelial cell interactions with granulocytes: tethering and signaling molecules. Immunol Today 1992; 13:93–100.

49. Mantovani A, Dejana E. Cytokines as communication signals between leukocytes and endothelial cells. Immunol Today 1989; 10:370–375.

50. Hingorani AD, Cross J, Kharbanda RK et al. Acute systemic inflammation impairs endothelium-dependent dilatation in humans. Circulation 2000; 102:994–999.

51. Faas MM, Schuiling GA, Baller JF et al. A new animal model for human preeclampsia: ultra-low-dose endotoxin infusion in pregnant rats. Am J Obstet Gynecol 1994; 171:158–164.

52. Alexander BT, Cockrell KL, Massey MB et al. Tumor necrosis factor-alpha-induced hypertension in pregnant rats results in decreased renal neuronal nitric oxide synthase expression. Am J Hypertens 2002; 15:170–175.

53. Impey L, Greenwood C, Sheil O et al. The relation between pre-eclampsia at term and neonatal encephalopathy. Arch Dis Child Fetal Neonatal Ed 2001; 85:F170–172.

54. Sakai M, Tsuda H, Tanebe K et al. Interleukin-12 secretion by peripheral blood mononuclear cells is decreased in normal pregnant subjects and increased in preeclamptic patients. Am J Reprod Immunol 2002; 47:91–97.

55. Hubel CA. Dyslipidemia, iron, and oxidative stress in preeclampsia, assessment of maternal and feto–placental interactions. Semin Reprod Endocrinol 1998; 16,75–92.

56. Wickens D, Wilkins MH, Lunec J et al. Free radical oxidation (peroxidation) products in plasma in normal and abnormal pregnancy. Ann Clin Biochem 1981; 18:158–162.

57. Raijmakers MT, Dechend R, Poston L. Oxidative stress and preeclampsia: rationale for antioxidant clinical trials. Hypertension 2004; 44:374–380.

58. Terrone DA, Rinehart BK, May WL et al. Leukocytosis is proportional to HELLP syndrome severity: evidence for an inflammatory form of preeclampsia. South Med J 2000; 93:768–771.

59. Haeger M, Bengtson A, Karlsson K et al. Complement activation and anaphylatoxin (C3a and C5a) formation in preeclampsia and by amniotic fluid. Obstet Gynecol 1989; 73:551–556.

60. Perry KGJ, Martin JNJ. Abnormal hemostasis and coagulopathy in preeclampsia and eclampsia. Clin Obstet Gynecol 1992; 35:338–350.

61. Konijnenberg A, Stokkers EW, van der Post J et al. Extensive platelet activation in preeclampsia compared with normal pregnancy, enhanced expression of cell adhesion molecules. Am J Obstet Gynecol 1997; 176:461–469.

62. Taylor RN, Crombleholme WR, Friedman SA et al. High plasma cellular fibronectin levels correlate with biochemical and clinical features of preeclampsia but cannot be attributed to hypertension alone. Am J Obstet Gynecol 1991; 165:895–901.

63. Gratacos E, Casals E, Deulofeu R et al. Lipid peroxide and vitamin E patterns in pregnant women with different types of hypertension in pregnancy Am J Obstet Gynecol 1989; 178:1072–1076.

64. Vince GS, Starkey PM, Austgulen R et al. Interleukin-6, tumour necrosis factor and soluble tumour necrosis factor receptors in women with pre-eclampsia. Br J Obstet Gynaecol 1995; 102:20–25.

65. Greer IA, Lyall F, Perera T et al. Increased concentrations of cytokines interleukin-6 and interleukin-1 receptor antagonist in plasma of women with preeclampsia: a mechanism for endothelial dysfunction? Obstet Gynecol 1994; 84:937–940.

66. Stallmach T, Hebisch G, Joller H et al. Expression pattern of cytokines in the different compartments of the feto–maternal unit under various conditions. Reprod Fertil Dev 1995; 7:1573–1580.

67. Vitoratos N, Salamalekis E, Dalamaga N et al. Defective antioxidant mechanisms via changes in serum ceruloplasmin and total iron binding capacity of serum in women with pre-eclampsia. Eur J Obstet Gynecol Reprod Biol 1999; 84:63–67.

68. Johansen KA, Williams JH, Stark JM. Acute-phase C56-forming ability and concentrations of complement components in normotensive and hypertensive pregnancies. Br J Obstet Gynaecol 1981; 88:504–512.

69. Teran E, Escudero C, Moya W et al. Elevated C-reactive protein and pro-inflammatory cytokines in Andean women with pre-eclampsia. Int J Gynaecol Obstet 2001; 75:243–249.

70. Kaaja R, Laivuori H, Laakso M et al. Evidence of a state of increased insulin resistance in preeclampsia. Metabolism 1999; 48:892–896.

71. Roberts RN, Henriksen JE, Hadden DR. Insulin sensitivity in pre-eclampsia. Br J Obstet Gynaecol 1998; 105:1095–1100.

72. Kendall RL, Wang G, Thomas KA et al. Identification of a natural soluble form of the vascular endothelial growth factor receptor, FLT-1, and its heterodimerization with KDR. Biochem Biophys Res Commun 1996; 226:324–328.

73. Kabbinavar F, Hurwitz HI, Fehrenbacher L et al. Phase II, randomized trial comparing bevacizumab plus fluorouracil (FU)/leucovorin (LV) with FU/LV alone in patients with metastatic colorectal cancer. J Clin Oncol 2003; 21:60–65.

74. Maynard SE, Min JY, Merchan J et al. Excess placental soluble fms-like tyrosine kinase 1 (sFlt1) may contribute to endothelial dysfunction, hypertension, and proteinuria in preeclampsia. J Clin Invest 2003; 111:649–658.

75. Hornig C, Barleon B, Ahmad S et al. Release and complex formation of soluble VEGFR-1 from endothelial cells and biological fluids. Lab Invest 2000; 80:443–454.

76. Barleon B, Reusch P, Totzke F et al. Soluble VEGFR-1 secreted by endothelial cells and monocytes is present in human serum and plasma from healthy donors. Angiogenesis 2001; 4:143–154.

77. Li H, Gu B, Zhang Y et al. Hypoxia-induced increase in soluble Flt-1 production correlates with enhanced oxidative stress in trophoblast cells from the human placenta. Placenta 2005; 26:210–217.

78. Zabriskie JR. Effect of cigarette smoking during pregnancy. Study of 2000 cases. Obstet Gynecol 1963; 21:405–411.

79. Belgore FM, Lip GY, Blann AD. Vascular endothelial growth factor and its receptor, Flt-1, in smokers and non-smokers. Br J Biomed Sci 2000; 57:207–213.

80. Belgore FM, Blann AD, Lip GY. Measurement of free and complexed soluble vascular endothelial growth factor receptor, Flt-1, in fluid samples: development and application of two new immunoassays. Clin Sci (Lond) 2001; 100:567–575.

81. Felmeden DC, Spencer CG, Belgore FM et al. Endothelial damage and angiogenesis in hypertensive patients: relationship to cardiovascular risk factors and risk factor management. Am J Hypertens 2003; 16:11–20.

82. Benyo DF, Smarason A, Redman CWG et al. Expression of inflammatory cytokines in placentas from women with preeclampsia. J Clin Endocrinol Metab 2001; 86:2505–2512.

83. Mellembakken JR, Aukrust P, Olafsen MK et al. Activation of leukocytes during the uteroplacental passage in preeclampsia. Hypertension 2002; 39:155–160.

84. Redman CWG, Sargent IL. Placental debris, oxidative stress and pre-eclampsia. Placenta 2000; 21:597–602.

85. Knight M, Redman CW, Linton EA et al. Shedding of syncytiotrophoblast microvilli into the maternal circulation in pre-eclamptic pregnancies. Br J Obstet Gynaecol 1998; 105:632–640.

86. Huppertz B, Frank HG, Kingdom JC et al. Villous cytotrophoblast regulation of the syncytial apoptotic cascade in the human placenta. Histochem Cell Biol 1998; 110:495–508.

87. Nelson DM. Apoptotic changes occur in syncytiotrophoblast of human placental villi where fibrin type fibrinoid is deposited at discontinuities in the villous trophoblast. Placenta 1996; 17: 387–391.

88. Ishihara N, Matsuo H, Murakoshi H et al. Increased apoptosis in the syncytiotrophoblast in human term placentas complicated by either preeclampsia or intrauterine growth retardation. Am J Obstet Gynecol 2002; 186:158–166.

89. Levy R, Smith SD, Chandler K, Sadovsky Y, Nelson DM. Apoptosis in human cultured trophoblasts is enhanced by hypoxia and diminished by epidermal growth factor. Am J Physiol Cell Physiol 2000; 278: C982–988.

90. Schrocksnadel H, Daxenbichler G, Artner E, Steckel-Berger G, Dapunt O. Tumor markers in hypertensive disorders of pregnancy. Gynecol Obstet Invest 1993; 35:204–208.

91. Lo YM, Leung TN, Tein MS et al. Quantitative abnormalities of fetal DNA in maternal serum in preeclampsia. Clin Chem 1999; 45:184–188.

92. Johansen M, Redman CWG, Wilkins T et al. Trophoblast deportation in human pregnancy – its relevance for pre-eclampsia. Placenta 1999; 20:531–539.

93. Cester N, Staffolani R, Rabini RA et al. Pregnancy induced hypertension: a role for peroxidation in microvillus plasma membranes. Mol Cell Biochem 1994; 131:151–155.

94. Smarason AK, Sargent IL, Starkey PM et al. The effect of placental syncytiotrophoblast microvillous membranes from normal and pre-eclamptic women on the growth of endothelial cells in vitro. Br J Obstet Gynaecol 1993; 100: 943–949.

95. Von Dadelszen P, Hurst G, Redman CW. The supernatants from co-cultured endothelial cells and syncytiotrophoblast microvillous membranes activate peripheral blood leukocytes in vitro. Hum Reprod 1999; 14:919–924.

96. Aly AS, Khandelwal M, Zhao J et al. Neutrophils are stimulated by syncytiotrophoblast microvillous membranes to generate superoxide radicals in women with preeclampsia. Am J Obstet Gynecol 2004; 190:252–258.

97. Rodie VA, Freeman DJ, Sattar N et al. Pre-eclampsia and cardiovascular disease: metabolic syndrome of pregnancy? Atherosclerosis 2004; 175:189–202.

98. Ros HS, Cnattingius S, Lipworth L. Comparison of risk factors for preeclampsia and gestational hypertension in a population-based cohort study. Am J Epidemiol 1998; 147:1062–1070

99. Garner PR, D'Alton ME, Dudley DK et al. Preeclampsia in diabetic pregnancies. Am J Obstet Gynecol 1990; 163:505–508.

100. Sibai BM, Gordon T, Thom E et al. Risk factors for preeclampsia in healthy nulliparous women: a prospective multicenter study. The National Institute of Child Health and Human Development Network of Maternal-Fetal Medicine Units. Am J Obstet Gynecol 1995; 172:642–648.

101. Yudkin JS, Kumari M, Humphries SE et al. Inflammation, obesity, stress and coronary heart disease: is interleukin-6 the link? Atherosclerosis. 1999; 148:209–214.

102. Sattar N, Greer IA. Pregnancy complications and maternal cardiovascular risk: opportunities for intervention and screening? BMJ 2002; 325:157–160.

10. The fetal inflammatory response syndrome

Roberto Romero, Jimmy Espinoza, Luís F Gonçalves, Juan Pedro Kusanovic, and Ricardo Gomez

INTRODUCTION

Fetal infection/inflammation has been implicated in the pathophysiology of both preterm parturition and that of short- and long-term fetal and neonatal injury[1,2] predisposing to cerebral palsy (CP)[3] and chronic lung disease.[4] Intrauterine infection/inflammation is now recognized as a frequent and important cause of preterm parturition[1,2,5–12] and is the only pathological process for which both a firm causal link with prematurity is established and a defined molecular pathophysiology is known.[13] In this chapter, we review the fetal inflammatory response syndrome and the contribution of fetal infection/inflammation to short- and long-term neonatal morbidity and mortality.

LOCAL VERSUS SYSTEMIC INFLAMMATION

Inflammation has been traditionally defined by the five Latin words *calor, dolor, rubor, tumor,* and *functio laesa,* which translate to heat, pain, redness, swelling, and loss of function. All of which reflect the effects of chemokines, cytokines, and other inflammatory mediators on the local blood vessels and tissues.[14,15] Dilation and enhanced permeability of the blood vessels during inflammation lead to increased local blood flow and the leakage of fluid. This explains the increased temperature, redness, and swelling, while the migration of cells into the tissue and the action of their mediators on the nerve endings account for pain.[14] Whereas the traditional definition of inflammation describes 'localized inflammation,' the diagnosis of systemic inflammation requires a different set of criteria now referred to as the 'systemic inflammatory response syndrome.' This condition, originally described in adults, is often referred to by the acronym SIRS. The concept of SIRS was introduced in 1992 by the American College of Chest Physicians and the Society of Critical Care Medicine to describe a complex set of findings that often involve cardiovascular abnormalities and are thought to be the result of systemic activation of the innate immune system.[16] The changes, which include fever, tachycardia, hyperventilation, and an elevated white blood cell count,[16] have been attributed to the effects of cytokines and other proinflammatory mediators.[17] In 2001, the same organizations noted that the elevation of certain mediators, such as interleukin-6 (IL-6), may be associated with SIRS, and that this observation may bring about a new definition of the syndrome in adult patients, as the clinical and laboratory findings originally proposed to characterize SIRS were non-specific.[18] We defined the fetal counterpart of SIRS for the first time in 1997, using precisely the same parameter that is now being proposed for use in adults: an elevated IL-6 concentration.[19] We coined the term, 'fetal inflammatory response syndrome' (FIRS), to refer to this fetal counterpart of SIRS.[1]

WHAT CAUSES INFLAMMATION?

Inflammation is a host response to various insults, including infection, trauma, toxins, and neoplasia.[15] In adults, an excessive inflammatory response has been implicated in the pathogenesis of diabetes, atherosclerosis, Alzheimer's disease, cataracts, cancer, rheumatic fever, systemic lupus erythematosus, and rheumatoid arthritis.[15]

In the fetus, the only described cause of systemic inflammation is infection,[1] whereas the classic signs of local inflammation (e.g. heat, pain, redness, swelling, and loss of function) have not been directly observed in the fetus while in utero. In the next sections of this chapter, we will review the evidence indicating that the fetus can mount an inflammatory response, as well as the short- and long-term consequences of FIRS.

INNATE AND ADAPTIVE IMMUNE RESPONSE

The immune system evolved primarily as a host defense against infection. Host defense is accomplished by means of the innate and adaptive limbs of the immune system, (which are discussed in more detail in earlier chapters). The innate component is non-specific, whereas the acquired or adaptive response improves with repeated exposure to a specific antigen.[14] The cells of the immune system are derived from pluripotential hematopoietic stem cells (HSCs), which are first present in the yolk sack and then migrate to the liver, spleen, and bone marrow. In response to inductive signals, these HSCs undergo differentiation along two major pathways:

- the innate immune system, whose cellular components include phagocytes (neutrophils, monocytes, macrophages), cells that release inflammatory mediators (e.g. basophils, mast cells, eosinophils), and natural killer cells
- the adaptive immune system, composed of two major classes of lymphocytes (B and T cells).[15]

A key feature of the adaptive immune system is the recognition of 'self'. Seminal studies performed by the group of Sir Peter Medawar, published over 50 years ago, suggested that antigen presentation in the fetus induces tolerance rather than immunity, and that embryonic and neonatal lymphocytes are hyporesponsive.[20] However, recent reports indicate that tolerance is not an intrinsic property of the newborn immune system, but that the nature of the antigen-presenting cell determines whether the outcome is neonatal tolerance or immunization.[21] Indeed, mature virgin T cells from newborn mice can be immunized, made tolerant, or switched to Th1 or Th2 responses, according to the dose of the antigen, the type of adjuvant, and the type of antigen-presenting cells.[21–23]

The ability to mount an immune response to pathogens while remaining tolerant to self-antigens is a critical feature of the immune system. Developing T cells that recognize self-antigens with a high affinity undergo clonal deletion in the thymus.[24] This process, however, does not remove all of these T cells. Thus, other mechanisms besides clonal deletion prevent T cells from inducing immune pathology, including function inactivation, as well as tolerance mediated by a subset of T regulatory cells or CD4+ CD25+ T_R cells.[24] This subset of T cells has the ability to inhibit T-cell proliferation in vitro[25,26] and is present in both the human thymus and peripheral blood.[27] The role of regulatory cells in preventing autoimmunity is supported by the following observations:

- defective T regulatory cells have been described in multiple sclerosis,[28] autoimmune polyglandular syndrome,[29] and arthritis[30]
- neonatal thymectomy at day 3 induces auto-immune disease in susceptible mouse strains, which, in turn, can be prevented by the administration of adult-derived CD4+ CD5+ T_R cells.[31]

Recently, it has been reported that functional regulatory cells are present in the thymus and secondary lymphoid organs of the human fetus from 14 to 17 weeks of gestation.[32]

Collectively, this evidence indicates that newborns are capable of mounting an immune response and that T regulatory cells may modulate this immune response.

CAN THE FETUS MOUNT AN INFLAMMATORY RESPONSE?

Evidence that the fetus can mount an inflammatory response was communicated by Gomez et al to the Society of Maternal-Fetal Medicine in 1997.[19] The authors reported that a fetal plasma concentration of IL-6 >11 pg/ml among pregnancies complicated by preterm labor and preterm premature rupture of membranes (PROM) was associated with severe neonatal morbidity[1] and a shorter cordocentesis-to-delivery interval.[2]

A growing body of evidence indicates that fetuses can also mount an adaptive immune response.[27] Indeed, in mice, fetal T lymphocytes can mount Th1 (cell-mediated) and Th2 (antibody-mediated) immune responses when challenged with adjuvants, appropriate antigen-presenting cells, or a suitable amount of antigens.[21] In humans, Matsuoka et al reported a high proportion of Th1 cells – interferon-γ (IFN-γ)-producing CD3+ T cells – in the cord blood of neonates with clinical evidence of intrauterine infection, and that the proportion of Th1 cells correlated with the timing of the rupture of membranes before the onset of labor.[33] Similar results were reported by Yoneyama et al in neonates exposed to PROM without clinical evidence of neonatal infection.[34] Presumably, these fetuses mounted an adequate inflammatory response that prevented the clinical manifestation of neonatal infection.

THE FETAL INFLAMMATORY RESPONSE SYNDROME

The term 'fetal inflammatory response syndrome' was coined to define a subclinical condition originally described in fetuses of women presenting with preterm labor and intact membranes, as well as preterm PROM.[1,2] The operational definition was an elevation of fetal plasma IL-6 concentration >11 pg/ml.[2] IL-6, a major mediator of the host response to infection and tissue damage, is capable of eliciting biochemical, physiological, and immunological changes in the host, including stimulation of the production of C-reactive protein by liver cells, the acute phase plasma protein response, and activation of T and natural killer cells.

The original work describing FIRS was based on fetal blood samples obtained by cordocentesis.[1,2] Many of these findings have since been confirmed by studying umbilical cord blood at the time of birth, including the elevation of proinflammatory cytokines and the relationship between these cytokines, and the likelihood of clinical and suspected sepsis.[4,35,36]

Pathological examination of the umbilical cord is an easy approach to determine whether fetal inflammation was present before birth. Funisitis and chorionic vasculitis are the histopathological hallmarks of FIRS.[37] Funisitis is associated with endothelial activation, a key mechanism in the development of organ damage,[38] and neonates with funisitis are at increased risk for neonatal sepsis[39] and long-term handicaps, such as bronchopulmonary dysplasia (BPD)[4] and CP.[3]

Another approach to detect FIRS is to measure C-reactive protein concentration in umbilical cord blood, which has been shown to be elevated in patients with amniotic fluid infection, funisitis, and congenital neonatal sepsis.[40] In addition, since neutrophils in the amniotic fluid are predominantly of fetal origin,[41] the amniotic fluid white blood cell count can also be used as an indirect index of fetal inflammation.[41] Intra-amniotic inflammation is a risk factor for impending preterm delivery and adverse perinatal outcome in women with preterm PROM, even in the absence of documented intra-amniotic infection.[42]

FETAL TARGET ORGANS DURING FIRS

Fetal microbial invasion or other insults result in a systemic fetal inflammatory response that can progress in the absence of timely delivery toward multiple organ dysfunction, septic shock, and perhaps death. Evidence of multisystemic involvement in cases of FIRS includes increased concentrations of fetal plasma metalloproteinase (MMP)9,[43] an enzyme involved in both the digestion of type IV collagen and in pathophysiology of preterm PROM.[44] Moreover, several fetal organs (including the hematopoietic system, the adrenals, heart, brain, lungs, and skin), have been proposed to be target organs during FIRS (Figure 10.1).

THE HEMATOPOIETIC SYSTEM

The hematological response of the human fetus to FIRS is characterized by significant changes in the

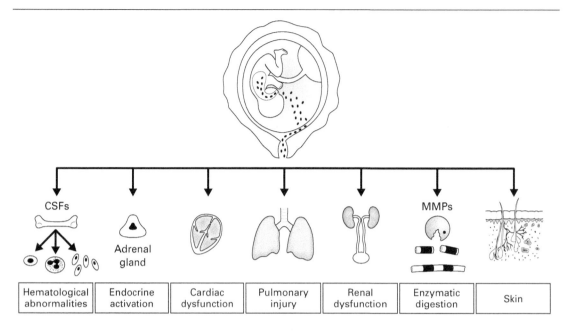

Hematological abnormalities	Endocrine activation	Cardiac dysfunction	Pulmonary injury	Renal dysfunction	Enzymatic digestion	Skin

Figure 10.1. Fetal target organs during the fetal inflammatory response syndrome. CSFs, colony-stimulating factors; MMPs, metalloproteinases.

granulocyte and red blood cell lineages.[45] Indeed, two-thirds of fetuses with FIRS have neutrophilia, defined as a neutrophil blood count above the 95th percentile for gestational age.[45] In contrast, neuturopenia is present in only approximately 7% of fetuses with FIRS.[45] The mechanisms responsible for fetal neutrophilia are not completely understood. However, it has been proposed that granulocyte colony-stimulating factor (G-CSF), the primary physiological regulator of neutrophil production, may participate in these mechanisms.[46] Indeed, it has been previously demonstrated that fetuses with FIRS have a higher median plasma concentration of G-CSF than those without FIRS (median 714.4 pg/ml, range 23.3–4229.2 vs median 55.7 pg/ml, range 7.7–411; $p < 0.01$).[46]

Fetuses with FIRS also have a higher median nucleated red blood cell count than those without FIRS (median 2.42, range 0–35 vs median 1.38, range 0–63.6; $p < 0.05$).[45] These changes are not associated with differences in the umbilical vein pH or pO_2

levels.[47] Thus, unlike fetuses with intrauterine growth restriction and abnormal Doppler velocimetry in the middle cerebral artery and ductus venosus (where metabolic acidemia may be the cause of the red cell shift),[48] the likelihood that elevated nucleated red blood cell counts are a consequence of FIRS should be considered. Evidence in favor of this possibility has been recently reported, indicating that the IL-6 concentration in umbilical cord blood may be an independent explanatory variable for the prediction of high nucleated red blood cell count.[49]

FIRS has also been associated with changes in markers of monocyte and neutrophil activation.[50] Indeed, fetuses that deliver within 72 hours of cordocentesis have a higher expression of CD11c, CD13, CD15, and CD67 than those that deliver at term. In contrast, no significant differences in the percentages of CD14 and CD63 have been observed between the two groups. Collectively, these results indicate that fetuses that deliver prematurely have activation of the monocyte–neutrophil system.[50]

THE ADRENAL GLANDS

Fetuses with FIRS have endocrine evidence of fetal stress, expressed as an abnormal cortisol/dehydroepiandrosterone ratio.[51] Indeed, Yoon et al reported a significant correlation between fetal plasma cortisol and fetal plasma IL-6 ($r = 0.3$, $p < 0.05$) as well as a significant association between fetal plasma cortisol/dehydroepiandrosterone sulfate ratio and a shorter interval from cordocentesis to deliver: (hazard ratio (HR) = 2.9, 95% confidence interval (CI) 1–8.4; $p < 0.05$).[51] Fetal plasma cortisol, but not maternal cortisol, was an independent predictor of the duration of pregnancy, after adjusting for gestational age and the results of amniotic fluid cultures (HR = 2.9, 95% CI 1.3–6.7; $p < 0.05$). Patients with preterm PROM who went into spontaneous labor and delivered within 7 days of cordocentesis had a significantly higher median fetal plasma concentration of cortisol, but not of dehydroepiandrosterone sulfate, than those who delivered after 7 days:

- for fetal plasma cortisol, median = 8.35 μg/dl, range = 4.7–12.4 μg/dl vs median = 4.75 μg/dl, range = 3.0–10.4 μg/dl; $p < 0.0001$
- for fetal plasma dehydroepiandrosterone sulfate, median = 154.4 μg/dl, range = 8.6–333.8 μg/dl vs median = 194.6 μg/dl, range = 96.7–402.5 μg/dl; $p = 0.09$.[51]

Collectively, these results indicate that an elevation in fetal plasma cortisol, but not dehydroepiandrosterone sulfate, is followed by the onset of spontaneous preterm labor in patients with preterm PROM.

THE FETAL SKIN

To determine if the fetal skin participates in FIRS, Kim et al[52] harvested skin from fetuses who died shortly after delivery due to extreme prematurity (21–24 weeks of gestation) and underwent autopsy ($n = 12$). The skin biopsies were grouped according to the presence of histological chorioamnionitis. Expression of toll-like receptors (TLR)-2 and TLR-4 was determined by immunohistochemistry with polyclonal antibodies and image analysis. The results of this study reported that:

1. The skin from fetuses born to mothers without chorioamnionitis expressed TLR-2 and TLR-4 in the epidermis: TLR-2, median 3%, range 0.4–7.2%; TLR-4, median 99.5%, range 91–100%.
2. There was a dramatic increase in the expression of TLR-2, but not in TLR-4, in the epidermis of fetuses born after chorioamnionitis: TLR-2, median 19.6%, range 10.3–89.6%; $p = 0.007$; TLR-4, median 100%, range 89.4–100%; $p = 0.5$.
3. TLR-2 and TLR-4 were also expressed in the mononuclear inflammatory infiltrate of the dermal–epidermal junction.

The authors proposed that the fetal skin is capable of recognizing the presence of microorganisms through the expression of 'pattern-recognition receptors', and thus participates in a fetal inflammatory response to microbial products.[52] The clinical manifestation of fetal skin involvement during FIRS would be fetal dermatitis.

THE FETAL KIDNEYS

Yoon et al reported that there is an inverse correlation between the amount of amniotic fluid and FIRS among patients with preterm PROM.[53] Patients with an amniotic fluid index ≤5 cm had: (1) significantly higher IL-6 concentrations in umbilical cord plasma at birth (*fetal response*); (2) higher concentrations of amniotic fluid proinflammatory cytokines such as IL-6, IL-1β, and tumor necrosis factor-α (TNF-α) (*intra-amniotic inflammatory response*); and (3) higher rates of histological and clinical chorioamnionitis (*maternal response*) than those with an amniotic fluid index >5 cm.[51,53] These observations are consistent with the report that fetuses with fetal bacteremia diagnosed by cordocentesis had oligohydramnios (amniotic fluid index <5 cm) more frequently than those with a sterile blood culture.[54]

The reasons why oligohydramnios in preterm PROM is associated with a higher rate of fetal infection/inflammation remain unclear. Yoon et al proposed that since the amniotic fluid has antimicrobial properties,[55] oligohydramnios may reduce the protective effect of this component of innate immunity. Alternatively, redistribution of blood flow away from the kidneys may take place as part of the host response to microbial products leading to oligohydramnios.[51,53]

THE FETAL HEART

A recent report indicates that fetuses with preterm PROM have changes in the parameters used to evaluate diastolic function of the heart when compared to fetuses of women with uncomplicated pregnancies.[56] The most common method used to assess diastolic function is pulsed Doppler fetal echocardiography, in which the sample volume is placed below the atrioventricular (AV) valves.[57,58] The parameters derived from this type of investigation do not measure ventricular diastolic function directly, but rely on the hemodynamic consequences of ventricular diastolic function on the Doppler velocity waveform, as there is evidence that parameters of diastolic function derived from Doppler studies correlate well with those obtained from invasive testing in adults.[59] The E wave reflects early diastolic filling, whereas the A wave represents changes in flow velocity during atrial contraction.[58] The E/A peak velocity ratio has been used to assess changes in ventricular diastolic function and is considered to reflect both ventricular compliance and preloading conditions.[60–62] Another parameter used to examine diastolic function is the velocity–time integral (VTI), which is the area under the curve of the E and A waves.[63]

The changes in the Doppler waveform characteristics in fetuses with preterm PROM are consistent with a high left ventricular compliance, particularly among those with proven intra-amniotic infection. These changes include a higher ratio between the early filling delta E/A ratio in both ventricles and a higher delta E/A VTI in the left ventricle, as compared with normal fetuses.

A pattern of myocardial depression, characterized by left ventricular dilatation, decreased left ventricular ejection fraction, and a normal or increased cardiac index, has been observed within the first few days of septic shock in adults.[64] Acute ventricular dilatation within the first days of septic shock is more frequent among survivors. This observation has been attributed to compensatory ventricular dilatation to maintain stroke volume, despite a profound loss in myocardial contractility.[64] Thus, it is possible that the changes in cardiac diastolic function seen in human fetuses represent a compensatory mechanism similar to the one observed in adults with sepsis. It is also possible that fetuses unable to change cardiac compliance in the context of a fetal systemic inflammatory response syndrome may not be able to maintain ventricular stroke volume and cardiac output and, hence, may not perfuse the brain adequately, predisposing to hypotension and brain ischemia in utero, which could create conditions for the development of periventricular leukomalacia (PVL). These changes in diastolic function may, therefore, have protective and even survival value. In cases of overwhelming fetal sepsis (the pathophysiological counterpart to septic shock in adults), myocardial depression may lead to fetal death, which we have observed in cases with preterm PROM.

The reason why fetuses without evidence of microbial invasion of the amniotic cavity (MIAC) also have changes in cardiac function remains unclear. One explanation is that a substantial number of fetuses with preterm PROM do not have microbiological evidence of infection, but rather intra-amniotic inflammation.[42] Thus, although culture results may be negative, these fetuses could still have an inflammatory response. There is now evidence that intra-amniotic inflammation is as good at predicting pregnancy and neonatal outcomes as proven MIAC with standard microbiological techniques.[65] Future studies need to examine the relationship between a fetal cytokine response and changes in cardiac function, regardless of the microbial state of the amniotic cavity. Similarly, studies with molecular microbiological techniques allowing for the detection of microorganisms that cannot be isolated with cultivation techniques may yield valuable information to address this question.[66,67]

The mechanism by which sepsis induces myocardial depression is not completely understood. The most likely explanation is that the myocardium is depressed by the action of soluble factors such as bacterial products and cytokines, which are elevated in the circulation of patients with septic shock.[68–70] There is now substantial evidence indicating that endotoxin and proinflammatory cytokines, such as TNF-α, IL-1β, and macrophage migration inhibitory factor (MIF), play a central role as myocardial depressants in the context of sepsis. Bacterial lipopolysaccharide (LPS) (or endotoxin), a component of the cell wall of Gram-negative bacteria, has been implicated in the pathophysiology of preterm labor,[71–75] preterm PROM,[76] and septic shock.[77] The mechanism by which LPS induces a cellular response has been partially defined. LPS binds to an acute phase reactant protein, known as LPS-binding protein (LBP), to form an LPS–LBP complex, which, in turn, binds to CD14, a receptor present on the surface of neutrophils, monocytes, and macrophages.[78–81] The interaction of CD14 with the LPS–LBP complex initiates signal transduction with the participation of TLR-4.[82] This eventually leads to activation of the mitogen-activated protein kinase (MAP kinase) and nuclear factor (NF)-κB pathway.[83] These events result in the production of proinflammatory cytokines such as TNF-α and IL-1β.[84,85]

Animal models of endotoxin-induced cardiac dysfunction indicate that this proinflammatory cascade may play an important role in the pathogenesis of cardiac dysfunction in septic patients. The evidence in support of this view includes:

1. LPS impairs myocardial contractility and relaxation, increasing the proportion of isovolumetric relaxation and contraction times.[86]
2. CD14-deficient mice are protected against LPS-induced left ventricular dysfunction.[87]
3. TLR-4 mRNA and protein are constitutively present in the fetal myocardium,[86] and TLR-4-deficient mice do not experience left ventricular diastolic and systolic dysfunction after intraperitoneal injection of LPS.[88]

4. LPS up-regulates the production of TNF-α and IL-1β mRNA transcripts and protein in the fetal and adult myocardium.[86,87]
5. An intraperitoneal injection of LPS in mice induced the myocardial expression of mRNA and protein of TNF-α, IL-1β, IL-6, and monocyte chemotactic protein-1.[89]

The observation that fetuses with preterm PROM and intra-amniotic infection undergo changes in cardiac function are consistent with the findings of Yanowitz et al,[90] who recently reported that neonates born with histological chorioamnionitis had several hemodynamic abnormalities (including a decreased mean and diastolic blood pressure), and that there was a correlation between mean blood pressure and umbilical cord IL-6 concentrations.[90] It is possible that some of these hemodynamic changes are present in utero and may contribute to the pathophysiology of PVL and cerebral palsy.[91] Those conditions were originally considered to be due to ischemia/hypoxia and have recently been linked to chorioamnionitis, infection, and fetal inflammation. In the context of FIRS, the combination of inflammatory changes in the brain and fetal systemic hypotension may increase the likelihood of brain injury.

Monoclonal antibodies against TNF-α have recently been shown to prevent both LPS-induced ventricular dilatation and the reduction in myocardial contractility in an animal model of sepsis.[92] Furthermore, phase III clinical trials with an anti-TNF-α monoclonal antibody therapy in patients with septic shock reported an improvement in the left ventricular function, although this did not improve survival.[93,94] Since some neonates are born with very high concentrations of TNF-α, approaches aimed at modulating the innate immunoresponse with the use of anti-TNF, IL-10, and anti-MIF deserve consideration for the neonate with early sepsis. The recent development of a mouse model of fetal inflammation where fetal cardiac dysfunction was achieved by the intra-amniotic injection of LPS[86] provides a potential tool to explore these therapeutic options.

WHY DOES THE FETUS MOUNT AN INFLAMMATORY RESPONSE?

When FIRS was originally described, we proposed that in the context of intrauterine infection, the onset of preterm labor would have survival value and that it would be part of the repertoire of host defense mechanisms against infection.[1,2] The fetus would use the effector limb of the immune response via the secretion of proinflammatory cytokines to signal the onset of labor and exit a hostile intrauterine environment. Evidence in support of this hypothesis has been recently reported by Lahra and Jeffery,[95] who compared the frequency of a histological fetal response to chorioamnionitis (umbilical vasculitis with or without funisitis) between infants who survived the neonatal period and cases of perinatal death. Neonatal survivors had a higher prevalence of histological chorioamnionitis (95% CI 1.02–1.21; $p = 0.02$) and a higher rate of umbilical vasculitis/funisitis at 25–29 weeks of gestation (95% CI 0.33–0.86; $p = 0.01$) and 30–34 weeks of gestation (95% CI 0.18–0.85; $p = 0.02$) than infants who died in the perinatal period.

SHORT-TERM CONSEQUENCES OF FETAL INFLAMMATORY RESPONSE SYNDROME

NEONATAL MORBIDITY

Fetuses with FIRS have a higher rate of neonatal complications, including respiratory distress syndrome, suspected or proved neonatal sepsis, pneumonia, intraventricular hemorrhage, periventricular leukomalacia, and necrotizing enterocolitis,[1] and are frequently born to mothers with subclinical MIAC.[1]

PRETERM PARTURITION

Among women with preterm PROM, FIRS is associated with the impending onset of preterm labor, regardless of the inflammatory state of the amniotic fluid 1,2 (Figure 10.2).[2] This suggests that the human fetus plays a role in initiating the onset of labor. However, maternal cooperation must occur for parturition. Fetal inflammation is linked to the onset of labor in association with ascending intrauterine infection. Systemic fetal inflammation

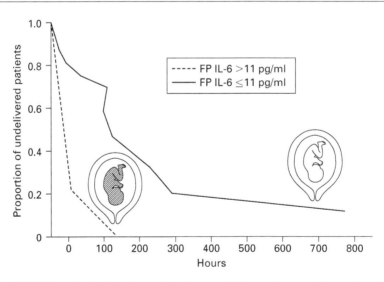

Figure 10.2. Fetuses with fetal plasma interleukin-6 (FP IL-6) levels >11 pg/ml have a shorter cordocentesis-to-delivery interval than those with FP IL-6 concentrations ≤11 pg/ml (median 0.8 days, range 0.1–5 vs median 6 days, range 0.2–33.6, respectively; $p <0.05$). (Reproduced with permission from Romero et al.[2]).

may take place in the absence of labor when the inflammatory process does not involve the chorioamniotic membranes and decidua. Such instances occur in the context of hematogenous viral infections or other disease processes (i.e. alloimmunization).

PERINATAL DEATH

An association between placental inflammation and perinatal death has been reported by several investigators.[96–101] Moyo et al[99] compared the frequency of vasculitis in the placental chorionic plate between stillbirths and live neonates in a case–control study. The investigators showed that 9% (6/66) of the stillbirths, but none of the live births (0/66), had evidence of vasculitis in the chorionic plate [odds ratio (OR 14, 95% CI 2.8–72)]. In a larger cohort study, Mwanyumba et al[100] correlated placental pathology and adverse perinatal outcomes in 701 unselected consecutive infants delivered in Kenya, and found that acute placental inflammation, defined as inflammation involving the membranes, decidua, villi, or umbilical cord, was an independent risk factor for low birth weight [adjusted relative risk (ARR) 3.8, 95% CI 1.7–8.9; $p < 0.01$], stillbirth (ARR 2.3, 95% CI 1.1–5.0; $p = 0.03$), and perinatal death (ARR 2.8, 95% CI 1.4–5.4; $p < 0.01$).

Blackwell et al[102] proposed that failure of the fetus to mount an inflammatory response sufficient to signal the onset of preterm labor may account for some cases of fetal death. Indeed, histological chorioamnionitis (a maternal host response) is nine times more frequent than funisitis [20.9% (9/43) vs 2.3% (1/43); $p = 0.008$] in cases of fetal death. Changes in the adaptive limb of the maternal immune response are also associated with unexplained fetal death. Evidence in support of this concept includes the finding that an increased proportion of 'memory-like' T cells (CD45RO+ isoform) was observed in the maternal blood of pregnancies complicated by unexplained fetal death, suggesting that prior maternal exposure to microbial products (bacterial or viral) or other unidentified antigens occurred in these cases.[103]

CONTRIBUTION OF FETAL INFECTION/INFLAMMATION TO LONG-TERM HANDICAP

WHITE MATTER DAMAGE AND CEREBRAL PALSY

Cerebral palsy is a symptom complex characterized by the aberrant control of movement or posture that appears in early life and can lead to costly, life-long disability.[104] The estimated annual prevalence of CP ranges from 1.5 to 2.5 per 1000 live births, depending on the studied cohort.[105,106]

There is strong evidence linking brain injury and infant exposure to perinatal infection and inflammation.[104,107–110] In 1955, Eastman and DeLeon observed that intrapartum maternal fever was associated with a sevenfold increase in the risk of CP.[111] In 1978, Nelson and Ellenberg,[112] using data from the Collaborative Perinatal Project, showed that among low-birth-weight infants, chorioamnionitis increased the risk of CP from 12 per 1000 to 39 per 1000 live births. These observations were independently confirmed by several other studies.[104,107,113–116] The general view is that an initiator event (either pre-pregnancy infection or intrauterine infection) leads to maternal and fetal inflammatory responses, which, in turn, contribute to adverse outcomes such as preterm delivery, intraventricular hemorrhage (IVH), white matter damage (WMD), and neurodevelopment disability (mainly CP).[117] The following evidence supports this concept:

- a fetal inflammatory response precedes spontaneous preterm delivery[1,2]
- chorioamnionitis is associated with an increased risk of CP[104,107,113–116,118,119]
- white matter lesions are associated with spontaneous preterm labor[114,120–124]
- infection is causally linked to WMD[108,113,114,122]
- fetal cytokinemia is associated with IVH, WMD, and CP[109,117,125–131]
- chorionic and umbilical cord vessel inflammation (fetal vasculitis) is associated with an increased risk for IVH, WMD, and CP.[3,132–135]

Prematurity and CP are strongly associated.[122] Indeed approximately one-third of all neonates who later have signs of CP weigh less than 2500 g at birth.[136] Newborns whose birth weights are <1500 g have a rate of CP 25–31 times higher than those with a normal birth weight.[136] A possible mechanism contributing to the increased risk of CP among extremely premature infants is their inability to produce an adequate amount of proteins that either modulate the synthesis of inflammatory cytokines[110,137–143] or help to minimize oxidative stress.[143,144] Moreover, some fetuses may have an increased genetic susceptibility to develop CP in the setting of intrauterine infection/inflammation. Nelson et al[145] have recently examined the association of genetic polymorphisms and CP in premature infants. In a case–control study of 96 infants with CP and 119 control children delivered before 32 weeks, an association with CP was observed in heterozygotes for the following single nucleotide polymorphisms (SNPs):

- endothelial nitric oxide synthase (eNOS) A-922G (OR = 3.0, 95% CI 1.4–6.4)
- factor 7 (F7) arg353gln and del[-323]10bp-ins (OR = 2.7, 95% CI 1.1–6.5)
- plasminogen activation inhibitor factor-1 (PAI-1) 4G(-675)5G and G11053T (OR = 3.2, 95% CI 1.2–8.7)
- lymphotoxin A (LTA) thr26asn (OR = 2.1, 95% CI 1.0–4.6).

These SNPs are related to nitric oxide, thrombosis or thrombolysis, and cytokine function, respectively.

The association between chorioamnionitis and subsequent development of CP has been extensively investigated.[3,109,146–153] A recent meta-analysis reporting on the association of chorioamnionitis and CP concluded that clinical chorioamnionitis is associated with an increased risk of both CP and WMD, with RR 1.9 (95% CI 1.5–2.5) and RR 2.6 (95% CI 1.7–3.9) for each of these outcomes, respectively.[154] Evidence supporting a role for the fetus in the process of chorioamnionitis comes from studies comparing IL-6 concentrations in umbilical venous blood obtained from pregnancies with ($n = 26$) and without ($n = 111$) clinical chorioamnionitis.[35] The median concentration of venous plasma IL-6 was higher in neonates born to mothers with clinical chorioamnionitis than in neonates born to women in the control group. Sixty-two percent (16/26) of the neonates born to women with clinical chorioamnionitis had elevated plasma concentrations of IL-6 >11 pg/ml in the umbilical vein. The observation that the concentration of IL-6 was higher in the blood from the umbilical artery than in the blood from the umbilical vein suggests a fetal origin of the excess plasma IL-6.

Further evidence that a fetal inflammatory response is involved in the pathophysiology of CP comes from a study of Yoon et al,[3] who followed 123 preterm children to the age of 3, observing that the odds of developing CP were higher in the presence of funisitis (OR = 5.5, 95% CI 1.2–24.5), increased amniotic fluid IL-6 concentrations (OR = 6.4, 95% CI 1.3–33.0), and increased amniotic fluid IL-8 concentrations (OR = 5.9, 95% CI 1.1–30.7). All 14 children who subsequently developed CP had evidence of WMD, while 11 had evidence of intrauterine inflammation. Fifty percent (7/14) of the children had positive amniotic fluid cultures. Although histological chorioamnionitis was associated with subsequent development of CP, this association disappeared after adjusting for gestational age at birth. The findings of this study suggest that it is the fetal rather than maternal inflammatory response that predisposes to CP. Nonetheless, neither infection nor inflammation were considered sufficient causal factors for WMD or CP, as the latter did not develop in 82% (23/28) of fetuses with documented MIAC and in 76% (34/45) of those with evidence of intrauterine inflammation. Other studies supporting a link between fetal inflammation and brain injury have documented higher concentrations of IL-6,[124,155,156] TNF-α,[155] and MMP8[157] in the umbilical cord blood and amniotic fluid[3,109] of fetuses with WMD who subsequently developed CP. Recently, Kaukola et al[158] performed a case–control study that comprised 19 children with CP and 19 controls matched by gestational age at birth.

They measured the serum concentrations of eight cytokines (ciliary neurotrophic factor, IL-5, IL-12p40, IL-12p70, IL-13, IL-15, MIF, and TNF-related apoptosis inducing ligand), that were found to be higher in the cord blood samples of neonates who subsequently developed CP. Similarly, serum concentrations of epidermal growth factor and three chemokines [B-lymphocyte chemoattractant, monocyte chemotactic protein (MCP)-3, and monokine induced by IFN-γ] were higher in the cord blood samples from infants with CP than in controls. Infants with CP that were born preterm had a different pattern of cytokines in the cord blood than infants with CP who delivered at term, suggesting that the pathophysiology of CP may vary according to the gestational age at birth.

White matter damage identified by neonatal brain ultrasound is currently considered the best predictor of long-term disability in preterm infants.[143,159] Adverse outcomes associated with WMD include cognitive limitations,[160] behavioral problems,[161] visuospatial difficulties,[162] and CP.[163] WMD is more common among children of pregnancies complicated by chorioamnionitis[114] and purulent amniotic fluid,[113] as well as among neonates with bacteremia.[122]

Experimental evidence indicates that intra-uterine infection results in WMD and neuronal lesions.[108,164–169] Yoon et al[108] experimentally induced ascending intrauterine infection with *Escherichia coli* in 31 pregnant rabbits and inoculated 14 controls with sterile saline solution. Histological evidence of brain WMD was identified in 12 fetuses born to 10 *E. coli*-inoculated rabbits, compared with none in the control group (p <0.05). All cases with WMD had evidence of intrauterine inflammation. Similar findings were reported by Debillon et al.[165,166] Increased cytokine expression in the white matter (mainly TNF-α[125,170–172] and, to a lesser extent, IL-6,[125] IL-1β,[125,172] and IL-2[173]) has been demonstrated by immunohistochemistry studies performed in neonatal brains with PVL. Moreover, increased immunoreactivity for TNF-α has been reported in the neocortex, hippocampus, basal ganglia, and thalamus of neonatal brains with PVL.[174]

Leviton[128] proposed that inflammatory cytokines (TNF-α) released during the course of intrauterine infection could participate in the pathogenesis of PVL by four different mechanisms:

1. Induction of fetal hypotension and brain ischemia.[129]
2. Stimulation of the tissue factor production and release, which activates the hemostatic system and contributes to coagulation necrosis of white matter.[175]
3. Induction of the release of platelet activating factor, which could act as a membrane detergent causing direct brain damage.[130]
4. A direct cytotoxic effect of TNF-α on oligodendrocytes and myelin.[126,127]

Yoon et al[109] proposed a mechanism by which inflammatory cytokines could lead to WMD and CP. MIAC, which occurs in approximately 25% of preterm births, results in congenital fetal infection/inflammation that stimulates fetal mononuclear cells to produce IL-1β and TNF-α. These cytokines increase the permeability of the blood–brain barrier, facilitating the passage of microbial products and cytokines into the brain.[176,177] Microbial products then stimulate the human fetal microglia to produce IL-1 and TNF-α, with subsequent activation of astrocyte proliferation and production of TNF-α. TNF-α damages oligodendrocytes, which are the cells responsible for the deposition of myelin. IFN-γ and LPS also increase the permeability of the blood–brain barrier, and this increase in permeability is, at least in part, dependent on cGMP and nitric oxide.[177] For a detailed review of the evidence linking prenatal exposure to LPS and brain injury, the reader is referred to the excellent review by Hagberg and Mallard.[178]

Evidence for involvement of the adaptive arm of the immune system in the pathogenesis of WMD comes from the study of Duggan et al,[155] who proposed that activated memory T cells may be involved in brain injury among neonates born between 23 and 29 weeks. These investigators found that the percentage of CD45RO+ cells is higher among neonates with cerebral lesions detected by magnetic resonance imaging (MRI), when compared to neonates with normal MRI results. MRI abnormalities included germinal layer or intraventricular hemorrhage, discrete periventricular lesions, and/or cystic lesions in the caudate nucleus. The authors proposed that high fetal cytokinemia may be due to antigen exposure and is not secondary to the brain injury, hypoxia, or parturition.[155]

BRONCHOPULMONARY DYSPLASIA

Bronchopulmonary dysplasia is operationally defined as oxygen dependence at 36 weeks postmenstrual age plus a total oxygen exposure for ≥28 days.[179] It is one of the most frequent and clinically significant complications of prematurity, as it is associated with an increased risk of bronchial hyperresponsiveness and asthma.[180]

A substantial body of evidence links a fetal inflammatory response with the subsequent development of BPD. This data is summarized below and includes associations between elevated cytokine concentrations in the amniotic and tracheal fluids, as well as umbilical cord blood of fetuses/infants who subsequently developed BPD.[4,181–183]

Watterberg et al[182] studied the association between lung inflammation and chorioamnionitis in 53 low-birth-weight infants who required intubation. Lung inflammation was evaluated on days 1, 2, and 4 of intubation, by measuring the concentration of IL-1β, thromboxane B_2, leukotriene B_4 (LT-B_4), and prostaglandin E_2 (PGE$_2$) in tracheal lavage samples. Infants exposed to chorioamnionitis had a higher concentration of IL-1β in their tracheal fluid from the first day of intubation forward and were more likely to develop BPD. It is noteworthy that the authors also reported that these very low-birth-weight infants had fewer instances of respiratory distress syndrome (RDS) than controls. Thus, fetuses exposed to chorioamnionitis appear to have less RDS but more BPD than controls.[184]

Antenatal exposure to proinflammatory cytokines is also a risk factor for the development of BPD.[181] Ghezzi et al[181] measured IL-8 in the amni-

otic fluid of women with preterm labor with intact membranes or preterm PROM ($n = 47$) who delivered between 24 and 28 weeks of gestation. BPD was diagnosed in 23.4% (11/47) of the cases. The prevalence of a positive amniotic fluid culture was 44.7% (21/47). IL-8 concentrations were higher in the amniotic fluid of neonates who subsequently developed BPD, compared to those who did not develop BPD. The majority of mothers whose fetuses developed BPD had an amniotic fluid IL-8 concentration level >11.5 ng/ml, and this relationship remained significant even after correction for the effect of gestational age and birth weight (OR = 11.9; p <0.05). The relationship between amniotic fluid IL-6, TNF-α, IL-1β and IL-8 and the occurrence of BPD was further examined in a subsequent study[185] of 69 neonates who delivered preterm (≤33 weeks) within 5 days of amniocentesis. BPD was diagnosed in 19% (13/69) of the neonates, and the median amniotic fluid concentrations of IL-6, IL-1β and IL-8 were each significantly higher in the amniotic fluid of infants who developed BPD than that of those who did not develop BPD.

Yoon et al[4] studied the relationship between IL-6 concentration in umbilical cord plasma at birth and the occurrence of BPD in 203 preterm births (25–34 weeks). BPD was diagnosed in 17% (34/203) of the cases. Neonates who developed BPD had a significantly higher median IL-6 concentration in umbilical cord plasma at birth than those who did not develop BPD (median = 68.3 pg/ml, 95% CI 0.3–6150.0 pg/ml vs median = 6.9 pg/ml, 95% CI 0–19 230.0 pg/ml; p <0.001). This difference remained significant even after adjusting for gestational age at birth (OR = 4.2, 95% CI 1.6–11.2). This same group[183] has also observed an association between a fetal inflammatory response (defined as the presence of funisitis or umbilical cord plasma IL-6 concentration >17.5 pg/ml or amniotic fluid MMP8 concentration >23 ng/ml) and the development of atypical chronic lung disease (defined as chronic lung disease in the absence of RDS). Among 70 newborns with chronic lung disease, a fetal inflammatory response was present in 76% (53/70) of the cases and was more common among those with atypical chronic lung disease [90% (27/30) vs 65% (26/40); $p < 0.05$].

Although prematurity and antenatal infection/inflammation are considered risk factors for both WMD and BPD, there is no evidence that BPD or other adverse neonatal respiratory outcomes are more common among infants with an ultrasonographic diagnosis of WMD than among those without such a diagnosis.[183,186–188] In contrast, an association between BPD and CP has been reported in five of six studies.[186,189–194] Dammann et al coined the term 'tip-of-the-iceberg' effect to describe this paradox: BPD is associated with CP, but not with its predecessor (WMD).[189] The hypothesis is that what is seen on the brain ultrasound represents only a small portion of all the WMD that occurs in preterm infants. Specifically, ultrasound would not be sufficiently sensitive to detect all WMD lesions associated with later developmental disabilities.[186] For example, whereas ultrasound is capable of determining gross necrotic lesions of the cerebral white matter, it does not perform as well as diffusion-weighted MRI in the identification of early diffuse WMD.[186]

INTRAUTERINE INFECTION/INFLAMMATION AS A CHRONIC PROCESS

Although intrauterine infection is traditionally considered an acute complication of pregnancy, accumulating evidence suggests it may be a chronic condition. The evidence in support of this view is derived from studies of the microbiological state of the amniotic fluid, as well as the concentration of inflammatory mediators at the time of genetic amniocentesis.

CHRONIC INTRA-AMNIOTIC INFLAMMATION/INFECTION AND PRETERM BIRTH

Amniotic fluid IL-6 concentration is a marker of intra-amniotic inflammation and is frequently associated with microbiological infection in either the amniotic fluid or chorioamniotic space.[195–198] Romero et al[199] conducted a case–control study in which IL-6 was measured in the stored amniotic fluid of women who had a pregnancy loss after a midtrimester amniocentesis, and compared the IL-6 concentration with samples from a control group who delivered at term. Patients who lost their pregnancies had a significantly higher median amniotic fluid IL-6 concentration than those with a normal outcome. Similar findings were reported by Wenstrom et al.[200] In contrast, maternal plasma IL-6 concentration is not associated with adverse pregnancy outcome. Chaiworapongsa et al[201] compared amniotic fluid MCP-1 concentration at the time of genetic amniocentesis in 10 patients who had a pregnancy loss after the procedure with MCP-1 concentration in a control group of 84 patients. MCP-1 concentrations were higher among those who had a spontaneous pregnancy loss after the procedure than in those with a normal pregnancy outcome. An amniotic fluid MCP-1 concentration >765 pg/ml was strongly associated with pregnancy loss (OR = 7.35, 95% CI 1.7–31).

There is also an association between markers of inflammation in midtrimester amniotic fluid of asymptomatic women and preterm delivery. The concentrations of MMP8,[202] IL-6,[203] TNF-α,[204] angiogenin,[205] and C-reactive protein[206] in amniotic fluid samples obtained at midtrimester amniocentesis were each elevated in patients who subsequently delivered preterm.

Collectively, the evidence suggests that a chronic intra-amniotic inflammatory process is associated with both spontaneous abortion and spontaneous preterm delivery. Whether intra-amniotic inflammation is detectable non-invasively remains to be determined. Goldenberg et al[207] demonstrated that the maternal plasma concentration of G-CSF at 24 and 28 weeks of gestation was associated with early preterm birth. To the extent that G-CSF may reflect an inflammatory process, this finding suggests that a chronic inflammatory process identifiable in the maternal compartment is associated with early preterm birth.

MOLECULAR MECHANISMS FOR PRETERM PARTURITION IN THE CONTEXT OF INTRAUTERINE INFLAMMATION/INFECTION

A considerable body of evidence supports a role for inflammatory mediators in the mechanisms of preterm parturition associated with infection. These factors may also play a part in spontaneous labor at term, although the evidence for it is less compelling. Much attention has been placed on proinflammatory cytokines (such as IL-1β and TNF-α), and chemokines (such as IL-8). However, other proinflammatory and anti-inflammatory cytokines may be relevant, including platelet activating factor, prostaglandins, and arachidonate lipoxygenase metabolites.[13] The current understanding of the pathophysiology of preterm parturition in the context of intrauterine infection is summarized below. The interested reader is referred to the references for a comprehensive discussion.[13]

PROSTAGLANDINS AND LIPOXYGENASE PRODUCTS

Intrauterine prostaglandins are considered by many to be the key mediators of the biochemical mechanisms regulating the onset of labor. They can induce myometrial contractility,[208–211] as well as changes in the extracellular matrix metabolism associated with cervical ripening.[212–216] In addition, they are thought to participate in decidual/fetal membrane activation.[13]

The evidence traditionally invoked in support of a role for prostaglandins in the initiation of human labor includes:

- administration of prostaglandins induces early and late termination of pregnancy (abortion or labor)[217–225]
- treatment with indomethacin or aspirin delays the spontaneous onset of parturition in animals[226–228]
- concentrations of prostaglandins in plasma and amniotic fluid increase during labor[229–235]
- intra-amniotic injection of arachidonic acid can induce abortion.[236]

Infection can increase prostaglandin production by amnion, chorion, or decidua through the activity of bacterial products, proinflammatory cytokines, growth factors, and other inflammatory mediators. Indeed, amniotic fluid concentrations of prostaglandins PGE_2 and $PGF_{2\alpha}$ and their stable metabolites, PGEM and PGFM, are significantly higher in women with preterm labor and MIAC than in those with preterm labor without infection. Moreover, amnion obtained from women with histological chorioamnionitis produces higher amounts of prostaglandins than amnion obtained from patients without histological chorioamnionitis.

Metabolites of arachidonic acid derived through the lipoxygenase pathway, including leukotrienes (LTs) and hydroxyeicosatetraenoic acids (HETEs), are also implicated in the mechanisms of spontaneous preterm and term parturition. Concentrations of 5-HETE, LT-B_4, and 15-HETE are increased in the amniotic fluid of women with preterm labor and MIAC. Similarly, amnion from patients with histological chorioamnionitis releases more LT-B_4 in vitro than amnion from women delivering preterm without inflammation. However, the precise role of arachidonate lipoxygenase metabolites in human parturition remains to be determined. 5-HETE and LT-C_4 can stimulate uterine contractility, and LT-B_4 is thought to play a role in the recruitment of neutrophils to the site of infection as well as regulation of the specific arachidonic acid metabolite of the cyclooxygenase (COX) pathway. Additionally, LT-B_4 can act as a calcium ionophore in human intrauterine tissues (i.e. it increases phospholipase activity and enhances the rate of prostaglandin biosynthesis).[237] A role for oxygen-derived free radicals is also proposed in the mechanism of preterm parturition.[238,239] Exposure of chorioamniotic membranes to superoxide anion in vitro results in increased activity of MMP9, a matrix-degrading enzyme involved in the pathogenesis of PROM. Administration of the antioxidant N-acetylcysteine inhibits MMP9 activity and the generation of superoxide within the membranes.[238]

PROINFLAMMATORY CYTOKINES

Evidence for the participation of IL-1 and TNF-α in preterm parturition includes:

1. IL-1β and TNF-α stimulate prostaglandin production by amnion, decidua, and myometrium,[240–242] whereas prostaglandins are considered a central mediator for the onset of labor.
2. Human decidua produces IL-1β and TNF-α in response to bacterial products.[240,243,244]
3. Amniotic fluid IL-1β and TNF-α bioactivity and concentrations are elevated in women with preterm labor and intra-amniotic infection.[245–248]
4. In women with preterm PROM and intra-amniotic infection, IL-1β and TNF-α concentrations are higher in the presence of labor.[237,240–242]
5. IL-1β and TNF-α induce preterm parturition when administered systemically to pregnant animals.[249,250]
6. Pre-treatment with the natural IL-1 receptor antagonist prior to the administration of IL-1 to pregnant animals prevents preterm parturition.[251]
7. Fetal plasma IL-β is elevated in the context of preterm labor with intrauterine infection.[19]
8. Placental tissue obtained from patients in labor, particularly those with chorioamnionitis, produces larger amounts of IL-1β than that obtained from women not in labor.[252]

However, there is considerable redundancy in the cytokine network, and it remains unclear whether a particular cytokine signals the onset of labor. Experimental studies in which anti-TNF and the natural IL-1 receptor antagonist (IL-1ra) were administered to pregnant animals with intrauterine infection did not prevent preterm delivery.[253] The results of knockout animal experiments suggest that infection-induced preterm labor and delivery occurs in subjects lacking a particular cytokine.[254]

The precise mechanisms of action by which IL-1 and TNF participate in the activation of the myometrium have been the subject of intensive research, and some evidence suggests that they involve the participation of cytosolic phospholipase A_2 (PLA$_2$), cyclooxygenase-2 (COX-2),[255,256] MAP kinases,[257] and NF-κB. Thrombin, an enzyme with oxytocin-like properties that is generated during the course of inflammation, is also postulated to have a role.[258–262] A novel observation is that labor is associated with increased activity of NF-κB, a transcription factor responsible for many of the actions of IL-1 and TNF-α. NF-κβ may affect uterine function by generating a functional progesterone withdrawal.[263]

MATRIX DEGRADING ENZYMES

Preterm PROM accounts for 30–40% of all preterm deliveries. The mechanisms responsible for PROM are only partially understood. Since the tensile strength and elasticity of the chorioamniotic membranes are attributed to extracellular matrix proteins, matrix-degrading enzymes have been implicated in preterm PROM. There is now compelling evidence that preterm PROM is associated with increased availability of MMP1,[264] MMP8,[265–267] MMP9,[268–270] and neutrophil elastase,[271] but not MMP2,[268,272] MMP3,[273] MMP7,[274] and MMP13.[275] Proposed mechanisms to regulate the expression and activity of matrix-degrading enzymes in fetal membranes include programmed cell death (apoptosis)[276] and increased availability of superoxide anions (redox state),[238] respectively.

Since intrauterine infection is present in 30% of patients with preterm PROM and proinflammatory cytokines can stimulate the production of MMP1, MMP9, and MMP8, a genetic predisposition to overproduction of MMPs in response to microorganisms has been implicated in the genesis of PROM. Fetal carriage of two functional polymorphisms for MMP1 and MMP9 have been associated with preterm PROM.[277,278]

A polymorphism at nt-1607 in the MMP1 promoter [an insertion of a guanine (G)] creates a core Ets binding site and increases promoter activity.[278] The 2G promoter has an activity more than two times greater than the 1G allele in amnion mesenchymal cells and a cloned amnion cell line. Phorbol 12-myristate 13-acetate (PMA) increased mesenchymal cell nuclear protein binding with greater affinity to the 2G allele. Induction of MMP1 mRNA by PMA is significantly greater in cells with a 1G/2G or 2G/2G genotype than in cells homozygous for the 1G allele. After treatment with PMA, the 1G/2G and 2G/2G cells produce greater amounts of MMP1 protein than 1G/1G cells. A significant association was found between the presence of a 2G allele in the fetus and preterm PROM. Thus, the 2G allele has stronger promoter activity in amnion cells and confers increased responsiveness of amnion cells to stimuli that induce MMP1. Carriage of this polymorphism augments the risk of preterm PROM.[278]

A second polymorphism implicated in preterm PROM is located within the MMP9 gene.[277] Functional studies of the 14 CA-repeat allele indicate the allele is a stronger promoter than the 20 CA-repeat allele in both amnion epithelial cells and WISH amnion-derived cells (yet the 14 and 20 CA-repeat alleles have similar activities in monocyte/macrophage cell lines). A case–control study concluded that the 14 CA-repeat allele was more common in newborns delivered to mothers who had preterm PROM than in those who delivered at term. Thus, differences in MMP9 promoter activity related to the CA-repeat number and fetal carriage of the 14 CA-repeat allele appeared to be associated with preterm PROM.[277]

MANAGEMENT OF FETAL INFLAMMATORY RESPONSE SYNDROME

Three approaches can be used to interrupt the course of FIRS:

- delivery
- antimicrobial treatment of women in whom the FIRS is due to microbial invasion of susceptible bacteria
- administration of agents that down-regulate the inflammatory response.

Preterm delivery places the unborn child at risk for complications of prematurity. Therefore, the risks of prematurity and intrauterine infection must be balanced.

The administration of antimicrobial agents may eradicate MIAC in cases of preterm PROM.[43,279] The results of the ORACLE I trial suggest that antibiotic administration may not only delay the onset of labor but may also improve neonatal outcome.[279] These findings are supported by recent experimental evidence in pregnant rabbits inoculated with *E coli*.[280] Antibiotic administration within 12 hours of microbial inoculation (but not after 18 hours) effectively prevented maternal fever, reduced the rate of preterm delivery, and improved neonatal survival. It is tempting to postulate that this was accomplished by modulating the fetal inflammatory response.

Agents that down-regulate the inflammatory response, such as anti-inflammatory cytokines (i.e. IL-10),[281,282] antibody to MIF,[283,284] and antioxidants, may also play a role in preventing preterm delivery, neonatal injury, and long-term perinatal morbidity.[238,285,286] A combination of antibiotics and immunomodulators (dexamethasone and indomethacin) was effective in non-human pregnant primates to eradicate infection, suppress the inflammatory response, and prolong gestation in experimental premature labor induced by intra-amniotic inoculation with group B streptococci.[287] Collectively, this evidence indicates that immunomodulation may be an effective intervention in preventing fetal injury and prolonging gestation among patients with inflammation/infection-induced preterm labor.

REFERENCES

1. Gomez R, Romero R, Ghezzi F et al. The fetal inflammatory response syndrome. Am J Obstet Gynecol 1998; 179:194–202.
2. Romero R, Gomez R, Ghezzi F et al. A fetal systemic inflammatory response is followed by the spontaneous onset of preterm parturition. Am J Obstet Gynecol 1998; 179:186–193.
3. Yoon BH, Romero R, Park JS et al. Fetal exposure to an intra-amniotic inflammation and the development of cerebral palsy at the age of three years. Am J Obstet Gynecol 2000; 182:675–681.

4. Yoon BH, Romero R, Kim KS et al. A systemic fetal inflammatory response and the development of bronchopulmonary dysplasia. Am J Obstet Gynecol 1999; 181:773–779.

5. Brocklehurst P. Infection and preterm delivery. BMJ 1999; 318:548–549.

6. Gibbs RS, Romero R, Hillier SL, Eschenbach DA, Sweet RL. A review of premature birth and subclinical infection. Am J Obstet Gynecol 1992; 166:1515–1528.

7. Goldenberg RL, Hauth JC, Andrews WW. Intrauterine infection and preterm delivery. N Engl J Med 2000; 342:1500–1507.

8. Ledger WJ. Infection and premature labor. Am J Perinatol 1989; 6:234–236.

9. Minkoff H. Prematurity: infection as an etiologic factor. Obstet Gynecol 1983; 62:137–144.

10. Naeye RL, Ross SM. Amniotic fluid infection syndrome. Clin Obstet Gynaecol 1982; 9:593–607.

11. Romero R, Mazor M. Infection and preterm labor. Clin Obstet Gynecol 1988; 31:553–584.

12. Romero R, Mazor M, Wu YK et al. Infection in the pathogenesis of preterm labor. Semin Perinatol 1988; 12:262–279.

13. Romero R, Mazor M, Munoz H et al. The preterm labor syndrome. Ann NY Acad Sci 1994; 734:414–429.

14. Janeway CA, Travers P, Walport M, Shlomchik M. Basic concepts in immunology. In: Janeway CA, Travers P, Walport M, Shlomchik M, eds. Immunobiology: The Immune System in Health and Disease. New York: Garland; 2001: 1–34.

15. Gallin JI, Snyderman R. Inflammation: Historical Perspective. In: Fearon DT, Haynes BF, Nathan C, eds. Inflammation Basic Principles and Clinical Correlates. Philadelphia: Lippincott, Williams & Wilkins; 1999: 5–12.

16. American College of Chest Physicians/Society of Critical Care Medicine Consensus Conference. Definitions for sepsis and organ failure and guidelines for the use of innovative therapies in sepsis. Crit Care Med 1992; 20:864–874.

17. Weiss M, Moldawer LL, Schneider EM. Granulocyte colony-stimulating factor to prevent the progression of systemic nonresponsiveness in systemic inflammatory response syndrome and sepsis. Blood 1999; 93:425–439.

18. Levy MM, Fink MP, Marshall JC et al. 2001 SCCM/ESICM/ACCP/ATS/SIS International Sepsis Definitions Conference. Intensive Care Med 2003; 29:530–538.

19. Gomez R, Ghezzi F, Romero R et al. Two thirds of human fetuses with microbial invasion of the amniotic cavity have a detectable systemic cytokine response before birth. Am J Obstet Gynecol 1997; 176:514.

20. Billingham RE, Brent L, Medawar PB. Activity acquired tolerance of foreign cells. Nature 1953; 172:603–606.

21. Ridge JP, Fuchs EJ, Matzinger P. Neonatal tolerance revisited: turning on newborn T cells with dendritic cells. Science 1996; 271: 1723–1726.

22. Sarzotti M, Robbins DS, Hoffman PM. Induction of protective CTL responses in newborn mice by a murine retrovirus. Science 1996; 271:1726–1728.

23. Forsthuber T, Yip HC, Lehmann PV. Induction of TH1 and TH2 immunity in neonatal mice. Science 1996; 271:1728–1730.

24. Van Parijs L, Abbas AK. Homeostasis and self-tolerance in the immune system: turning lymphocytes off. Science 1998; 280:243–248.

25. Sakaguchi S. Naturally arising CD4+ regulatory t cells for immunologic self-tolerance and negative control of immune responses. Annu Rev Immunol 2004; 22:531–562.

26. Shevach EM. CD4+ CD25+ suppressor T cells: more questions than answers. Nat Rev Immunol 2002; 2:389–400.

27. Izcue A, Powrie F. Prenatal tolerance – a role for regulatory T cells? Eur J Immunol 2005; 35:379–382.

28. Viglietta V, Baecher-Allan C, Weiner HL, Hafler DA. Loss of functional suppression by CD4+CD25+ regulatory T cells in patients with multiple sclerosis. J Exp Med 2004; 199:971–979.

29. Kriegel MA, Lohmann T, Gabler C et al. Defective suppressor function of human CD4+ CD25+ regulatory T cells in autoimmune polyglandular syndrome type II. J Exp Med 2004; 199:1285–1291.

30. Ehrenstein MR, Evans JG, Singh A et al. Compromised function of regulatory T cells in rheumatoid arthritis and reversal by anti-TNFalpha therapy. J Exp Med 2004; 200:277–285.

31. Asano M, Toda M, Sakaguchi N, Sakaguchi S. Autoimmune disease as a consequence of developmental abnormality of a T cell subpopulation. J Exp Med 1996; 184:387–396.

32. Cupedo T, Nagasawa M, Weijer K, Blom B, Spits H. Development and activation of regulatory T cells in the human fetus. Eur J Immunol 2005; 35:383–390.

33. Matsuoka T, Matsubara T, Katayama K et al. Increase of cord blood cytokine-producing T cells in intrauterine infection. Pediatr Int 2001; 43:453–457.

34. Yoneyama Y, Suzuki S, Sawa R et al. Changes in the proportion of T helper 1 and T helper 2 cells in cord blood after premature rupture of membranes. Arch Gynecol Obstet 2003; 267:217–220.

35. Chaiworapongsa T, Romero R, Kim JC et al. Evidence for fetal involvement in the pathologic process of clinical chorioamnionitis. Am J Obstet Gynecol 2002; 186:1178–1182.

36. Witt A, Berger A, Gruber CJ et al. IL-8 concentrations in maternal serum, amniotic fluid and cord blood in relation to different pathogens within the amniotic cavity. J Perinat Med 2005; 33:22–26.

37. Pacora P, Chaiworapongsa T, Maymon E et al. Funisitis and chorionic vasculitis: the histological counterpart of the fetal inflammatory response syndrome. J Matern Fetal Neonatal Med 2002; 11: 18–25.

38. D'Alquen D, Kramer BW, Seidenspinner S et al. Activation of umbilical cord endothelial cells and fetal inflammatory response in preterm infants with chorioamnionitis and funisitis. Pediatr Res 2005; 57:263–269.

39. Yoon BH, Romero R, Park JS et al. The relationship among inflammatory lesions of the umbilical cord (funisitis), umbilical cord plasma interleukin 6 concentration, amniotic fluid infection, and neonatal sepsis. Am J Obstet Gynecol 2000; 183:1124–1129.

40. Yoon BH, Romero R, Shim JY et al. C-reactive protein in umbilical cord blood: a simple and widely available clinical method to assess the risk of amniotic fluid infection and funisitis. J Matern Fetal Neonatal Med 2003; 14:85–90.

41. Sampson JE, Theve RP, Blatman RN et al. Fetal origin of amniotic fluid polymorphonuclear leukocytes. Am J Obstet Gynecol 1997; 176:77–81.

42. Shim SS, Yoon BH, Romero R et al. The frequency and clinical significance on intra-amniotic inflammation in patients with preterm premature rupture of the membranes. Am J Obstet Gynecol 2003; 189:S83.

43. Romero R, Athayde N, Gomez R et al. The fetal inflammatory response syndrome is characterized by the outpouring of a potent extracellular matrix degrading enzyme into the fetal circulation. Am J Obstet Gynecol 1998; 178:S3.

44. Romero R, Chaiworapongsa T, Espinoza J et al. Fetal plasma MMP-9 concentrations are elevated in preterm premature rupture of the membranes. Am J Obstet Gynecol 2002; 187:1125–1130.

45. Gomez R, Berry S, Yoon BH et al. The hematologic profile of the fetus with systemic inflammatory response syndrome. Am J Obstet Gynecol 1998; 178:S202.

46. Berry SM, Gomez R, Athayde N et al. The role of granulocyte colony stimulating factor in the neutrophilia observed in the fetal inflammatory response syndrome. Am J Obstet Gynecol 1998; 178: S202.

47. Gomez R, Romero R, Ghezzi F et al. Are fetal hypoxia and acidemia causes of preterm labor and delivery? Am J Obstet Gynecol 1997; 176:S115.

48. Baschat AA, Gembruch U, Reiss I et al. Neonatal nucleated red blood cell counts in growth-restricted fetuses: relationship to arterial and venous Doppler studies. Am J Obstet Gynecol 1999; 181:190–195.

49. Ferber A, Minior VK, Bornstein E, Divon MY. Fetal 'nonreassuring status' is associated with elevation of nucleated red blood cell counts and interleukin-6. Am J Obstet Gynecol 2005; 192:1427–1429.

50. Berry SM, Romero R, Gomez R et al. Premature parturition is characterized by in utero activation of the fetal immune system. Am J Obstet Gynecol 1995; 173:1315–1320.

51. Yoon BH, Romero R, Jun JK et al. An increase in fetal plasma cortisol but not dehydroepiandrosterone sulfate is followed by the onset of preterm labor in patients with preterm premature rupture of the membranes. Am J Obstet Gynecol 1998; 179:1107–1114.

52. Kim YM, Kim GJ, Kim MR et al. Skin: an active component of the fetal innate immune system. Am J Obstet Gynecol 2003; 189(6): S74.

53. Yoon BH, Kim YA, Romero R et al. Association of oligohydramnios in women with preterm premature rupture of membranes with an inflammatory response in fetal, amniotic, and maternal compartments. Am J Obstet Gynecol 1999; 181:784–788.

54. Carroll SG, Papaioannou S, Nicolaides KH. Assessment of fetal activity and amniotic fluid volume in the prediction of intrauterine infection in preterm prelabor amniorrhexis. Am J Obstet Gynecol 1995; 172:1427–1435.

55. Heine RP, Wiesenfeld H, Mortimer L, Greig PC. Amniotic fluid defensins: potential markers of subclinical intrauterine infection. Clin Infect Dis 1998; 27:513–518.

56. Romero R, Espinoza J, Goncalves LF et al. Fetal cardiac dysfunction in preterm premature rupture of membranes. J Matern Fetal Neonatal Med 2004; 16:146–157.

57. Naqvi TZ. Diastolic function assessment incorporating new techniques in Doppler echocardiography. Rev Cardiovasc Med 2003; 4: 81–99.

58. Nishimura RA, Tajik AJ. Evaluation of diastolic filling of left ventricle in health and disease: Doppler echocardiography is the clinician's Rosetta Stone. J Am Coll Cardiol 1997; 30:8–18.

59. Stoddard MF, Pearson AC, Kern MJ et al. Left ventricular diastolic function: comparison of pulsed Doppler echocardiographic and hemodynamic indexes in subjects with and without coronary artery disease. J Am Coll Cardiol 1989; 13:327–336.

60. Labovitz AJ, Pearson AC. Evaluation of left ventricular diastolic function: clinical relevance and recent Doppler echocardiographic insights. Am Heart J 1987; 114:836–851.

61. Stoddard MF, Pearson AC, Kern MJ et al. Influence of alteration in preload on the pattern of left ventricular diastolic filling as assessed by Doppler echocardiography in humans. Circulation 1989; 79: 1226–1236.

62. Rizzo G, Arduini D, Romanini C. Fetal Doppler echocardiography: principles, technique and reference limits. In: Arduini D, Rizzo G, Romanini C, eds. Fetal Cardiac Function. London: Parthenon; 1995: 33–41.

63. Veille JC, Smith N, Zaccaro D. Ventricular filling patterns of the right and left ventricles in normally grown fetuses: a longitudinal follow-up study from early intrauterine life to age 1 year. Am J Obstet Gynecol 1999; 180:849–858.

64. Parker MM, Shelhamer JH, Bacharach SL et al. Profound but reversible myocardial depression in patients with septic shock. Ann Intern Med 1984; 100:483–490.

65. Yoon BH, Romero R, Moon JB et al. Clinical significance of intra-amniotic inflammation in patients with preterm labor and intact membranes. Am J Obstet Gynecol 2001; 185:1130–1136.

66. Yoon BH, Romero R, Lim JH et al. The clinical significance of detecting Ureaplasma urealyticum by the polymerase chain reaction in the amniotic fluid of patients with preterm labor. Am J Obstet Gynecol 2003; 189:919–924.

67. Yoon BH, Romero R, Kim M et al. Clinical implications of detection of Ureaplasma urealyticum in the amniotic cavity with the polymerase chain reaction. Am J Obstet Gynecol 2000; 183:1130–1137.

68. Court O, Kumar A, Parrillo JE, Kumar A. Clinical review: myocardial depression in sepsis and septic shock. Crit Care 2002; 6:500–508.

69. Kumar A, Krieger A, Symeonides S, Kumar A, Parrillo JE. Myocardial dysfunction in septic shock: Part II. Role of cytokines and nitric oxide. J Cardiothorac Vasc Anesth 2001; 15:485–511.

70. Kumar A, Haery C, Parrillo JE. Myocardial dysfunction in septic shock: Part I. Clinical manifestation of cardiovascular dysfunction. J Cardiothorac Vasc Anesth 2001; 15:364–376.

71. Romero R, Sirtori M, Oyarzun E et al. Infection and labor. V. Prevalence, microbiology, and clinical significance of intraamniotic infection in women with preterm labor and intact membranes. Am J Obstet Gynecol 1989; 161:817–824.

72. Romero R, Hobbins JC, Mitchell MD. Endotoxin stimulates prostaglandin E2 production by human amnion. Obstet Gynecol 1988; 71:227–228.

73. Romero R, Kadar N, Hobbins JC, Duff GW. Infection and labor: the detection of endotoxin in amniotic fluid. Am J Obstet Gynecol 1987; 157:815–819.

74. Romero R, Mazor M, Wu YK et al. Bacterial endotoxin and tumor necrosis factor stimulate prostaglandin production by human decidua. Prostaglandins Leukot Essent Fatty Acids 1989; 37:183–186.

75. Fidel PI Jr, Romero R, Maymon E, Hertelendy F. Bacteria-induced or bacterial product-induced preterm parturition in mice and rabbits is preceded by a significant fall in serum progesterone concentrations. J Matern Fetal Med 1998; 7:222–226.

76. Romero R, Roslansky P, Oyarzun E et al. Labor and infection. II. Bacterial endotoxin in amniotic fluid and its relationship to the onset of preterm labor. Am J Obstet Gynecol 1988; 158:1044–1049.

77. Van Amersfoort ES, Van Berkel TJ, Kuiper J. Receptors, mediators, and mechanisms involved in bacterial sepsis and septic shock. Clin Microbiol Rev 2003; 16:379–414.

78. Schumann RR, Leong SR, Flaggs GW et al. Structure and function of lipopolysaccharide binding protein. Science 1990; 249:1429–1431.

79. Schumann RR. Function of lipopolysaccharide (LPS)-binding protein (LBP) and CD14, the receptor for LPS/LBP complexes: a short review. Res Immunol 1992; 143:11–15.

80. Schumann RR, Zweigner J. A novel acute-phase marker: lipopolysaccharide binding protein (LBP). Clin Chem Lab Med 1999; 37:271–274.

81. Tobias PS, Soldau K, Ulevitch RJ. Isolation of a lipopolysaccharide-binding acute phase reactant from rabbit serum. J Exp Med 1986; 164:777–793.

82. Hoshino K, Takeuchi O, Kawai T et al. Cutting edge: Toll-like receptor 4 (TLR4)-deficient mice are hyporesponsive to lipopolysaccharide:

evidence for TLR4 as the Lps gene product. J Immunol 1999; 162:3749–3752.

83. Downey JS, Han J. Cellular activation mechanisms in septic shock. Front Biosci 1998; 3:d468–d476.

84. Fenton MJ, Golenbock DT. LPS-binding proteins and receptors. J Leukoc Biol 1998; 64:25–32.

85. Schumann RR, Latz E. Lipopolysaccharide-binding protein. Chem Immunol 2000; 74:42–60.

86. Rounioja S, Rasanen J, Glumoff V et al Intra-amniotic lipopolysaccharide leads to fetal cardiac dysfunction. A mouse model for fetal inflammatory response. Cardiovasc Res 2003; 60:156–164.

87. Knuefermann P, Nemoto S, Misra A et al. CD14-deficient mice are protected against lipopolysaccharide-induced cardiac inflammation and left ventricular dysfunction. Circulation 2002; 106:2608–2615.

88. Nemoto S, Vallejo JG, Knuefermann P et al. Escherichia coli LPS-induced LV dysfunction: role of toll-like receptor-4 in the adult heart. Am J Physiol Heart Circ Physiol 2002; 282:H2316–H2323.

89. Kadokami T, McTiernan CF, Kubota T et al. Effects of soluble TNF receptor treatment on lipopolysaccharide-induced myocardial cytokine expression. Am J Physiol Heart Circ Physiol 2001; 280:H2281–H2291.

90. Yanowitz TD, Jordan JA, Gilmour CH et al. Hemodynamic disturbances in premature infants born after chorioamnionitis: association with cord blood cytokine concentrations. Pediatr Res 2002; 51:310–316.

91. Garnier Y, Coumans AB, Jensen A, Hasaart TH, Berger R. Infection-related perinatal brain injury: the pathogenic role of impaired fetal cardiovascular control. J Soc Gynecol Investig 2003; 10:450–459.

92. Kraut EJ, Chen S, Hubbard NE, Erickson KL, Wisner DH. Tumor necrosis factor depresses myocardial contractility in endotoxemic swine. J Trauma 1999; 46:900–906.

93. Abraham E, Anzueto A, Gutierrez G et al. Double-blind randomised controlled trial of monoclonal antibody to human tumour necrosis factor in treatment of septic shock. NORASEPT II Study Group. Lancet 1998; 351:929–933.

94. Vincent JL, Bakker J, Marecaux G et al. Administration of anti-TNF antibody improves left ventricular function in septic shock patients. Results of a pilot study. Chest 1992; 101:810–815.

95. Lahra MM, Jeffery HE. A fetal response to chorioamnionitis is associated with early survival after preterm birth. Am J Obstet Gynecol 2004; 190:147–151.

96. Olding L. Bacterial infection in cases of perinatal death. A morphological and bacteriological study based on 264 autopsies. Acta Paediatr Scand 1966; Suppl.

97. Madan E, Meyer MP, Amortequi A. Chorioamnionitis: a study of organisms isolated in perinatal autopsies. Ann Clin Lab Sci 1988; 18:39–45.

98. Osman NB, Folgosa E, Gonzales C, Bergstrom S. Genital infections in the aetiology of late fetal death: an incident case-referent study. J Trop Pediatr 1995; 41:258–266.

99. Moyo SR, Hagerstrand I, Nystrom L et al. Stillbirths and intrauterine infection, histologic chorioamnionitis and microbiological findings. Int J Gynaecol Obstet 1996; 54:115–123.

100. Mwanyumba F, Inion I, Gaillard P et al. Placental inflammation and perinatal outcome. Eur J Obstet Gynecol Reprod Biol 2003; 108:164–170.

101. Quinn PA, Butany J, Taylor J, Hannah W. Chorioamnionitis: its association with pregnancy outcome and microbial infection. Am J Obstet Gynecol 1987; 156:379–387.

102. Blackwell S, Romero R, Chaiworapongsa T et al. Maternal and fetal inflammatory responses in unexplained fetal death. J Matern Fetal Neonatal Med 2003; 14:151–157.

103. Blackwell S, Romero R, Chaiworapongsa T et al. Unexplained fetal death is associated with changes in the adaptive limb of the maternal immune response consistent with prior antigenic exposure. J Matern Fetal Neonatal Med 2003; 14:241–246.

104. Grether JK, Nelson KB. Maternal infection and cerebral palsy in infants of normal birth weight. JAMA 1997; 278:207–211.

105. Paneth N, Kiely J. The frequency of cerebral palsy: a review of population studies in industrialized nations since 1950. In: Stanley F, Alberman E, eds. The Epidemiology of the Cerebral Palsies. Oxford: Blackwell Scientific Publications; 1984: 46–56.

106. Stanley FJ, Watson L. Trends in perinatal mortality and cerebral palsy in Western Australia, 1967 to 1985. BMJ 1992; 304:1658–1663.

107. Murphy DJ, Sellers S, MacKenzie IZ, Yudkin PL, Johnson AM. Case-control study of antenatal and intrapartum risk factors for cerebral palsy in very preterm singleton babies. Lancet 1995; 346:1449–1454.

108. Yoon BH, Kim CJ, Romero R et al. Experimentally induced intrauterine infection causes fetal brain white matter lesions in rabbits. Am J Obstet Gynecol 1997; 177:797–802.

109. Yoon BH, Jun JK, Romero R et al. Amniotic fluid inflammatory cytokines (interleukin-6, interleukin-1beta, and tumor necrosis factor-alpha), neonatal brain white matter lesions, and cerebral palsy. Am J Obstet Gynecol 1997; 177:19–26.

110. Nelson KB, Dambrosia JM, Grether JK, Phillips TM. Neonatal cytokines and coagulation factors in children with cerebral palsy. Ann Neurol 1998; 44:665–675.

111. Eastman NJ, DeLeon M. The etiology of cerebral palsy. Am J Obstet Gynecol 1955; 69:950–961.

112. Nelson KB, Ellenberg JH. Epidemiology of cerebral palsy. Adv Neurol 1978; 19:421–435.

113. Bejar R, Wozniak P, Allard M et al. Antenatal origin of neurologic damage in newborn infants. I. Preterm infants. Am J Obstet Gynecol 1988; 159:357–363.

114. Verma U, Tejani N, Klein S et al. Obstetric antecedents of intraventricular hemorrhage and periventricular leukomalacia in the low-birth-weight neonate. Am J Obstet Gynecol 1997; 176:275–281.

115. O'Shea TM, Klinepeter KL, Dillard RG. Prenatal events and the risk of cerebral palsy in very low birth weight infants. Am J Epidemiol 1998; 147:362–369.

116. Alexander JM, Gilstrap LC, Cox SM, McIntire DM, Leveno KJ. Clinical chorioamnionitis and the prognosis for very low birth weight infants. Obstet Gynecol 1998; 91:725–729.

117. Dammann O, Leviton A. Role of the fetus in perinatal infection and neonatal brain damage. Curr Opin Pediatr 2000; 12:99–104.

118. Nelson KB. The epidemiology of cerebral palsy in term infants. Ment Retard Dev Disabil Res Rev 2002; 8:146–150.

119. Shea KG, Coleman SS, Carroll K, Stevens P, Van Boerum DH. Pemberton pericapsular osteotomy to treat a dysplastic hip in cerebral palsy. J Bone Joint Surg Am 1997; 79:1342–1351.

120. DeReuck J, Chattha AS, Richardson EP Jr. Pathogenesis and evolution of periventricular leukomalacia in infancy. Arch Neurol 1972; 27:229–236.

121. Johnston MV, Trescher WH, Taylor GA. Hypoxic and ischemic central nervous system disorders in infants and children. Adv Pediatr 1995; 42:1–45.

122. Leviton A, Paneth N. White matter damage in preterm newborns – an epidemiologic perspective. Early Hum Dev 1990; 24:1–22.

123. Tamisari L, Vigi V, Fortini C, Scarpa P. Neonatal periventricular leukomalacia: diagnosis and evolution evaluated by real-time ultrasound. Helv Paediatr Acta 1986; 41:399–407.

124. Yoon BH, Romero R, Yang SH et al. Interleukin-6 concentrations in umbilical cord plasma are elevated in neonates with white matter lesions associated with periventricular leukomalacia. Am J Obstet Gynecol 1996; 174:1433–1440.

125. Yoon BH, Romero R, Kim CJ et al. High expression of tumor necrosis factor-alpha and interleukin-6 in periventricular leukomalacia. Am J Obstet Gynecol 1997; 177:406–411.

126. Selmaj KW, Raine CS. Tumor necrosis factor mediates myelin and oligodendrocyte damage in vitro. Ann Neurol 1988; 23:339–346.

127. Robbins DS, Shirazi Y, Drysdale BE et al. Production of cytokine profile in plasma of baboons challenged with lethal and sublethal *Escherichia coli*. Circ Schock 1992; 33:84–91.

128. Leviton A. Preterm birth and cerebral palsy: is tumor necrosis factor the missing link? Dev Med Child Neurol 1993; 35:553–558.

129. Iida K, Takashima S, Takeuchi Y. Etiologies and distribution of neonatal leukomalacia. Pediatr Neurol 1992; 8:205–209.

130. Camussi G, Bussolino F, Salvidio G, Baglioni C. Tumor necrosis factor/cachectin stimulates peritoneal macrophages, polymorphonuclear neutrophils, and vascular endothelial cells to synthesize and release platelet-activating factor. J Exp Med 1987; 166:1390–1404.

131. Benett JC. Approach to the patient with immune disease. In: Benett JC, Plum F, eds. Cecil Textbook of Medicine. Philadephila: WB Saunders; 1996: 1993–1998.

132. Stuber F, Petersen M, Bokelmann F, Schade U. A genomic polymorphism within the tumor necrosis factor locus influences plasma tumor necrosis factor-alpha concentrations and outcome of patients with severe sepsis. Crit Care Med 1996; 24:381–384.

133. McGuire W, Hill AV, Allsopp CE, Greenwood BM, Kwiatkowski D. Variation in the TNF-alpha promoter region associated with susceptibility to cerebral malaria. Nature 1994; 371:508–510.

134. Monzon-Bordonaba F, Parry S, Holder J et al. A genetic marker for preterm delivery. J Soc Gynecol Investig 1998; 5:71A.

135. Wilson AG, Symons JA, McDowell TL, McDevitt HO, Duff GW. Effects of a polymorphism in the human tumor necrosis factor alpha promoter on transcriptional activation. Proc Natl Acad Sci USA 1997; 94:3195–3199.

136. Hagberg B, Hagberg G, Olow I, von Wendt L. The changing panorama of cerebral palsy in Sweden. V. The birth year period 1979–82. Acta Paediatr Scand 1989;78:283–290.

137. Brus F, Van Oeveren W, Okken A, Oetomo SB. Activation of the plasma clotting, fibrinolytic, and kinin–kallikrein system in preterm infants with severe idiopathic respiratory distress syndrome. Pediatr Res 1994; 36:647–653.

138. Chheda S, Palkowetz KH, Garofalo R, Rassin DK, Goldman AS. Decreased interleukin-10 production by neonatal monocytes and T cells: relationship to decreased production and expression of tumor necrosis factor-alpha and its receptors. Pediatr Res 1996; 40: 475–483.

139. Jones CA, Cayabyab RG, Kwong KY et al. Undetectable interleukin (IL)-10 and persistent IL-8 expression early in hyaline membrane disease: a possible developmental basis for the predisposition to chronic lung inflammation in preterm newborns. Pediatr Res 1996; 39:966–975.

140. Brus F, Van Oeveren W, Okken A, Oetomo SB. Disease severity is correlated with plasma clotting and fibrinolytic and kinin–kallikrein activity in neonatal respiratory distress syndrome. Pediatr Res 1997; 41:120–127.

141. Grether JK, Nelson KB, Dambrosia JM, Phillips TM. Interferons and cerebral palsy. J Pediatr 1999; 134:324–332.

142. Blahnik MJ, Ramanathan R, Riley CR, Minoo P. Lipopolysaccharide-induced tumor necrosis factor-alpha and IL-10 production by lung macrophages from preterm and term neonates. Pediatr Res 2001; 50:726–731.

143. Dammann O, Leviton A, Gappa M, Dammann CE. Lung and brain damage in preterm newborns, and their association with gestational age, prematurity subgroup, infection/inflammation and long term outcome. BJOG 2005; 112 (Suppl 1):4–9.

144. Rogers S, Witz G, Anwar M, Hiatt M, Hegyi T. Antioxidant capacity and oxygen radical diseases in the preterm newborn. Arch Pediatr Adolesc Med 2000; 154:544–548.

145. Nelson KB, Dambrosia JM, Iovannisci DM et al. Genetic polymorphisms and cerebral palsy in very preterm infants. Pediatr Res 2005; 57:494–499.

146. O'Shea TM, Klinepeter KL, Meis PJ, Dillard RG. Intrauterine infection and the risk of cerebral palsy in very low-birthweight infants. Paediatr Perinat Epidemiol 1998; 12:72–83.

147. Redline RW, Wilson-Costello D, Borawski E, Fanaroff AA, Hack M. Placental lesions associated with neurologic impairment and cerebral palsy in very-low-birth-weight infants. Arch Pathol Lab Med 1998; 122:1091–1098.

148. Grether JK, Nelson KB. Intrauterine infection and cerebral palsy in preterm children. Am J Obstet Gynecol 2000; 182:S95.

149. Jacobsson B, Hagberg G, Hagberg B et al. Cerebral palsy in preterm infants: a population based analysis of antenatal risk factors. Am J Obstet Gynecol 2000; 182:S29.

150. Matsuda Y, Kouno S, Hiroyama Y et al. Intrauterine infection, magnesium sulfate exposure and cerebral palsy in infants born between 26 and 30 weeks of gestation. Eur J Obstet Gynecol Reprod Biol 2000; 91:159–164.

151. Ng E, Asztalos E, Rose T et al. The association of clinical and histologic chorioamnionitis (CA) with cystic periventricular leukomalacia (cPVL) and cerebral palsy (CP) in preterm infants. Pediatr Res 2000; 47:318A.

152. Roland EH, Magee JF, Rodriguez E, Lupton BA, Hill A. Placental abnormalities: insights into pathogenesis of cystic periventricular leukomalacia. Ann Neurol 1996; 40:3213.

153. Leviton A, Paneth N, Reuss ML et al. Maternal infection, fetal inflammatory response, and brain damage in very low birth weight infants. Developmental Epidemiology Network Investigators. Pediatr Res 1999; 46:566–575.

154. Wu YW. Systematic review of chorioamnionitis and cerebral palsy. Ment Retard Dev Disabil Res Rev 2002; 8:25–29.

155. Duggan PJ, Maalouf EF, Watts TL et al. Intrauterine T-cell activation and increased proinflammatory cytokine concentrations in preterm infants with cerebral lesions. Lancet 2001; 358: 1699–1700.

156. Viscardi RM, Muhumuza CK, Rodriguez A et al. Inflammatory markers in intrauterine and fetal blood and cerebrospinal fluid compartments are associated with adverse pulmonary and neurologic outcomes in preterm infants. Pediatr Res 2004; 55: 1009–1017.

157. Moon JB, Kim JC, Yoon BH et al. Amniotic fluid matrix metalloproteinase-8 and the development of cerebral palsy. J Perinat Med 2002; 30:301–306.

158. Kaukola T, Satyaraj E, Patel DD et al. Cerebral palsy is characterized by protein mediators in cord serum. Ann Neurol 2004; 55:186–194.

159. de Vries LS, Groenendaal F. Neuroimaging in the preterm infant. Ment Retard Dev Disabil Res Rev 2002; 8:273–280.

160. Dammann O, Kuban KC, Leviton A. Perinatal infection, fetal inflammatory response, white matter damage, and cognitive limitations in children born preterm. Ment Retard Dev Disabil Res Rev 2002; 8:46–50.

161. Hagberg B, Hagberg G, Beckung E, Uvebrant P. Changing panorama of cerebral palsy in Sweden. VIII. Prevalence and origin in the birth year period 1991–94. Acta Paediatr 2001; 90:271–277.

162. Stewart AL, Rifkin L, Amess PN et al. Brain structure and neurocognitive and behavioural function in adolescents who were born very preterm. Lancet 1999; 353:1653–1657.

163. Kuban KC, Leviton A. Cerebral palsy. N Engl J Med 1994; 330: 188–195.

164. Bell MJ, Hallenbeck JM. Effects of intrauterine inflammation on developing rat brain. J Neurosci Res 2002; 70:570–579.

165. Debillon T, Gras-Leguen C, Verielle V et al. Intrauterine infection induces programmed cell death in rabbit periventricular white matter. Pediatr Res 2000; 47:736–742.

166. Debillon T, Gras-Leguen C, Leroy S et al. Patterns of cerebral inflammatory response in a rabbit model of intrauterine infection-mediated brain lesion. Brain Res Dev Brain Res 2003; 145:39–48.

167. Duncan JR, Cock ML, Scheerlinck JP et al. White matter injury after repeated endotoxin exposure in the preterm ovine fetus. Pediatr Res 2002; 52:941–949.

168. Hagberg H, Peebles D, Mallard C. Models of white matter injury: comparison of infectious, hypoxic-ischemic, and excitotoxic insults. Ment Retard Dev Disabil Res Rev 2002; 8:30–38.

169. Mallard C, Welin AK, Peebles D, Hagberg H, Kjellmer I. White matter injury following systemic endotoxemia or asphyxia in the fetal sheep. Neurochem Res 2003; 28:215–223.

170. Deguchi K, Mizuguchi M, Takashima S. Immunohistochemical expression of tumor necrosis factor alpha in neonatal leukomalacia. Pediatr Neurol 1996; 14:13–16.

171. Deguchi K, Oguchi K, Takashima S. Characteristic neuropathology of leukomalacia in extremely low birth weight infants. Pediatr Neurol 1997; 16:296–300.

172. Kadhim H, Tabarki B, Verellen G et al. Inflammatory cytokines in the pathogenesis of periventricular leukomalacia. Neurology 2001; 56: 1278–1284.

173. Kadhim H, Tabarki B, De Prez C, Rona AM, Sebire G. Interleukin-2 in the pathogenesis of perinatal white matter damage. Neurology 2002; 58:1125–1128.

174. Kadhim H, Tabarki B, De Prez C, Sebire G. Cytokine immunoreactivity in cortical and subcortical neurons in periventricular leukomalacia: are cytokines implicated in neuronal dysfunction in cerebral palsy? Acta Neuropathol (Berl) 2003; 105:209–216.

175. van der PT, Buller HR, ten Cate H et al. Activation of coagulation after administration of tumor necrosis factor to normal subjects. N Engl J Med 1990; 322:1622–1627.

176. Sharief MK, Thompson EJ. In vivo relationship of tumor necrosis factor-alpha to blood–brain barrier damage in patients with active multiple sclerosis. J Neuroimmunol 1992; 38:27–33.

177. Wong D, Dorovini-Zis K, Vincent SR. Cytokines, nitric oxide, and cGMP modulate the permeability of an in vitro model of the human blood–brain barrier. Exp Neurol 2004; 190:446–455.

178. Hagberg H, Mallard C. Effect of inflammation on central nervous system development and vulnerability. Curr Opin Neurol 2005; 18:117–123.

179. Shennan AT, Dunn MS, Ohlsson A, Lennox K, Hoskins EM. Abnormal pulmonary outcomes in premature infants: prediction from oxygen requirement in the neonatal period. Pediatrics 1988; 82:527–532.

180. Jobe AH, Bancalari E. Bronchopulmonary dysplasia. Am J Respir Crit Care Med 2001; 163:1723–1729.

181. Ghezzi F, Gomez R, Romero R et al. Elevated interleukin-8 concentrations in amniotic fluid of mothers whose neonates subsequently develop bronchopulmonary dysplasia. Eur J Obstet Gynecol Reprod Biol 1998; 78:5–10.

182. Watterberg KL, Demers LM, Scott SM, Murphy S. Chorioamnionitis and early lung inflammation in infants in whom bronchopulmonary dysplasia develops. Pediatrics 1996; 97:210–215.

183. Yoon BH, Romero R, Shim JY et al. 'Atypical' chronic lung disease of the newborn is linked to fetal systemic inflammation. Am J Obstet Gynecol 2002; 187:S129.

184. Jobe AH. Antenatal associations with lung maturation and infection. J Perinatol 2005; 25(Suppl 2):S31–S35.

185. Yoon BH, Romero R, Jun JK et al. Amniotic fluid cytokines (interleukin-6, tumor necrosis factor-alpha, interleukin-1 beta, and interleukin-8) and the risk for the development of bronchopulmonary dysplasia. Am J Obstet Gynecol 1997; 177:825–830.

186. Dammann O, Allred EN, Van Marter LJ, Dammann CE, Leviton A. Bronchopulmonary dysplasia is not associated with ultrasound-defined cerebral white matter damage in preterm newborns. Pediatr Res 2004; 55:319–325.

187. O'Shea TM, Goldstein DJ, deRegnier RA et al. Outcome at 4 to 5 years of age in children recovered from neonatal chronic lung disease. Dev Med Child Neurol 1996; 38:830–839.

188. Rojas MA, Gonzalez A, Bancalari E et al. Changing trends in the epidemiology and pathogenesis of neonatal chronic lung disease. J Pediatr 1995; 126:605–610.

189. Dammann O, Leviton A, Bartels DB, Dammann CE. Lung and brain damage in preterm newborns. Are they related? How? Why? Biol Neonate 2004; 85:305–313.

190. Gray PH, Burns YR, Mohay HA, O'Callaghan MJ, Tudehope DI. Neurodevelopmental outcome of preterm infants with bronchopulmonary dysplasia. Arch Dis Child Fetal Neonatal Ed 1995; 73:F128–F134.

191. Majnemer A, Riley P, Shevell M et al. Severe bronchopulmonary dysplasia increases risk for later neurological and motor sequelae in preterm survivors. Dev Med Child Neurol 2000; 42:53–60.

192. Skidmore MD, Rivers A, Hack M. Increased risk of cerebral palsy among very low-birthweight infants with chronic lung disease. Dev Med Child Neurol 1990; 32:325–332.

193. Vohr BR, Coll CG, Lobato D et al. Neurodevelopmental and medical status of low-birthweight survivors of bronchopulmonary dysplasia at 10 to 12 years of age. Dev Med Child Neurol 1991; 33: 690–697.

194. Vrlenich LA, Bozynski ME, Shyr Y et al. The effect of bronchopulmonary dysplasia on growth at school age. Pediatrics 1995; 95: 855–859.

195. Romero R, Avila C, Santhanam U, Sehgal PB. Amniotic fluid interleukin 6 in preterm labor. Association with infection. J Clin Invest 1990; 85:1392–1400.

196. Romero R, Sepulveda W, Kenney JS et al. Interleukin 6 determination in the detection of microbial invasion of the amniotic cavity. Ciba Found Symp 1992; 167:205–220.

197. Romero R, Yoon BH, Kenney JS et al. Amniotic fluid interleukin-6 determinations are of diagnostic and prognostic value in preterm labor. Am J Reprod Immunol 1993; 30:167–183.

198. Yoon BH, Romero R, Kim CJ et al. Amniotic fluid interleukin-6: a sensitive test for antenatal diagnosis of acute inflammatory lesions of preterm placenta and prediction of perinatal morbidity. Am J Obstet Gynecol 1995; 172:960–970.

199. Romero R, Munoz H, Gomez R et al. Two thirds of spontaneous abortion/fetal deaths after genetic amniocentesis are the result of a pre-existing sub-clinical inflammatory process of the amniotic cavity. Am J Obstet Gynecol 1995; 172:S261.

200. Wenstrom KD, Andrews WW, Tamura T et al. Elevated amniotic fluid interleukin-6 levels at genetic amniocentesis predict subsequent pregnancy loss. Am J Obstet Gynecol 1996; 175: 830–833.

201. Chaiworapongsa T, Romero R, Tolosa JE et al. Elevated monocyte chemotactic protein-1 in amniotic fluid is a risk factor for pregnancy loss. J Matern Fetal Neonatal Med 2002; 12:159–164.

202. Yoon BH, Oh SY, Romero R et al. An elevated amniotic fluid matrix metalloproteinase-8 level at the time of mid-trimester genetic amniocentesis is a risk factor for spontaneous preterm delivery. Am J Obstet Gynecol 2001; 185:1162–1167.

203. Wenstrom KD, Andrews WW, Hauth JC et al. Elevated second-trimester amniotic fluid interleukin-6 levels predict preterm delivery. Am J Obstet Gynecol 1998; 178:546–550.

204. Ghidini A, Eglinton GS, Spong CY et al. Elevated mid-trimester amniotic fluid tumor necrosis alpha levels: a predictor of preterm delivery. Am J Obstet Gynecol 1996; 174:S307.

205. Spong CY, Ghidini A, Sherer DM et al. Angiogenin: a marker for preterm delivery in midtrimester amniotic fluid. Am J Obstet Gynecol 1997; 176:415–418.

206. Ghezzi F, Franchi M, Raio L et al. Elevated amniotic fluid C-reactive protein at the time of genetic amniocentesis is a marker for preterm delivery. Am J Obstet Gynecol 2002; 186:268–273.

207. Goldenberg RL, Andrews WW, Mercer BM et al. The preterm prediction study: granulocyte colony-stimulating factor and spontaneous preterm birth. National Institute of Child Health and Human Development Maternal-Fetal Medicine Units Network. Am J Obstet Gynecol 2000; 182:625–630.

208. Bennett PR, Elder MG, Myatt L. The effects of lipoxygenase metabolites of arachidonic acid on human myometrial contractility. Prostaglandins 1987; 33:837–844.

209. Carraher R, Hahn DW, Ritchie DM, McGuire JL. Involvement of lipoxygenase products in myometrial contractions. Prostaglandins 1983; 26:23–32.

210. Ritchie DM, Hahn DW, McGuire JL. Smooth muscle contraction as a model to study the mediator role of endogenous lipoxygenase products of arachidonic acid. Life Sci 1984; 34:509–513.

211. Wiqvist N, Martin JN, Bygdeman M, Green K. Prostaglandin analogues and uterotonic potency: a comparative study of seven compounds. Prostaglandins 1975; 9:255–269.

212. Calder AA. Pharmacological management of the unripe cervix in the human. In: Naftolin F, Stubblefield P, eds. Dilatation of the Uterine Cervix. New York: Raven Press; 1980: 317.

213. Greer I. Cervical ripening. In: Drife J, Calder AA, eds. Prostaglandins and the Uterus. London: Springer-Verlag; 1992: 191.

214. Ellwood DA, Mitchell MD, Anderson AB, Turnbull AC. The in vitro production of prostanoids by the human cervix during pregnancy: preliminary observations. Br J Obstet Gynaecol 1980; 87:210–214.

215. Rajabi M, Solomon S, Poole AR. Hormonal regulation of interstitial collagenase in the uterine cervix of the pregnant guinea pig. Endocrinology 1991; 128:863–871.

216. Calder AA, Greer IA. Pharmacological modulation of cervical compliance in the first and second trimesters of pregnancy. Semin Perinatol 1991; 15:162–172.

217. Karim SM, Filshie GM. Therapeutic abortion using prostaglandin F_{2alpha}. Lancet 1970; 1:157–159.

218. Embrey MP. Induction of abortion by prostaglandins E_1 and E_2. Br Med J 1970; 1:258–260.

219. Husslein P. Use of prostaglandins for induction of labor. Semin Perinatol 1991; 15:173–181.

220. Macer J, Buchanan D, Yonekura ML. Induction of labor with prostaglandin E_2 vaginal suppositories. Obstet Gynecol 1984; 63:664–668.

221. MacKenzie IZ. Prostaglandins and midtrimester abortion. In: Drife J, Calder AA, eds. Prostaglandins and the Uterus. London: Springer-Verlag; 1992: 119.

222. World Health Organization Task Force. Repeated vaginal administration of 15-methyl PGF_{2a} for termination of pregnancy in the 13th to 20th week of gestation. Contraception 1977; 16:175.

223. World Health Organization Task Force. Comparision of intra-amniotic prostaglanding F_{2a} and hypertonic saline for second trimester abortion. BMJ 1976; 1:1373.

224. World Health Organization Task Force. Termination of second trimester pregnancy by intramuscular injection of 16-phenoxy-ω-17,18,19,20-tetranor-PGE_2 methyl sulphonylamide. Int J Gynaecol Obstet 1982; 20:383–386.

225. Ekman G, Forman A, Marsal K, Ulmsten U. Intravaginal versus intracervical application of prostaglandin E_2 in viscous gel for cervical priming and induction of labor at term in patients with an unfavorable cervical state. Am J Obstet Gynecol 1983; 147: 657–661.

226. Giri SN, Stabenfeldt GH, Moseley TA et al. Role of eicosanoids in abortion and its prevention by treatment with flunixin meglumine in cows during the first trimester of pregnancy. Zentralbl Veterinarmed A 1991; 38:445–459.

227. Keirse MJ, Turnbull AC. E prostaglandins in amniotic fluid during late pregnancy and labour. J Obstet Gynaecol Br Commonw 1973; 80:970–973.

228. Harper MJ, Skarnes RC. Inhibition of abortion and fetal death produced by endotoxin or prostaglandin F_{2alpha}. Prostaglandins 1972; 2:295–309.

229. Romero R, Wu YK, Mazor M, Hobbins JC, Mitchell MD. Increased amniotic fluid leukotriene C4 concentration in term human parturition. Am J Obstet Gynecol 1988; 159:655–657.

230. Sellers SM, Mitchell MD, Anderson AB, Turnbull AC. The relation between the release of prostaglandins at amniotomy and the subsequent onset of labour. Br J Obstet Gynaecol 1981; 88:1211–1216.

231. Romero R, Emamian M, Quintero R et al. Amniotic fluid prostaglandin levels and intra-amniotic infections. Lancet 1986; 1:1380.

232. Romero R, Emamian M, Wan M et al. Prostaglandin concentrations in amniotic fluid of women with intra-amniotic infection and preterm labor. Am J Obstet Gynecol 1987; 157:1461–1467.

233. Romero R, Wu YK, Mazor M, Hobbins JC, Mitchell MD. Amniotic fluid prostaglandin E_2 in preterm labor. Prostaglandins Leukot Essent Fatty Acids 1988; 34:141–145.

234. Keirse MJ. Endogenous prostaglandins in human parturition. In: Keirse MJ, Gravenhorst J, eds. Human Parturition. The Netherlands: Martinus Nijhoff; 1979: 101.

235. Romero R, Wu YK, Mazor M, Hobbins JC, Mitchell MD. Amniotic fluid concentration of 5-hydroxyeicosatetraenoic acid is increased in human parturition at term. Prostaglandins Leukot Essent Fatty Acids 1989; 35:81–83.

236. MacDonald PC, Schultz FM, Duenhoelter JH et al. Initiation of human parturition. I. Mechanism of action of arachidonic acid. Obstet Gynecol 1974; 44:629–636.

237. Serhan CN, Fridovich J, Goetzl EJ, Dunham PB, Weissmann G. Leukotriene B4 and phosphatidic acid are calcium ionophores. Studies employing arsenazo III in liposomes. J Biol Chem 1982; 257:4746–4752.

238. Buhimschi IA, Kramer WB, Buhimschi CS, Thompson LP, Weiner CP. Reduction-oxidation (redox) state regulation of matrix metalloproteinase activity in human fetal membranes. Am J Obstet Gynecol 2000; 182:458–464.

239. Buhimschi IA, Buhimschi CS, Pupkin M, Weiner CP. Beneficial impact of term labor: nonenzymatic antioxidant reserve in the human fetus. Am J Obstet Gynecol 2003; 189:181–188.

240. Romero R, Wu YK, Brody DT et al. Human decidua: a source of interleukin-1. Obstet Gynecol 1989; 73:31–34.

241. Romero R, Mazor M, Manogue K, Oyarzun E, Cerami A. Human decidua: a source of cachectin-tumor necrosis factor. Eur J Obstet Gynecol Reprod Biol 1991; 41:123–127.

242. Romero R, Durum SK, Dinarello CA et al. Interleukin-1: a signal for the initiation of labor in chorioamnionitis. 1986. 33rd Annual Meeting for the Society for Gynecologic Investigation, Toronto, Ontario, Canada.

243. Casey ML, Cox SM, Beutler B, Milewich L, MacDonald PC. Cachectin/tumor necrosis factor-alpha formation in human decidua. Potential role of cytokines in infection-induced preterm labor. J Clin Invest 1989; 83:430–436.

244. Gauldie J, Richards C, Harnish D, Lansdorp P, Baumann H. Interferon beta 2/B-cell stimulatory factor type 2 shares identity with monocyte-derived hepatocyte-stimulating factor and regulates the major acute phase protein response in liver cells. Proc Natl Acad Sci USA 1987; 84:7251–7255.

245. Romero R, Manogue KR, Mitchell MD et al. Infection and labor. IV. Cachectin-tumor necrosis factor in the amniotic fluid of women with intraamniotic infection and preterm labor. Am J Obstet Gynecol 1989; 161:336–341.

246. Romero R, Brody DT, Oyarzun E et al. Infection and labor. III. Interleukin-1: a signal for the onset of parturition. Am J Obstet Gynecol 1989; 160:1117–1123.

247. Romero R, Mazor M, Sepulveda W et al. Tumor necrosis factor in preterm and term labor. Am J Obstet Gynecol 1992; 166: 1576–1587.

248. Romero R, Mazor M, Brandt F et al. Interleukin-1 alpha and interleukin-1 beta in preterm and term human parturition. Am J Reprod Immunol 1992; 27:117–123.

249. Romero R, Mazor M, Tartakovsky B. Systemic administration of interleukin-1 induces preterm parturition in mice. Am J Obstet Gynecol 1991; 165:969–971.

250. Silver RM. Tumor necrosis factor-alpha mediates LPS-induced abortion: evidence from the LPS-resistant murine strain C3H/HeJ. J Soc Gynecol Investig 1993.

251. Romero R, Tartakovsky B. The natural interleukin-1 receptor antagonist prevents interleukin-1-induced preterm delivery in mice. Am J Obstet Gynecol 1992; 167:1041–1045.

252. Taniguchi T, Matsuzaki N, Kameda T et al. The enhanced production of placental interleukin-1 during labor and intrauterine infection. Am J Obstet Gynecol 1991; 165:131–137.

253. Fidel PL Jr, Romero R, Cutright J et al. Treatment with the interleukin-1 receptor antagonist and soluble tumor necrosis factor receptor Fc fusion protein does not prevent endotoxin-induced preterm parturition in mice. J Soc Gynecol Investig 1997; 4:22–26.

254. Hirsch E, Muhle RA, Mussalli GM, Blanchard R. Bacterially induced preterm labor in the mouse does not require maternal interleukin-1 signaling. Am J Obstet Gynecol 2002; 186:523–530.

255. Molnar M, Romero R, Hertelendy F. Interleukin-1 and tumor necrosis factor stimulate arachidonic acid release and phospholipid metabolism in human myometrial cells. Am J Obstet Gynecol 1993; 169:825–829.

256. Hertelendy F, Rastogi P, Molnar M, Romero R. Interleukin-1beta-induced prostaglandin E_2 production in human myometrial cells: role of a pertussis toxin-sensitive component. Am J Reprod Immunol 2001; 45:142–147.

257. Molnar M, Rigo J Jr, Romero R, Hertelendy F. Oxytocin activates mitogen-activated protein kinase and up-regulates cyclooxygenase-2 and prostaglandin production in human myometrial cells. Am J Obstet Gynecol 1999; 181:42–49.

258. Elovitz MA, Saunders T, Ascher-Landsberg J, Phillippe M. Effects of thrombin on myometrial contractions in vitro and in vivo. Am J Obstet Gynecol 2000; 183:799–804.

259. Elovitz MA, Ascher-Landsberg J, Saunders T, Phillippe M. The mechanisms underlying the stimulatory effects of thrombin on myometrial smooth muscle. Am J Obstet Gynecol 2000; 183:674–681.

260. Elovitz MA, Baron J, Phillippe M. The role of thrombin in preterm parturition. Am J Obstet Gynecol 2001; 185:1059–1063.

261. Phillippe M, Elovitz M, Saunders T. Thrombin-stimulated uterine contractions in the pregnant and nonpregnant rat. J Soc Gynecol Investig 2001; 8:260–265.

262. Chaiworapongsa T, Espinoza J, Yoshimatsu J et al. Activation of coagulation system in preterm labor and preterm premature rupture of membranes. J Matern Fetal Neonatal Med 2002; 11:368–373.

263. Allport VC, Pieber D, Slater DM et al. Human labour is associated with nuclear factor-kappaB activity which mediates cyclooxygenase-2 expression and is involved with the 'functional progesterone withdrawal'. Mol Hum Reprod 2001; 7:581–586.

264. Maymon E, Romero R, Pacora P et al. Evidence for the participation of interstitial collagenase (matrix metalloproteinase 1) in preterm premature rupture of membranes. Am J Obstet Gynecol 2000; 183:914–920.

265. Maymon E, Romero R, Pacora P et al. Human neutrophil collagenase (matrix metalloproteinase 8) in parturition, premature rupture of the membranes, and intrauterine infection. Am J Obstet Gynecol 2000; 183:94–99.

266. Maymon E, Romero R, Chaiworapongsa T et al. Value of amniotic fluid neutrophil collagenase concentrations in preterm premature rupture of membranes. Am J Obstet Gynecol 2001; 185: 1143–1148.

267. Maymon E, Romero R, Chaiworapongsa T et al. Amniotic fluid matrix metalloproteinase-8 in preterm labor with intact membranes. Am J Obstet Gynecol 2001; 185:1149–1155.

268. Maymon E, Romero R, Pacora P et al. Evidence of in vivo differential bioavailability of the active forms of matrix metalloproteinases 9 and 2 in parturition, spontaneous rupture of membranes, and intra- amniotic infection. Am J Obstet Gynecol 2000; 183:887–894.

269. Athayde N, Edwin SS, Romero R et al. A role for matrix metalloproteinase-9 in spontaneous rupture of the fetal membranes. Am J Obstet Gynecol 1998; 179:1248–1253.

270. Athayde N, Romero R, Gomez R et al. Matrix metalloproteinases-9 in preterm and term human parturition. J Matern Fetal Med 1999; 8:213–219.

271. Helmig BR, Romero R, Espinoza J et al. Neutrophil elastase and secretory leukocyte protease inhibitor in prelabor rupture of membranes, parturition and intra-amniotic infection. J Matern Fetal Neonatal Med 2002; 12:237–246.

272. Maymon E, Romero R, Pacora P et al. A role for the 72 kDa gelatinase (MMP-2) and its inhibitor (TIMP-2) in human parturition, premature rupture of membranes and intraamniotic infection. J Perinat Med 2001; 29:308–316.

273. Park KH, Chaiworapongsa T, Kim YM et al. Matrix metalloproteinase 3 in parturition, premature rupture of the membranes, and microbial invasion of the amniotic cavity. J Perinat Med 2003; 31:12–22.

274. Maymon E, Romero R, Pacora P et al. Matrilysin (matrix metalloproteinase 7) in parturition, premature rupture of membranes, and intrauterine infection. Am J Obstet Gynecol 2000; 182: 1545–1553.

275. Fortunato SJ, LaFleur B, Menon R. Collagenase-3 (MMP-13) in fetal membranes and amniotic fluid during pregnancy. Am J Reprod Immunol 2003; 49:120–125.

276. Fortunato SJ, Menon R, Bryant C, Lombardi SJ. Programmed cell death (apoptosis) as a possible pathway to metalloproteinase activation and fetal membrane degradation in premature rupture of membranes. Am J Obstet Gynecol 2000; 182:1468–1476.

277. Ferrand PE, Parry S, Sammel M et al. A polymorphism in the matrix metalloproteinase-9 promoter is associated with increased risk of preterm premature rupture of membranes in African Americans. Mol Hum Reprod 2002; 8:494–501.

278. Fujimoto T, Parry S, Urbanek M et al. A single nucleotide polymorphism in the matrix metalloproteinase-1 (MMP-1) promoter influences amnion cell MMP-1 expression and risk for preterm premature rupture of the fetal membranes. J Biol Chem 2002; 277: 6296–6302.

279. Kenyon SL, Taylor DJ, Tarnow-Mordi W. Broad-spectrum antibiotics for preterm, prelabour rupture of fetal membranes: the ORACLE I randomised trial. ORACLE Collaborative Group. Lancet 2001; 357:979–988.

280. Fidel P, Ghezzi F, Romero R et al. The effect of antibiotic therapy on intrauterine infection-induced preterm parturition in rabbits. J Matern Fetal Neonatal Med 2003; 14:57–64.

281. Rodts-Palenik S, Barrilleaux P, Thigpen B et al. Intravenous interleukin-10/antibiotic therapy prolongs gestation, improves birthweight, and reduces fetal wastage in E. coli-mediated preterm labor. Am J Obstet Gynecol 2002; 186:S65.

282. Terrone DA, Rinehart BK, Granger JP et al. Interleukin-10 administration and bacterial endotoxin-induced preterm birth in a rat model. Obstet Gynecol 2001; 98:476–480.

283. Chaiworapongsa T, Espinoza J, Kim YM et al. A novel mediator of septic shock, macrophage migration inhibitory factor, is increased in intra-amniotic infection. Am J Obstet Gynecol 2002; 187:S73.

284. Calandra T, Echtenacher B, Roy DL et al. Protection from septic shock by neutralization of macrophage migration inhibitory factor. Nat Med 2000; 6:164–170.

285. Ben Haroush A, Harell D, Hod M et al. Plasma levels of vitamin E in pregnant women prior to the development of preeclampsia and other hypertensive complications. Gynecol Obstet Invest 2002; 54:26–30.

286. Buhimschi IA, Buhimschi CS, Weiner CP. Protective effect of N-acetylcysteine against fetal death and preterm labor induced by maternal inflammation. Am J Obstet Gynecol 2003; 188:203–208.

287. Gravett MG, Sadowsky D, Witkin M, Novy M. Immunomodulators plus antibiotics to prevent preterm delivery in experimental intra-amniotic infection (IAI). Am J Obstet Gynecol 2003; 189:S56.

11. Amniotic fluid inflammation and fetal lung development

Timothy JM Moss and Alan H Jobe

CHORIOAMNIONITIS: ACUTE vs CHRONIC

Amniotic fluid inflammation, defined as increased inflammatory cells and mediators of inflammation such as interleukins IL-1, IL-6 and IL-8, is thought to result from a spectrum of colonization/infection of the endometrium, fetal membranes and placenta, and/or the amniotic fluid and the fetus.[1,2] Traditionally, chorioamnionitis was diagnosed as a symptomatic, acute, and progressive infection, which primarily occurred in late gestation or at term and was often associated with ruptured membranes. The associated microorganisms were highly pathogenic microorganisms such as *Escherichia coli*, group B streptococcus, and *Listeria monocytogenes*. Anaerobes also caused an acute chorioamnionitis that less frequently resulted in fetal infection. Infants delivered after acute chorioamnionitis often had symptoms of a systemic inflammatory response and pneumonia from systemic seeding of the lungs with microorganisms or from aspiration of infected amniotic fluid. Acute chorioamnionitis resulting in infectious lung disease in infants is less frequent now because of the widespread use of antibiotics prior to delivery.

The focus of this chapter is on the fetal effects of chronic/indolent chorioamnionitis, such as that associated with early preterm delivery, because of its clinically relevant effects on the fetal lung.[3,4] Other chapters in this book extensively review the associations between chorioamnionitis, preterm labor, and preterm birth. The majority of infants born prior to 30 weeks of gestation have been exposed to chorioamnionitis that can be diagnosed by culture or by histopathology.[2,5,6] This infection/inflammation is caused by multiple different organisms of low pathogenicity such as *Ureaplasma* and *Mycoplasma* species. The colonization/infection of

the fetal compartment (membranes, placenta, amniotic fluid, fetus) has often been present for weeks or months.[7,8] There is seldom information available that calibrates the duration, location, or intensity of the fetal exposure to infection/inflammation prior to preterm birth. Finally, most of the pregnancies at risk of preterm birth are treated with tocolytic agents, antibiotics, and antenatal corticosteroids, which further complicate an understanding of the pulmonary effects of chronic/indolent chorioamnionitis.[9]

LUNG OUTCOMES AFTER VERY PRETERM BIRTH

Lung immaturity and lung injury are major contributors to the morbidity and mortality of infants with birth weights <1 kg.[10] The two major adverse outcomes are respiratory distress syndrome (RDS)/structural lung immaturity causing early death, and bronchopulmonary dysplasia (BPD). BPD is a progressive lung inflammation and injury syndrome in very preterm infants that results from disrupted development of the saccular fetal lung.[11,12] Secondary septation (alveolarization) and microvascular development of the lung is delayed as the lung develops from a saccular structure to an alveolarized structure after about 32 weeks of gestation. Traditionally, BPD was thought to result primarily from the inflammatory effects of mechanical ventilation and increased oxygen concentrations on the immature lung with RDS.[13] However, very-low-birth-weight infants born with minimal RDS and no supplemental oxygen or ventilation requirements can develop severe BPD.[14]

The normal fetus does not have a mature lecithin/sphingomyelin (L/S) ratio until after 36 weeks of gestation,[15] but few infants born after spontaneous labor at gestations greater than 32 weeks have RDS, presumably because of 'induced lung maturation'. The human fetus can 'induce' lung maturation in response to fetal stresses, and this induced lung maturation is thought to result from increased fetal cortisol production.[16] Antenatal treatments with corticosteroids are used to induce lung maturation in infants at risk for preterm delivery before 32–34 weeks gestation.[17] Infants exposed to histological chorioamnionitis have higher cord plasma cortisol levels than comparison groups of infants, indicating increased adrenal function presumably because of the stress related to the chronic exposure to inflammation.[18,19] In animal experiments, maternal corticosteroids have relatively modest maturational effects on the fetal lungs.[20] Antenatal corticosteroids decrease lung mesenchyme tissue and increase the potential lung gas volume, with modest effects on the surfactant system. We do not think that increases in cortisol alone or short-term maternal corticosteroid treatments would be sufficient to induce much lung maturation in very-low-birth-weight infants.

Few large studies have correlated chorioamnionitis with lung outcomes. Analysis of outcomes for all infants born before 26 weeks in the United Kingdom and Ireland in 1995 showed that the major cause of death was pulmonary insufficiency, and survival was increased with antenatal corticosteroids and when clinical chorioamnionitis was diagnosed.[21] Clinical chorioamnionitis occurred in 18% of the population, which certainly underestimated the total amount of chorioamnionitis. In another report, increased survival of infants born at 25–29 weeks of gestation was observed in a population of infants with an incidence of histological chorioamnionitis greater than 50%.[5] In contrast, histological chorioamnionitis was not associated with decreased death in a recent trial of cortisol to prevent BPD.[22] Of note, although chorioamnionitis is frequent, only about 2% of preterm infants with birth weights of <1 kg have positive blood cultures at birth.[23] Despite the clinical bias that infection should severely compromise the fetus, preterm

infants exposed to chorioamnionitis are seldom septic and may have decreased mortality.

A number of clinical reports indicate that chorioamnionitis can have large effects on the lung outcomes of preterm infants. Ventilated preterm infants exposed to histological chorioamnionitis had a decreased incidence of RDS but an increased risk of BPD[24] (Table 11.1). Increased levels of IL-1, IL-6, and IL-8 in amniotic fluid sampled within 5 days of preterm delivery were associated with an increased risk of BPD.[3] Similarly, many reports correlate increased indicators of inflammation in tracheal aspirates taken shortly after birth, a surrogate for prenatal inflammation/chorioamnionitis,[6] with the development of BPD.[25] In a recent study, 64% of placentae from infants with gestational ages at birth of less than 32 weeks had histological chorioamnionitis and only 40% of the cases with histological chorioamnionitis were detected clinically.[6] Severity of chorioamnionitis was correlated with the incidence and severity of BPD; moderate-to-severe BPD was associated with histological indicators of more severe chorioamnionitis (Figure 11.1). In contrast, another study showed that histological chorioamnionitis decreased the risk of BPD;[4] however, chorioamnionitis increased the risk if the infant required ventilation for greater than 7 days. The inconsistent association of chorioamnionitis with mortality and lung outcomes (RDS or BDP) probably results from the imprecise diagnosis of chorioamnionitis (clinical vs histological), minimal information on the duration and severity of the chorioamnionitis, and different care strategies of the infants that can increase the risk of BPD.

Table 11.1 Correlation of chorioamnionitis with respiratory distress syndrome (RDS) and bronchopulmonary dysplasia (BPD) in ventilated preterm infants

	Chorioamnionitis	No chorioamnionitis
RDS (%)	33	67
BPD (%)	67	33

Data from Watterberg et al.[24]

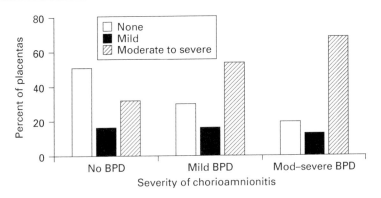

Figure 11.1 Relationship between the severity of chorioamnionitis and severity of bronchopulmonary dysplasia (BPD). Maternal stages of histological chorioamnionitis are indicated on the *x*-axis. None is no evidence of chorioamnionitis. Mild is neutrophils in the subchorionic plate and/or the chorionic laevae. Moderate to severe is neutrophils in the chorionic laevae and adjacent amnion or neutrophil karyorrhexis or eosinophilia of the basement membrane with or without epithelial sloughing. (Redrawn from data from Viscardi et al.[6]

UREAPLASMA AND CLINICAL OUTCOMES

Ureaplasmas are the microorganisms cultured most frequently from membranes or amniotic fluid of women who deliver very preterm infants.[2] Amniotic fluid that is positive for ureaplasmas contains high levels of proinflammatory mediators such as IL-6, IL-1β, and tumor necrosis factor-α (TNF-α), and increased numbers of white blood cells.[26] Levels of these proinflammatory mediators are similar to those reported for other culture-positive chorioamnionitis patients. Infants born from ureaplasma culture-positive pregnancies have elevated cord blood IL-6 levels, which is indicative of a fetal systemic inflammatory response.[27]

Ureaplasmas colonize the lungs of newborns and can be cultured from the lungs of infants with BPD. The controversial question is if antenatal ureaplasma exposure and/or persistent ureaplasma colonization/infection of the preterm lungs causes BPD. In 1995, meta-analysis of 17 reports indicated that ureaplasma-positive preterm infants had a 1.7-fold increased risk of developing BPD.[28] Subsequently, ureaplasma colonization was associated with less RDS but an increased risk of BPD[29] (Table 11.2). Predictors of BPD identified by multivariate logistic regression analysis were gestational age and ureaplasma isolation: odds ratio (OR) = 3.0, CI 1.0–9.1.

Table 11.2 Comparison of outcomes for singleton preterm infants with ureaplasma-positive or -negative tracheal aspirate samples

	Ureaplasma-positive	Ureaplasma-negative	*p* value
Number of infants	30	69	
Mean birth weight (g)	850	825	
Mean gestational age (weeks)	25.7	25.8	
RDS (%)	47	81	0.001
BPD (%)	43	19	0.03
Death (%)	7	23	0.09

RDS, respiratory distress syndrome; BPD, bronchopulmonary dysplasia.
Data from Hannaford et al.[29]

Early reports of the association of ureaplasma with an increased risk of BPD are confounded by the poor resolution of cultures and the presence of chorioamnionitis caused by other microorganisms. Culture techniques miss 40% of cases detected by a polymerase chain reaction (PCR) diagnosis.[30] Castro-Alcaraz et al used polymerase chain reaction to identify the patterns of colonization of infants with ureaplasma. In a population of 125 infants <32 weeks' gestation, PCR demonstrated that 14% were persistently positive, 11% had early transient colonization, and 6.4% had late acquisition of *Ureaplasma urealyticum*.[31] Multivariate analysis – correcting for birth weight, gestational age, gender, and patent ductus arteriosis – yielded an adjusted OR of 34 for the association of persistent ureaplasma with BPD.

ANIMAL MODELS OF CHORIOAMNIONITIS

Although the effects of antenatal infection on prematurity have been explored in many animal experiments, the primary outcomes of interest have usually been the pathogenesis of premature labor

and adverse effects on the fetal brain.[32] The first report of an antenatal inflammatory effect other than pneumonia on the fetal lung was the observation that intra-amniotic injection of the pro-inflammatory cytokine IL-1α to pregnant rabbits improved lung function after preterm delivery.[33] The mRNA for the surfactant proteins SP-A and SP-B in the fetal lungs and surfactant lipids also increased as indicators of induced lung maturation. This initial experiment, together with clinical observations linking chorioamnionitis to fetal lung development, prompted us to explore how inflammation can alter lung development.

INTRA-AMNIOTIC ENDOTOXIN AS A MODEL OF CHORIOAMNIONITIS

Endotoxin (lipopolysaccharide from Gram-negative microorganisms) is used widely as a potent proinflammatory agonist to study shock and inflammatory responses. Endotoxin initiates inflammation in many cell types by signaling through toll-like receptor-4 (TLR-4) to activate nuclear factor-κB (NF-κB) and the inflammatory cascade. Empirically, endotoxin can induce

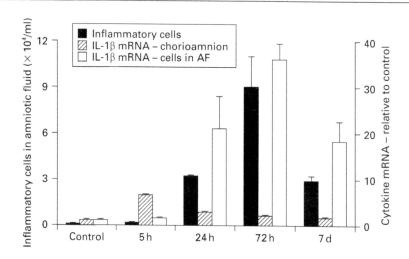

Figure 11.2 Time course of intrauterine inflammation induced by 4 mg endotoxin given by intra-amniotic injection. Inflammatory cells (granulocytes + monocytes) increase in amniotic fluid, interleukin IL-1β mRNA expression increases in the chorioamnion, and IL-1β mRNA expression increases and remains elevated in cells from the amniotic fluid (AF). (Redrawn from data from Kramer et al.[37])

chorioamnionitis and inflammatory responses in human pregnancies and preterm infants, and TLR-4 is expressed in the human chorioamnion.[34] Using ultrasound guidance, intra-amniotic injections of *E. coli* endotoxin in sheep induce chorioamnionitis, which is indicated by increased inflammatory cells in amniotic fluid, histological inflammation of the chorioamnion, and increased IL-1β, IL-6, and IL-8 mRNA in cells from amniotic fluid.[35,36] Proinflammatory cytokine mRNA expression in the chorioamnion is maximal 1 day after a 20 mg dose of intra-amniotic endotoxin and has returned to low baseline levels within several days. However, inflammatory cells in the amniotic fluid continue to express IL-1β and IL-8 cytokine mRNA for at least 1 week[37] (Figure 11.2).

LUNG INJURY FOLLOWING CHORIOAMNIONITIS

Intra-amniotic endotoxin induces lung inflammation, a lung injury response (apoptosis and cell proliferation), and morphological changes (Figure 11.3). Within 5 hours of injection of intra-amniotic endotoxin, the fetal airways express heat shock protein-70 and inflammatory cells are increased in bronchoalveolar washes.[38] Within 24 hours, monocytes and granulocytes are increased many fold in the bronchoalveolar lavage, and mRNA for proinflammatory cytokines IL-1β, IL-6, and IL-8 are strikingly increased in lung tissue. IP-10 and MIG, chemokines associated with inflammation and angiostasis, are expressed highly by inflammatory cells and the bronchioles.[39] Apoptosis of lung cells

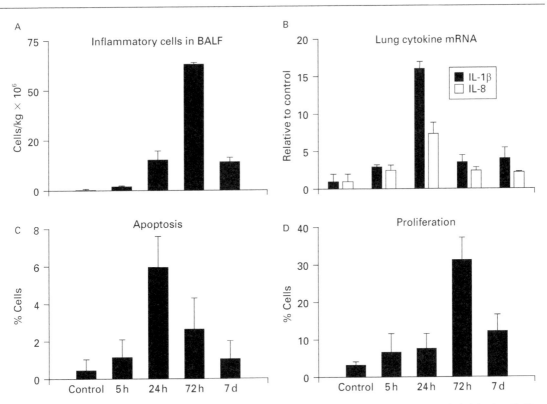

Figure 11.3 Indicators of inflammation and injury in the fetal lung after 4 mg endotoxin given by intra-amniotic injection. (A,B) Inflammatory cells in bronchoalveolar lavage fluid (BALF) and cytokine (interleukins IL-1β and IL-8) mRNA in lung parenchyma increase. (C,D) An increase in apoptosis precedes proliferation in the lung tissue. (Data redrawn from Kramer et al.[37,38])

increases 24 hours after intra-amniotic endotoxin, and lung cell proliferation increases by 72 hours.[38] The acute inflammatory responses of the fetal lung have resolved by 7 days; however, residual inflammatory cells remain in the bronchoalveolar lavage.

Inhibition of microvascular development is striking in the lungs of infants with BPD,[40] and parallel responses occur in the fetal sheep lungs. The lungs have decreased expression of multiple markers of vascular development – endothelial nitric oxide synthase, vascular endothelial growth factor (VEGF), platelet endothelial cell adhesion molecule, Tie-2, and VEGF receptor 2 – for 1–4 days after exposure to intra-amniotic endotoxin.[41] By day 7, the medial thickness of arteriolar walls has increased, alveolar size has increased, and alveolar number has decreased relative to controls.[42] Therefore, intra-amniotic endotoxin causes chorioamnionitis and alters the fetal lung anatomy similarly to the pathology of the lungs of infants with BPD.[43]

INTRA-AMNIOTIC ENDOTOXIN CAUSES LUNG MATURATION

Despite fetal lung injury, the functional outcome after intra-amniotic endotoxin is lung maturation.[44] The mRNAs for surfactant proteins A, B, C, and D are increased within 24 hours and the amounts of the surfactant proteins are increased by about 100-fold in bronchoalveolar lavages by 7 days (Figure 11.4). In parallel with the increases in surfactant, lung function of ventilated preterm lambs improves, with large increases in lung compliance, gas exchange, and oxygenation[45–47] (Figure 11.5). Of note, cord plasma cortisol does not increase in response to intra-amniotic endotoxin.

Endotoxin-induced increases in surfactant lipids and proteins are much greater than the increases achieved with corticosteroid treatments[20] (Figure 11.4). The clinically relevant response of the fetal lung to chorioamnionitis is induced lung maturation, which will result in a decreased incidence and severity of RDS. In our experimental sheep model, intra-amniotic doses of 1–100 mg *E. coli* endotoxin induce similar inflammatory and lung maturation responses.[47] In contrast, an intra-allantoic endo-

toxin injection causes no chorioamnionitis or lung responses.[47] The endotoxin injected into the amniotic fluid must not enter the circulation of the fetus, because intravascular doses as low as 1 µg will kill the fetus.[48] Thus, the fetal response to the inflammatory mediator is dependent on the compartment with the inflammation.

HOW ENDOTOXIN SIGNALS LUNG MATURATION

Endotoxin induces a cascade of proinflammatory mediators and recruits activated inflammatory cells to the chorioamnion. Diffuse inflammation of the chorioamnion could release effector molecules into the fetal systemic circulation and indirectly induce lung inflammation and maturation. However, intra-amniotic endotoxin has very modest effects on circulating white blood cells and platelets.[37,47] Proinflammatory cytokine mRNA in the fetal liver is inconsistently and minimally increased, and plasma interferon-γ (IFN-γ), IL-6, and IL-8 levels are minimally increased.[35,37] Also, cytokine mRNA levels in the placenta and gut do not increase appreciably. Therefore, a diffuse fetal inflammatory response does not explain the focal lung inflammation.

To identify the relationships between chorioamnionitis and the fetal lung, we surgically separated the fetal lungs from the amniotic fluid using tracheotomy and a silastic bag to collect lung fluid.[49] Endotoxin in the amniotic fluid caused chorioamnionitis but no lung inflammation or lung maturation (Figure 11.6). In contrast, a 24-hour infusion of endotoxin into the fetal trachea caused lung inflammation and subsequent lung maturation without chorioamnionitis. This result demonstrates that endotoxin can cause the inflammation/maturation sequence by direct contact with the fetal lung. Therefore, tidal fetal breathing must cause mixing of fetal lung fluid with amniotic fluid, which then signals the inflammation and maturation responses in the fetal lung.

In the clinical scenario, the mediator of inflammatory effects on the lungs could be the TLR-4 agonist endotoxin, some other TLR agonist, or an inflammatory product of chorioamnionitis. The mRNA for IL-1β is the cytokine which is most

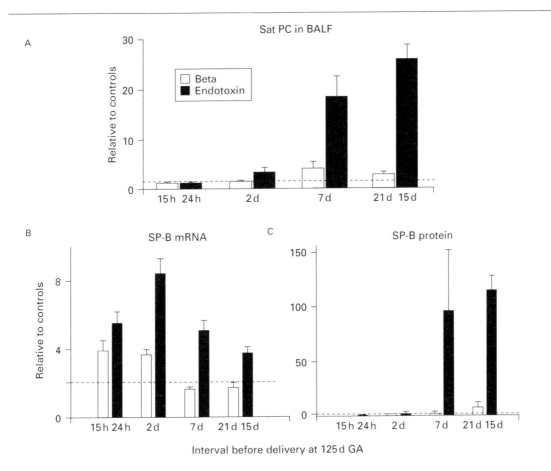

Figure 11.4 Comparison of increases in surfactant in response to intra-amniotic endotoxin and maternal betamethasone. (A) The amount of saturated phosphatidylcholine (Sat PC) increased more after endotoxin than betamethasone (Beta). (B) The mRNA for surfactant protein B (SP-B) increased persistently after intra-amniotic endotoxin. In contrast, there was a small and transient induction of SP-B mRNA with maternal betamethasone. (C) The recovery of SP-B protein in bronchoalveolar lavage increased strikingly with intra-amniotic endotoxin, but not maternal betamethasone. (Data redrawn from Ballard et al,[45] Tan et al,[46] and Jobe et al.[47])

increased in the chorioamnion after intra-amniotic endotoxin. The original description of lung maturation responses to intra-amniotic IL-1α in rabbits did not include an evaluation for chorioamnionitis.[33] Intra-amniotic injections of sheep recombinant IL-1α or IL-1β to ewes induced chorioamnionitis followed by striking lung maturation.[50] However, the fetus did not respond to either sheep recombinant TNF-α or IFN-γ with chorioamnionitis or lung inflammation/lung maturation.[51] Thus, the fetal compartment seems to be exquisitively sensitive to

IL-1β, the endogenously produced IL-1, and quite unresponsive to other normally potent proinflammatory cytokines.

To further explore if IL-1 is central to the cascade of inflammation/lung maturation, fetal sheep were given the IL-1 receptor antagonist (IL-ra) anakinra (Kineret; Amgen) into the amniotic fluid and intramuscularly to the fetus 3 hours prior to intra-amniotic endotoxin IL-1α.[52] The IL-1ra completely blocked IL-1-induced inflammation and lung maturation. It also blocked most of the lung

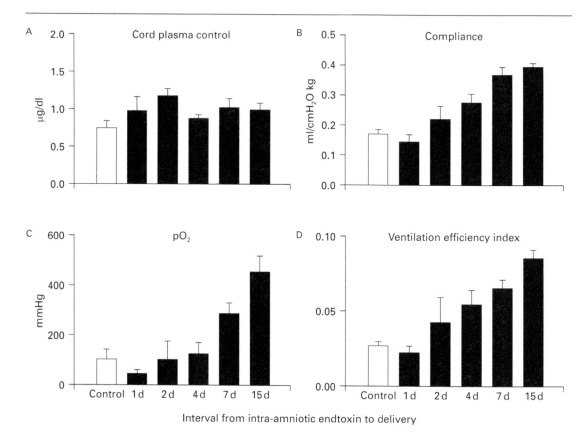

Figure 11.5 Cortisol and lung function after 20 mg intra-amniotic endotoxin and preterm delivery at 125 days' gestation. (A) Cord plasma cortisol was not changed by intra-amniotic endotoxin exposure of the fetus. (B) Lung compliance measured for ventilated preterm lambs increased following the fetal endotoxin exposure. (C) The highest pO_2 measured in preterm lambs ventilated with 100% O_2 increased 7 and 15 days after the intra-amniotic endotoxin. (D) Ventilation efficiency index, a measure of the integrated pressure requirements and pCO_2 levels achieved with mechanical ventilation, increased. (Data redrawn from Jobe et al.[47]).

inflammation/lung maturation induced by intra-amniotic endotoxin. Therefore, IL-1 is a major mediator of the fetal lung response to endotoxin-induced chorioamnionitis. In other experiments, an anti-CD-18 antibody blocked intra-amniotic endotoxin-mediated inflammatory cell recruitment to the fetal lungs and prevented lung maturation.[53] Our current understanding is that the fetal lung responds to proinflammatory mediators in amniotic fluid with a recruitment of inflammatory cells, which may be the major source of IL-1β, which in turn initiates the maturational signals.

The importance of IL-1 to lung maturation is supported by results in other models. IL-1 increased the mRNAs for surfactant proteins A, B, and C in explants of preterm fetal rabbit lungs.[54] In contrast, IL-1 suppressed these same mRNAs in explants from more mature rabbit fetuses. Endotoxin suppressed the surfactant protein mRNA species in lung explants from preterm and term rabbits.[55] These results demonstrate gestation-specific effects of IL-1 on the distal lung in the absence of inflammation (although resident inflammatory cells might be modulating the responses).

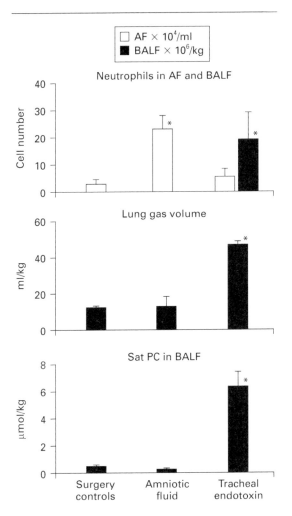

Figure 11.6 Inflammation induced by intra-amniotic or intratracheal administration of endotoxin after surgical isolation of the fetal respiratory tract. Increases in neutrophils occurred only at the site of endotoxin administration and lung maturation (increased lung gas volumes measured at 40 cmH₂O and saturated phosphatidylcholine (Sat PC)) increased only with direct infusion of endotoxin into the respiratory tract. AF, amniotic fluid; BALF, bronchoalveolar lavage fluid. *$p < 0.05$ between groups. (Data redrawn from Moss et al.[49])

In a mouse model of chorioamnionitis, intra-amniotic endotoxin increased the number of type II cells.[56] The effect of endotoxin on type II cell numbers was direct because endotoxin also increased type II cells in explants of fetal mouse lungs. The endotoxin effect was blocked by parthenolide, an inhibitor of NF-κB activation. The precise signaling pathways leading from chorioamnionitis to the multiple components of lung maturation – anatomic changes, induction of surfactant, and antioxidant enzymes – remain to be identified. If these pathways can be activated without inducing fetal lung inflammation/injury, there may be new therapeutic strategies for inducing lung maturation in the human fetus at risk of preterm delivery.

EFFECTS OF EARLY GESTATION AND PROLONGED ENDOTOXIN EXPOSURE

The responses of the fetal lung to chorioamnionitis induced by endotoxin described above resulted from single fetal exposures over the interval from about 110 days to 124 days' gestation, with delivery at about 125 days' gestation.[47] Chronic indolent chorioamnionitis may begin before 20 weeks of gestation and persist for weeks in the human.[2] Therefore, we gave ewes intra-amniotic injections of endotoxin at 60, 80, or 100 days of gestation and fetuses were delivered at 125 days.[57] Surprisingly, surfactant lipids in lung tissue, surfactant protein mRNAs, and the surfactant proteins were increased in all groups despite intervals from endotoxin exposure to delivery of up to 65 days, which represents 43% of the sheep's gestation period (Figure 11.7). Fetuses exposed to 28-day intra-amniotic endotoxin infusions from 80 to 108 days of gestation had improved lung function and increased amounts of surfactant at delivery at 125 days' gestation, but this prolonged exposure resulted in decreased alveolar numbers, the pathology seen in BPD.[47] These experiments demonstrate that the fetal lung responds at very early gestations to chorioamnionitis and the effects of that response can be detected many weeks later.

Chronic exposures to intra-amniotic endotoxin were also evaluated as the fetal sheep approached term to assess the residual effects of the inhibition of alveolar septation and microvascular injury. Groups of fetuses were exposed to either 28 days of intra-amniotic endotoxin delivered with an osmotic pump or four intra-amniotic injections given at

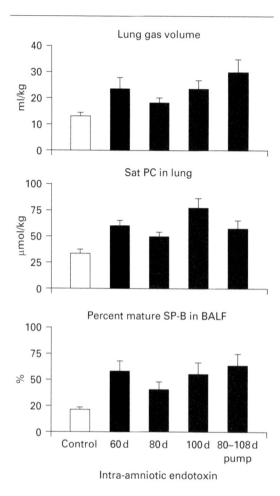

Figure 11.7 Effects of early–mid gestation exposure to intra-amniotic endotoxin on lung function and surfactant of preterm lambs delivered at 125 days' gestation. Lambs received 1 mg endotoxin at the indicated gestational ages. One group of lambs received 0.6 mg/day endotoxin for 28 days by an osmotic pump in the amniotic cavity. The endotoxin exposure increased lung gas volume measured at 40 cmH$_2$O pressure, increased the saturated phosphatidylcholine (Sat PC) in the fetal lungs, and increased the processing of surfactant protein B (SP-B) in the bronchoalveolar lavage fluid (BALF). Similar responses occurred for all exposure to delivery intervals. (Data redrawn from Moss et al.[57])

7-day intervals from 100 to 121 days' gestation.[58] When assessed at 130–145 days' gestation, the lungs had increased numbers of inflammatory cells in bronchoalveolar lavage and increased proinflam-

matory cytokine mRNA levels. However, despite the persistent mild inflammation, there was no anatomical evidence of decreased alveolar numbers or vascular injury. The only remaining effect of the prolonged endotoxin exposure was a large increase in surfactant lipids. The remarkable result was that the fetal lung repaired the early gestational lung injury induced by prolonged intra-amniotic endotoxin exposure despite persistent low-grade inflammation. Two-month-old lambs exposed to a single intra-amniotic dose of endotoxin at 119 days' gestation also had normal lungs.[59] The fetal lung is remarkably resistant to chorioamnionitis-induced lung injury, with the residual effect being induced lung maturation.

GLUCOCORTICOIDS AND CHORIOAMNIONITIS

The majority of women delivering before 30 weeks of gestation have clinically silent chorioamnionitis, and most of these women receive antenatal corticosteroids to induce lung maturation. The practice of corticosteroid treatment is supported by numerous clinical reports and a meta-analysis demonstrating decreased RDS, intraventricular hemorrhage (IVH), and death when corticosteroids are given to women with preterm rupture of membranes, a surrogate clinical indicator of chorioamnionitis.[60] In preterm fetal sheep, maternal corticosteroids given 7 days before delivery do not improve lung function as effectively as intra-amniotic endotoxin. The major difference is the much larger increase in surfactant induced by endotoxin[20,47] (see Figure 11.4). Maternal betamethasone causes fetal growth restriction and fetal thymic involution, but intra-amniotic endotoxin does not.[61] Surprisingly, intra-amniotic endotoxin prevents betamethasone-induced fetal growth restriction and thymic involution when these interventions are combined. Betamethasone suppressed the lung inflammation induced by endotoxin for about 2 days;[9] however, 5 and 15 days after both exposures, inflammatory cells and proinflammatory mediators were higher in the lungs exposed to both endotoxin and betamethasone than to endotoxin alone (Figure 11.8). A possible explanation for this result is suggested by the observation that mater-

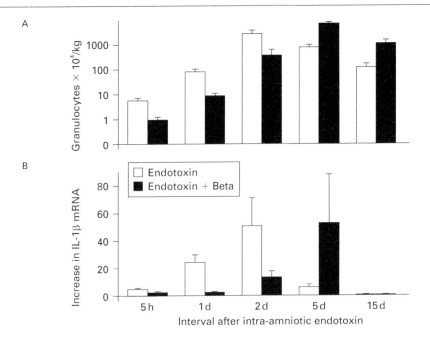

Figure 11.8 Maternal betamethasone modulation of fetal lung inflammation induced by intra-amniotic endotoxin. Fetal sheep were exposed to 10 mg endotoxin given by intra-amniotic injection or both 0.5 mg/kg maternal betamethasone and endotoxin given at the same time. (A) Granulocytes in bronchoalveolar lavage fluid initially were decreased by the maternal betamethasone (Beta) treatment, but granulocytes were increased at 5 and 15 days relative to the endotoxin group. (B) The mRNA for interleukin IL-1β showed the initial suppression by betamethasone with an increase at 5 days. Betamethasone alone did not increase granulocytes or IL-1β mRNA in separate groups of animals. (Data redrawn from Kallapur et al.[9])

nal betamethasone treatments initially suppress the inflammatory responses of fetal monocytes, but those responses are strikingly augmented 7 days after maternal betamethasone treatment.[62] Thus, maternal betamethasone may augment fetal lung inflammation induced by endotoxin by 'maturing' the inflammatory potential of fetal inflammatory cells. There is no experimental information about how the fetal lung will respond to betamethasone superimposed on chronic chorioamnionitis, the more usual clinical scenario.

UREAPLASMA COLONIZATION OF FETAL SHEEP

A criticism of studies of chorioamnionitis induced by endotoxin is that clinical chorioamnionitis results from live microorganisms that generally do not produce endotoxin. Therefore, the feasibility of coloniz-

ing the fetal sheep with clinical isolates of ureaplasma was evaluated using serovar 3 in one study and serovar 6 in a second study.[63] Serovar 3 (2×10^7 colony-forming units) was given by intra-amniotic injection at 55, 103, or 118 days' gestation, and fetal sheep were delivered at 125 days' gestation. The ureaplasma-exposed animals had culture-positive amniotic fluid and fetal lungs. The 7-day exposure had no effect on the fetus or the fetal lungs, but the 21-day and 68-day exposures caused fetal growth restriction in some animals and lung maturation (increased lung gas volumes and increased surfactant) (Figure 11.9). Ewes given injections with serovar 6 at 80 days' gestation had fetuses without growth restriction when delivered at 125 days. The amniotic fluid was culture-positive, proinflammatory cytokine mRNA expression was increased in the chorioamnion, and high levels of IL-8 protein were

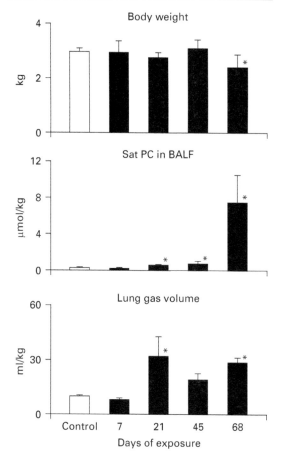

Figure 11.9 Effects of amniotic fluid colonization with ureaplasmas on fetal growth and lung development in preterm lambs. Short-term exposure did not affect fetal development but long-term exposure reduced fetal growth. Exposure to ureaplasmas for 3 weeks or more increased surfactant and lung compliance. Sat PC, saturated phosphatidylcholine; BALF, bronchoalveolar lavage fluid. *$p < 0.05$ vs control. (Data from Moss et al.[63])

in the amniotic fluid. Lung gas volumes and surfactant levels were strikingly increased, as were indicators of persistent lung inflammation. Therefore, ureaplasma colonizes the fetal sheep and causes persistent chorioamnionitis, lung inflammation, and lung maturation. This animal model may be ideal for exploring how chorioamnionitis impacts the fetus and the fetal lung.

SUMMARY

Chronic indolent chorioamnionitis associated with preterm birth can alter lung development. Very preterm infants may have induced lung maturation resulting in less RDS. Experiments in sheep demonstrate that endotoxin, the proinflammatory cytokine IL-1, or live ureaplasmas can cause striking lung maturation even at early gestational ages. Endotoxin-induced inflammation also decreases alveolar septation and causes microvascular injury, but the fetal lung can recover from that injury. Preterm lambs exposed to intra-amniotic endotoxin 30 days prior to delivery have an increased inflammatory response to ventilation.[64] The link between chorioamnionitis and BPD may result from the altered innate immune responses induced by chorioamnionitis and maternal betamethasone. BPD is clearly a multifactorial disease, with the primary risk factors being delivery at early gestation, mechanical ventilation, supplemental oxygen exposure, and postnatal sepsis. Other than gestational age, these risk factors are proinflammatory. Antenatal lung inflammation may initiate and potentiate a progressive inflammatory process that results in BPD. Any studies of lung outcomes of preterm infants should include information about chorioamnionitis.

ACKNOWLEDGMENTS

This work was supported in part by grants HD-12714 and HL-65397 from the National Institute of Health and by grants 139026 and 254502 from the NHMRC (Australia). TJMM is supported by an NHMRC Career Development Award.

REFERENCES

1. Romero R, Espinoza J, Chaiworapongsa T, Kalache K. Infection and prematurity and the role of preventive strategies. Semin Neonatol 2002; 7(4):259–274.
2. Goldenberg RL, Hauth JC, Andrews WW. Intrauterine infection and preterm delivery. N Engl J Med 2000; 342(20):1500–1507.
3. Yoon BH, Romero R, Jun JK et al. Amniotic fluid cytokines (interleukin-6, tumor necrosis factor-alpha, interleukin-1 beta, and interleukin-8) and the risk for the development of bronchopulmonary dysplasia. Am J Obstet Gynecol 1997; 177(4):825–830.

4. Van Marter LJ, Dammann O, Allred EN et al. Chorioamnionitis, mechanical ventilation, and postnatal sepsis as modulators of chronic lung disease in preterm infants. J Pediatr 2002; 140(2):171–176.

5. Lahra MM, Jeffery HE. A fetal response to chorioamnionitis is associated with early survival after preterm birth. Am J Obstet Gynecol 2004; 190(1):147–151.

6. Viscardi RM, Muhumuza CK, Rodriguez A et al. Inflammatory markers in intrauterine and fetal blood and cerebrospinal fluid compartments are associated with adverse pulmonary and neurologic outcomes in preterm infants. Pediatr Res 2004; 55(6):1009–1017.

7. Gerber S, Vial Y, Hohlfeld P, Witkin SS. Detection of *Ureaplasma urealyticum* in second-trimester amniotic fluid by polymerase chain reaction correlates with subsequent preterm labor and delivery. J Infect Dis 2003; 187(3):518–521.

8. Perni SC, Vardhana S, Korneeva I et al. *Mycoplasma hominis* and *Ureaplasma urealyticum* in midtrimester amniotic fluid: association with amniotic fluid cytokine levels and pregnancy outcome. Am J Obstet Gynecol 2004; 191(4):1382–1386.

9. Kallapur SG, Kramer BW, Moss TJ et al. Maternal glucocorticoids increase endotoxin-induced lung inflammation in preterm lambs. Am J Physiol Lung Cell Mol Physiol 2003; 284(4):L633–642.

10. Horbar JD, Badger GJ, Carpenter JH et al. Trends in mortality and morbidity for very low birth weight infants, 1991–1999. Pediatrics 2002; 110(1 Pt 1):143–151.

11. Albertine KH, Jones GP, Starcher BC et al. Chronic lung injury in preterm lambs. Disordered respiratory tract development. Am J Respir Crit Care Med 1999; 159:945–958.

12. O'Brodovich HM, Mellins RB. Bronchopulmonary dysplasia. Unresolved neonatal acute lung injury. Am Rev Respir Dis 1985; 132:694–709.

13. Northway WH. Bronchopulmonary dysplasia – then and now. Arch Dis Child 1990; 65:1076–1081.

14. Charafeddine L, D'Angio CT, Phelps DL. Atypical chronic lung disease patterns in neonates. Pediatrics 1999; 103(4 Pt 1):759–765.

15. Gluck L, Kulovich MV, Borer RC Jr, Keidel WN. The interpretation and significance of the lecithin–sphingomyelin ratio in amniotic fluid. Am J Obstet Gynecol 1974; 120(1):142–155.

16. Ballard PL. Hormones and Lung Maturation. New York: Springer-Verlag; 1986.

17. Crowley P. Prophylactic corticosteroids for preterm birth. The Cochrane Library, Issue 2, Oxford: Update Software 2001(3).

18. Gravett MG, Hitti J, Hess DL, Eschenbach DA. Intrauterine infection and preterm delivery: evidence for activation of the fetal hypothalamic–pituitary–adrenal axis. Am J Obstet Gynecol 2000; 182(6):1404–1413.

19. Watterberg KL, Scott SM, Naeye RL. Chorioamnionitis, cortisol, and acute lung disease in very low birth weight infants. Pediatrics 1997; 99:E6.

20. Jobe AH, Ikegami M. Fetal responses to glucocorticoids. In: Mendelson CR, ed. Endocrinology of the Lung. Totowa: Humana Press; 2000: 45–57.

21. Costeloe K, Hennessy E, Gibson AT, Marlow N, Wilkinson AR. The EPICure study: outcomes to discharge from hospital for infants born at the threshold of viability. Pediatrics 2000; 106(4): 659–671.

22. Watterberg KL, Gerdes JS, Cole CH et al. Prophylaxis of early adrenal insufficiency to prevent bronchopulmonary dysplasia: a multicenter trial. Pediatrics 2004; 114(6):1649–1657.

23. Stoll BJ, Hansen N, Fanaroff AA et al. Changes in pathogens causing early-onset sepsis in very-low-birth-weight infants. N Engl J Med 2002; 347(4):240–247.

24. Watterberg KL, Demers LM, Scott SM, Murphy S. Chorioamnionitis and early lung inflammation in infants in whom bronchopulmonary dysplasia develops. Pediatrics 1996; 97:210–215.

25. Speer CP. Inflammation and bronchopulmonary dysplasia. Semin Neonatol 2003; 8:29–38.

26. Yoon BH, Romero R, Park JS et al. Microbial invasion of the amniotic cavity with *Ureaplasma urealyticum* is associated with a robust host in fetal, amniotic, and maternal compartments. Am J Obstet Gynecol 1998; 179:1254–1260.

27. Chaiworapongsa T, Romero R, Kim JC et al. Evidence for fetal involvement in the pathologic process of clinical chorioamnionitis. Am J Obstet Gynecol 2002; 186(6):1178–1182.

28. Wang EE, Ohlsson A, Kellner J. Association of *Ureaplasma urealyticum* colonization with chronic lung disease of prematurity: results of a metaanalysis. J Pediatr 1995; 127:640–644.

29. Hannaford K, Todd DA, Jeffery H et al. Role of *Ureaplasma urealyticum* in lung disease of prematurity. Arch Dis Child Fetal Neonatal Ed 1999; 81(3):F162–167.

30. Yoon BH, Romero R, Kim M et al. Clinical implications of detection of *Ureaplasma urealyticum* in the amniotic cavity with the polymerase chain reaction. Am J Obstet Gynecol 2000; 183(5):1130–1137.

31. Castro-Alcaraz S, Greenberg EM, Bateman DA, Regan JA. Patterns of colonization with *Ureaplasma urealyticum* during neonatal intensive care unit hospitalizations of very low birth weight infants and the development of chronic lung disease. Pediatrics 2002; 110(4):e45.

32. Leviton A, Paneth N, Reuss ML et al. Maternal infection, fetal inflammatory response, and brain damage in very low birth weight infants. Developmental Epidemiology Network Investigators. Pediatr Res 1999; 46(5):566–575.

33. Bry K, Lappalainen U, Hallman M. Intraamniotic interleukin-1 accelerates surfactant protein synthesis in fetal rabbits and improves lung stability after premature birth. J Clin Invest 1997; 99:2992–2999.

34. Kim YM, Romero R, Chaiworapongsa T et al. Toll-like receptor-2 and -4 in the chorioamniotic membranes in spontaneous labor at term and in preterm parturition that are associated with chorioamnionitis. Am J Obstet Gynecol 2004; 191(4):1346–1355.

35. Kallapur SG, Willet KE, Jobe AH, Ikegami M, Bachurski C. Intra-amniotic endotoxin: chorioamnionitis precedes lung maturation in preterm lambs. Am J Physiol 2001; 280:L527–L536.

36. Jobe AH, Newnham JP, Willet KE et al. Effects of antenatal endotoxin and glucocorticoids on the lungs of preterm lambs. Am J Obstet Gynecol 2000; 182:401–408.

37. Kramer BW, Moss TJ, Willet K et al. Dose and time response after intra-amniotic endotoxin in preterm lambs. Am J Respir Crit Care Med 2001; 164:982–988.

38. Kramer BW, Kramer S, Ikegami M, Jobe A. Injury, inflammation, and remodeling in fetal sheep lung after intra-amniotic endotoxin. Am J Physiol Lung Cell Mol Physiol 2002; 283:L452–L459.

39. Kallapur SG, Jobe AH, Ikegami M, Bachurski CJ. Increased IP-10 and MIG expression after intra-amniotic endotoxin in preterm lamb lung. Am J Respir Crit Care Med 2003; 167:779–786.

40. Bhatt AJ, Pryhuber GS, Huyck H et al. Disrupted pulmonary vasculature and decreased vascular endothelial growth factor, Flt-1 and Tie-2 in human infants dying with bronchopulmonary dysplasia. Am J Respir Crit Care Med 2001; 164:1971–1980.

41. Kallapur SG, Bachurski CJ, Le Cras TD et al. Vascular changes following intra-amniotic endotoxin in preterm lamb lungs. Am J Physiol Lung Cell Mol Physiol 2004; 287(6):L1178–L1185.

42. Willet K, Jobe A, Ikegami M, Brennan S, Newnham J, Sly P. Antenatal endotoxin and glucocorticoid effects on lung morphometry in preterm lambs. Pediatr Res 2000; 48:782–788.

43. Coalson JJ. Pathology of chronic lung disease of early infancy. In: Bland RD, Coalson JJ, eds. Chronic Lung Disease in Early Infancy. New York: Marcel Dekker; 2000: 85–124.

44. Bachurski CJ, Ross GF, Ikegami M, Kramer BW, Jobe AH. Intra-amniotic endotoxin increases pulmonary surfactant components and induces SP-B processing in fetal sheep. Am J Physiol Lung Cell Mol Physiol 2001; 280:L279–L285.

45. Ballard PL, Ning Y, Polk D, Ikegami M, Jobe A. Glucocorticoid regulation of surfactant components in immature lambs. Am J Physiol 1997; 273:L1048–L1057.

46. Tan RC, Ikegami M, Jobe AH, Possmayer F, Ballard PL. Developmental and glucocorticoid regulation of surfactant protein mRNAs in preterm lambs. Am J Physiol 1999; 277:L1142–L1148.

47. Jobe AH, Newnham JP, Willet KE et al. Endotoxin-induced lung maturation in preterm lambs is not mediated by cortisol. Am J Respir Crit Care Med 2000; 162(5):1656–1661.

48. Duncan JR, Cock ML, Scheerlinck JP et al. White matter injury after repeated endotoxin exposure in the preterm ovine fetus. Pediatr Res 2002; 52(6):941–949.

49. Moss TJ, Nitsos I, Kramer BW et al. Intra-amniotic endotoxin induces lung maturation by direct effects on the developing respiratory tract in preterm sheep. Am J Obstet Gynecol 2002; 187: 1059–1065.

50. Willet K, Kramer BW, Kallapur SG et al. Intra-amniotic injection of IL-1 induces inflammation and maturation in fetal sheep lung. Am J Physiol Lung Cell Mol Physiol 2002; 282(3):L411–L420.

51. Ikegami M, Moss TJM, Kallapur SG et al. Minimal lung and systemic responses to TNFα in preterm sheep. Am J Physiol Lung Cell Mol Physiol 2003; 285(1):L121–L129.

52. Kallapur SG, Moss TJM, Ikegami M, et al. Recruited inflammatory cells mediate endotoxin-induced lung maturation in preterm fetal lambs. Am J Respir Crit Care Med 2005; 172:1315–1321.

53. Kallapur SG. IL-1 mediates endotoxin-induced lung maturation in preterm lambs. Abstracts of the Pediatric Academic Society 2005; in press.

54. Glumoff V, Vayrynen O, Kangas T, Hallman M. Degree of lung maturity determines the direction of the interleukin-1-induced effect on the expression of surfactant proteins. Am J Respir Cell Mol Biol 2000; 22(3):280–288.

55. Vayrynen O, Glumoff V, Hallman M. Regulation of surfactant proteins by LPS and proinflammatory cytokines in fetal and newborn lung. Am J Physiol Lung Cell Mol Physiol 2002; 282(4):L803–810.

56. Prince LS, Okoh VO, Moninger TO, Matalon S. Lipopolysaccharide increases alveolar type II cell number in fetal mouse lungs through Toll-like receptor 4 and NF-kappaB. Am J Physiol Lung Cell Mol Physiol 2004; 287(5):L999–1006.

57. Moss TM, Newnham J, Willet K et al. Early gestational intra-amniotic endotoxin: lung function, surfactant and morphometry. Am J Respir Crit Care Med 2002; 165:805–811.

58. Kallapur SG, Nitsos I, Moss TJ et al. Chronic endotoxin exposure does not cause sustained structural abnormalities in the fetal sheep lung. Am J Physiol Lung Cell Mol Physiol 2005.

59. Moss TJ, Harding R, Newnham JP. Lung function, arterial pressure and growth in sheep during early postnatal life following single and repeated prenatal corticosteroid treatments. Early Hum Dev 2002; 66(1):11–24.

60. Harding JE, Pang J, Knight DB, Liggins GC. Do antenatal corticosteroids help in the setting of preterm rupture of membranes? Am J Obstet Gynecol 2001; 184(2):131–139.

61. Newnham JP, Moss TJ, Padbury JF et al. The interactive effects of endotoxin with prenatal glucocorticoids on short-term lung function in sheep. Am J Obstet Gynecol 2001; 185:190–197.

62. Kramer BW, Ikegami M, Moss TJ et al. Antenatal betamethasone changes cord blood monocyte responses to endotoxin in preterm lambs. Pediatr Res 2004; 55(5):764–768.

63. Moss TJ, Nitsos I, Ikegami M, Jobe AH, Newnham JP. Experimental intrauterine Ureaplasma infection in sheep. Am J Obstet Gynecol 2005; 192(4):1179–1186.

64. Ikegami M, Jobe A. Postnatal lung inflammation increased by ventilation of preterm lambs exposed antenatally to E. coli endotoxin. Pediatr Res 2002; 52:356–362.

12. Infection, inflammation, and perinatal brain injury

Susern Tan, Donald M Peebles, and David Edwards

INTRODUCTION

Although the overall causes of significant neuro-developmental delay are often idiopathic, it is clear that perinatal brain injury plays an important role.[1–3]

Perinatal brain injury encompasses any damage sustained by the developing fetal and neonatal brain, and is therefore a consequence of diverse etiologies. Unfortunately, because of the inherent in-vivo complexity of these multifactorial causes, the etiology and pathophysiology often remain unclear.

Antenatal factors are critical in perinatal brain injury,[4] and include primary genetic and developmental anomalies as well as important conditions such as hypoxic ischemia and intrauterine infection.[5,6] This chapter will concentrate on epidemiological studies and animal models of brain injury associated with infection, specifically intrauterine infection, with particular emphasis on the role of inflammation.

OUTCOMES MEASURES IN PERINATAL BRAIN INJURY

It can be difficult to identify perinatal brain injury in the acute context, and most epidemiological studies have defined the condition using a combination of clinical signs, long-term neurodevelopmental outcome, or imaging abnormalities.[7–11] Unfortunately, there is potential inconsistency in these outcomes, which are not standardized or uniform, and inherent heterogeneity therefore exists under the umbrella of perinatal brain injury.

CEREBRAL PALSY

The diagnosis of perinatal brain injury is often a delayed one, as early signs may be non-specific rather than overtly neurological, or may initially be too subtle for detection in the normal clinical setting. This is especially true in preterm infants, where developmental immaturity may act as a further confounder. Because of the difficulties in acute diagnosis, many observational studies have utilized neurodevelopmental follow-up to assess brain damage. Epidemiological studies show that perinatal brain injury may be associated with a spectrum of adverse outcomes in later life, including cognitive delay, speech and language disorders, defective vision and hearing, neuropsychiatric conditions such as attention-deficit/hyperactivity disorder and schizophrenia, and cerebral palsy (CP).[10,12–15]

CP is a diverse syndrome, present from early life, of non-progressive central nervous system disorders characterized by abnormalities in control of movement or posture. The overall prevalence of CP is approximately 1–2.3 per 1000 live births. Term infants represent the majority of all births and thus still constitute the majority of infants with CP, although their overall individual risk for CP is low.

Premature birth accounts for only 5–10% of all deliveries, but is associated with significant neonatal mortality and morbidity, with infants born prematurely at the lower gestational ages (23–30 weeks) at particular risk of CP and impaired cognitive function.[16,17] Very low birth weight infants constitute around 1% of all liveborns, which, as a proportion of total births, has increased slightly over the last 30 years; these infants, particularly those weighing under 1500 g, are at highest risk of brain injury.[12,17]

Major medical advances in the developed world are reflected in lower perinatal mortality, but the incidence of CP has not shown a parallel decline.[12,18] The prevalence of CP in term infants is largely unchanged,[19] but there is now increasing survival of preterm and very low birth weight survivors, who are at highest risk of CP.[12,16,17] Preterm birth is in turn strongly associated with intrauterine infection, in which inflammation is crucial, and potential links between infection, inflammation, and perinatal brain injury therefore appear plausible.

NEONATAL ENCEPHALOPATHY

Neonatal encephalopathy is now increasingly used to replace the traditional term of hypoxic-ischemic encephalopathy, in recognition that it is often difficult to prove hypoxia or ischemia in the normal clinical setting using conventional clinical tools.[20] Although special neuroinvestigative techniques may help,[21,22] the signs of hypoxia and infection are non-specific.[1,23–25] Unfortunately, there is still no universally employed standard definition of neonatal encephalopathy, although a framework for clinical diagnosis has been suggested.[26,27] Nevertheless, neonatal encephalopathy is the best known predictor of neurodevelopmental disability in term or near-term infants, and up to 25% of affected infants may develop subsequent permanent neurodevelopmental deficits, and 15–20% may not survive the neonatal period.

NEUROPATHOLOGY

The immature brain demonstrates unique responses to injury, as well as a high degree of plasticity.[28] There are major differences in the responses of preterm and term infants which may be accounted for both by differences in the type of insult and in the stage of neural development.

Term infants typically demonstrate predominant gray matter injury, with neurons in the deep gray nuclei and perirolandic cortex most vulnerable to ischemic damage. Selective neuronal necrosis can occur, with the hippocampus, cerebellum, thalamus, putamen, and deep cerebral cortex being at highest risk of damage.[29] Mature oligodendrocytes have higher levels of expression of antioxidant enzymes, which may account for greater resistance to oxidative damage in term infants.[30]

The neuropathology of white matter damage in preterm infants includes hemorrhagic parenchymal infarction (HPI), cystic periventricular leukomalacia (PVL), diffuse white matter damage (DWMD), selective neuronal injury, and focal ischemic lesions. Historically, hemorrhagic lesions were the commonest pathologies, but now PVL, and in particular DWMD (thought by some to be a form of diffuse non-cystic PVL)[19] are much more common.[31]

Preterm infants thus appear to be particularly prone to white matter damage. Although cortical and deep gray matter are also affected, some clinicians have suggested that the gray matter abnormality is the consequence of previous white matter damage.[32] The clear link between significant respiratory disease, particularly pneumothorax, and HPI in the early days of neonatal medicine suggested a causal role for vascular instability and hypoxic ischemia, which would have improved with significant advances in respiratory management such as antenatal steroid therapy and exogenous surfactant treatment. That preterm infants now commonly develop DWMD suggests that other factors are relevant. Specific factors in preterm brain injury may include the selective vulnerability of oligodendrocyte precursors to oxidative damage, vascular and physiological immaturity, and a particular link with infection.[33,34]

Oligodendrocyte progenitors and immature oligodendrocytes constitute 90% of the cell population until 27 weeks' gestation, and demonstrate a particular susceptibility to oxidative stress and ischemic damage.[35–39] Late preoligodendrocytes, in particular, are at highest risk of oxidative stress damage, and predominate from 24 to 30 weeks' gestation, approximately coinciding with the clinical risk period for PVL, which is of highest incidence at 26–28 weeks' gestation.[34,35]

NEUROIMAGING

Much of the outcome data available from earlier observational studies have involved ultrasound scans (USS) to investigate brain injury and CP.

USS evidence of cystic PVL correlates with cerebral palsy in 60–100% of preterm infant USS,[40] and USS diagnosis of PVL has also been reported in 5–15% of very low birth weight infants.[41] Cystic PVL on USS predicts delayed or disrupted myelination on later magnetic resonance imaging (MRI).[42] The severity of defects on USS scan may predict the risk for significant clinical outcomes, with parietal–occipital abnormalities reflecting the risk of CP and the extent of white matter echolucencies corresponding to the risk of cognitive defects.[43]

However, USS is generally a poor measure of neurological outcome. USS is sensitive and specific in revealing cerebral hemorrhage, but has very low specificity for demonstrating hypoxic-ischemic lesions or DWMD.[44] DWMD is now the commonest form of preterm brain injury,[9] and diffuse changes are found in association with PVL in 90% of preterm infants who later developed cerebral palsy.[45]

It has been difficult, using USS, to distinguish antenatal damage, including perinatal hypoxic ischemia and intrauterine infection, from later events such as postnatal sepsis. MRI offers better detection of perinatal brain injury, and early MRI may also be instrumental in supporting an intrauterine timing of cerebral insult.[31,46]

MRI scanning detects diffuse abnormalities, and allows potentially more reliable assumptions to be made about the presence and timing of cerebral insult.[46] MRI also differentiates between cortical gray matter and cerebral white matter, and between myelinated and non-myelinated white matter, thus providing an in-vivo picture of actual brain maturation.

Besides conventional MRI, advances have also led to other techniques such as diffusion-weighted and functional MRI, and coinvestigative techniques such as magnetic resonance spectroscopy. These should now offer more accurate assessments about the pathogenesis of perinatal brain injury. However, definitive outcome studies showing that MRI reliably predicts neurodevelopmental function are still in progress.

MECHANISMS OF INJURY IN INFECTION

Hypoxic ischemia, cerebral hemorrhage, and infection are often not mutually exclusive. Synergy or multiple insult is likely, and observational data support this theory of additive insult.[47] Inflammatory mechanisms are part of the cerebral response to hypoxia–ischemia, and infection may lead to reduced perfusion and hypoxic-ischemic damage. It is thus not fruitful to attempt to fully distinguish infection and ischemic mechanisms.[6,48]

Perinatal brain injury involves complex pathways that may be systemic, such as pyrexia, or local, e.g. in direct cytokine neurotoxicity. Systemic and local effects again often display crossover: e.g. cytokines originating from both peripheral infection and the brain. Cellular actions may also be heterogeneous; cytokines appear to have a dual neurotrophic and detrimental role in hypoxic–ischemic injury.[49] Pathways leading to eventual damage may also be inextricably interlinked or exhibit symbiosis, thereby further confounding accurate in-vivo characterization of brain injury.

Cellular pathways with particular relevance to infection-related brain damage include the action of proinflammatory mediators, toxin-mediated cellular responses, circulatory and coagulation factors, circulatory redistribution, and pyrexia. In particular, there seems to be a central role of inflammation in perinatal brain injury and the damage directly attributable to cytokine action, which appears to apply both to preterm infants and term infants.[50–53]

INFLAMMATORY MEDIATORS

Both infection and hypoxic ischemia stimulate inflammatory responses, with production and release of varied pro- and anti-inflammatory mediators, and inflammatory activation is frequently associated with perinatal brain injury.[54] In preterm infants, a fetal inflammatory response is also frequently seen in association with brain injury.[52]

However, precise delineation of the role of infection and inflammation is difficult. The very large number of cytokines and growth factors induced during a cerebral inflammatory response have many and varied actions, and our understanding of this process is not complete. The role of cytokine activity, particularly the interleukins (ILs) and tumor necrosis factor (TNF), have been studied in the developing brain[55] and animal studies show that genetic manipulation of the cascade or exogenous administration of cytokines affect the severity of brain injury.[49,56]

Cytokines have been reported in the brain and cerebrospinal fluid of neonates with perinatal brain injury,[57] and increased expression of cytokines, including IL-1β, IL-2, IL-2R, IL-6 and TNF-α, has also been demonstrated in the brains of autopsied infants with PVL compared with controls.[58–60] The highest immunoreactivity appears in those who were infected.[61]

Cytokines may be of systemic origin and breach the blood–brain barrier or may be produced locally in the brain; they effect neurotoxicity or neuroprotection in various ways. Direct cytolysis of vulnerable myelinating oligodendrocytes may occur, hence interfering with the maturation process from precursor to mature oligodendrocyte.[62,63] Cytokines have also been shown to stimulate astrocyte mitosis and growth,[64] as well as activate microglia. These mechanisms reflect the pattern of preterm brain injury, which is characterized by focal necrosis and white matter abnormality. In addition, cytokines have also been shown to stimulate excitatory imbalance, increase apoptosis (probably via increased caspase-3 activity) and mediate coagulative and circulatory changes.[65]

However, cytokine action is complicated, and neuroprotective effects have also been demonstrated in experimental hypoxic ischemic injury, with knockout TNF mice exhibiting greater neuronal damage[66] than normal mice, and with the administration of exogenous IL-6 resulting in increased neuroprotection.[67] The complexity of proinflammatory mediator action makes it difficult to elucidate an exact in-vivo role for individual inflammatory agents, and the action of a single cytokine is only part of the complex inflammatory chain operative in brain injury.

It may be argued that the direct role of inflammation has mostly been implicated by circumstantial deduction, and it remains difficult to establish whether inflammation plays a causal or a modulatory role. Temporal proof of inflammation preceding cerebral damage is also elusive in most observational studies. Most studies associating brain injury with proinflammatory mediator action have been based on measuring blood and amniotic fluid cytokine levels or cytokine expression in brain tissue, and this may merely reflect preceding cell death, rather than confirm a causative association. Similar problems exist with measuring just TNF levels in fetal blood. Further work is required to define the exact role of systemic and local inflammation in the cascade of events leading to cerebral injury.

COAGULATIVE AND CIRCULATORY FACTORS

Cytokines and chemokines activate vascular and angiogenic factors in the brain following hypoxic ischemia, and cause lymphocyte recruitment,[68] polymorphonuclear cell accumulation in capillaries,[69] and microglial activation.[70]

Excess thrombin production has been demonstrated in preterm rupture of membranes and labor,[71] but it has been suggested that coagulation factors may mediate perinatal brain damage by the attenuation of general inflammatory response rather than by direct occlusion of cerebral circulation. This is supported by adult studies demonstrating that activated protein C, which is both anti-inflammatory and anticoagulative, reduces mortality and morbidity in systemic inflammation, whereas solely anticoagulative or inactivated therapies have been unsuccessful.[72]

As previously discussed, antigen-primed memory cells definitively reflect fetal infection, and evidence of their activation has been useful in confirming the direct role of infection in perinatal brain injury.[73] T cell CD45RO+ may spill over from the circulation into the fetal brain and prolong inflammatory neuronal damage.[51]

CARDIOVASCULAR FAILURE

Histological chorioamnionitis and raised fetal blood IL-6 and IL-1β levels have been associated with tachycardia and systemic hypotension in premature neonates, whereas non-specific indicators of sepsis, including maternal pyrexia and left-shift of neonatal white blood cells, have been associated with impaired left ventricular function.[74] Animal studies have provided evidence of endotoxemia-induced fetal circulatory redistribution in intrauterine infection, with systemic hypotension, loss of cerebral autoregulation, and subsequent hypoxic-ischemic brain injury.[75,76] Fetal circulatory changes associated with infection, including systemic hypotension, endothelial damage, and leukocyte aggregation, have thus been suggested to contribute to ischemic damage in vulnerable areas of the fetal brain,[33] and it has been suggested that endotoxemia or cytokine action may be the cause of secondary impairments in fetal cardiovascular control, resulting in hypotension, cerebral hypoperfusion, and hypoxic-ischemic brain injury.[77] These decreases in cerebral perfusion may be observed postnatally, or after large doses of endotoxin are administered experimentally to the fetus; however, the contribution of cerebral hypoperfusion to endotoxin-induced brain injury remains unclear, as low concentrations of endotoxin, sufficient to cause cystic PVL when injected systemically, do not lead to reductions in cerebral blood flow in fetal sheep.[78,79] The observation from these studies, that a fall in fetal oxygenation, probably occurring secondary to reduced placental perfusion, led to a prolonged fall in cerebral oxygen delivery, provides an alternative method by which endotoxin might damage the brain; although whether the degree of hypoxia alone was severe enough to independently cause PVL is doubtful, as the brain at this gestation is remarkably resistant to hypoxia. However, it is possible that, as in rodent studies, pre-exposure to lipopolysaccharide (LPS) sensitizes the brain to a hypoxic insult, occurring 4–6 hours later.

Understanding the role of circulatory failure in preterm brain injury is hindered by the lack of a definition of what constitutes a low cerebral blood flow state. Commonly used drugs, including aminophylline and indomethacin, significantly decrease cerebral blood flow yet have no demonstrable effect on outcome, and low cerebral blood flow of 5–10 ml/100 g/min has also been shown in infants with normal neurological outcome.[80,81] It seems very likely that low blood flow must damage the preterm brain, but the level of flow at which this happens has yet to be defined.

PYREXIA

Sheep studies demonstrate that, with exogenous maternal heat exposure, the fetus resists hyperthermia by increasing placental perfusion to effect heat loss, but is susceptible to hyperthermia generated by pyrexia in maternal infection.[82] A small increase of brain temperature also appears to strongly increase neuronal vulnerability to hypoxia–ischemia,[83] and relative fetal hyperthermia may reflect increased susceptibility to neurotoxic factors as a result of a higher metabolic requirement for oxygen. Hypothermia has been seen to be protective in neonatal animals, whereas hyperthermia increases brain injury in adult rats.[84,85]

Observational studies have reported intrapartum maternal pyrexia as an association of subsequent CP,[1] and maternal fever has been reported to have adverse effects peripartum and in the early neonatal period.[86,87] However, conflicting data showing that maternal and neonatal fever did not increase the risk of morbidity or encephalopathy also exist.[88]

EXCITOTOXIC DAMAGE

Excitotoxic damage results from the excessive concentration of the excitatory transmitter glutamate in the synaptic cleft. Glutamate interacts with a variety of receptors, including N-methyl-D-aspartate (NMDA) and α-amino-3-hydroxy-5-methyl-4-isoxazole propionic acid (AMPA) and kainate receptors.

NMDA agonists induce early microglial activation and astrocyte cell death,[89–91] and both AMPA–kainate and NMDA receptor agonists have been shown to induce murine white matter damage similar to preterm PVL.[91]

Previously, preoligodendrocytes were thought to possess AMPA and kainite receptors, but not NMDA receptors, so it was thought that the damage induced by NMDA was indirect.[91–94] However, it has recently been shown that NMDA receptors are present and capable of transducing preoligodendrocyte cell death; AMPA receptors are mainly expressed on the somas of preoligodendrocytes, whereas NMDA receptors are expressed on the cell processes.[95,96] Whereas AMPA–kainate receptors play a direct role in preoligodendritic cell death, NMDA receptors may also have an effect on cell maturation and survival by damaging the cell processes.

These important developments have now changed our understanding of the role of NMDA receptors in excitotoxic damage, but our knowledge is incomplete as many different receptor subtypes exist,[97] and there is uncertainty about their individual roles.[98] However, a role for glutaminergic damage must be considered as part of the injury cascade induced by hypoxia–ischemia and by infective processes.

DEFINING INTRAUTERINE INFECTION

Identifying the presence of intrauterine infection may itself present problems, given the potential for false results in microbiological investigation, and the mere presence or absence of bacteria cannot adequately define infection. Maternofetal inflammation, in the form of chorioamnionitis or an exaggerated inflammatory cascade response, has been demonstrated in association with infection, and the presence of this inflammatory response may offer a more valid confirmation of infection, particularly if pathogens are also demonstrable.

Chorioamnionitis may be identified in clinical or histological terms, and has a considerably higher incidence in preterm than in term births.[99–101] However, the diagnosis of chorioamnionitis on clinical grounds may be difficult, and moreover has been liberally applied in vague circumstances such as the mere presence of maternal pyrexia.[102] A strong association has been reported between immunohistological chorioamnionitis and the results of amniotic fluid culture in preterm infants, but some studies have also demonstrated that severe bacterial infection of the neonate can occur without evidence of chorioamnionitis,[103,104] and placental and cord inflammation may be histotopographically variable.[105] Qualifying criteria used to identify chorioamnionitis can therefore lack uniformity,[106] which may lead to heterogeneity in various studies and their subsequent conclusions.

In the absence of absolute histological evidence and with the inherent vagaries in clinical diagnosis, it may also be important to consider the inflammatory cascade when defining infection, and strong evidence exists of intrauterine infection inducing maternofetal host responses, in which the fetal inflammatory response syndrome appears to be of primary importance.[51,107–110]

EXPERIMENTAL STUDIES

Since the observation by Gilles in 1976, that prolonged exposure of neonatal kittens to LPS, a bacterial product, resulted in white matter damage, there have been many experiments demonstrating a link between perinatal administration of bacteria or endotoxin and brain injury[111] (for review see Hagberg et al[48]). These experiments establish some important principles:

1. A range of bacteria, including *Escherichia coli* and *Gardnerella vaginalis*, and endotoxins can

cause perinatal brain injury, mainly affecting white matter.[111–113]

2. This effect can be observed whether bacteria or LPS are administered intraperitoneally to the pregnant rat,[114] intracervically in rats and rabbits,[112] or systemically to the fetal sheep,[78,115] suggesting transplacental passage of neurotoxic mediators.

3. Almost identical cerebral histopathology can be arrived at by a variety of different insults, including hypoxia–ischemia, infection, and excitotoxicity.[116]

Maternofetal infection does not invariably cause neurological damage in these models; there is species specificity in that intraperitoneal LPS in mice and rat pups does not cause overt neural cell death. Route of administration may be important, as intra-amniotic administration of E. coli LPS in sheep is associated with much lower mortality rates and evidence of cerebral effects than when given systemically. It is relevant, considering the potential role of periodontal organisms in preterm labor, that, in fetal sheep, intra-amniotic LPS from Fusobacterium nucleatum and Porphyromonas gingivalis was associated with a much higher fetal mortality rate than E. coli.[117] Similar findings have been described with administration of P. gingivalis LPS to the pregnant hamster pig, even if the LPS was given prior to mating.[118]

Activation of systemic and cerebral inflammatory factors is likely to be an important factor in neural cell death. Several investigators have shown increased levels of mRNA and protein for the proinflammatory cytokines IL-1β and TNF-α within fetal brain, following maternal administration of LPS.[114,119] It is not clear whether these cytokines are produced in response to systemically produced cytokines crossing the blood–brain barrier (BBB), a direct action of endotoxin on microglia, or both. One of the effects of endotoxin is to increase BBB permeability, thereby allowing cytotoxic and proinflammatory substances to pass freely from the circulation into the brain following peripheral inflammatory stimulation.[120] The existence of a paracrine/autocrine feedback loop

whereby TNF-α increases microglial expression of the LPS receptor CD14 and induces the transcription factor NF-κB (nuclear factor-κB) suggests that LPS and TNF-α can work together to further increase levels of proinflammatory cytokines and cytotoxic oxygen free radicals.[121] Microglia appear to be the major LPS responsive cells within the central nervous system (CNS), and expression of a mutation that inactivates TLR4 (tlr4 mic) prevents LPS-mediated neural cell death, both in culture and in an in-vivo model of LPS-sensitized hypoxic-ischemic neuronal injury.[122] Whether produced as a result of glial cell activation or systemically, cytokines such as TNF-α have been shown to be directly cytotoxic, particularly effecting oligodendrocyte precursors, the major subtype of oligodendrocytes in the fetal brain premyelination;[123,124] sheep studies show that LPS results in fewer, morphologically abnormal oligodendrocytes.[115]

Studies using neonatal mice and rats suggest that another way in which LPS could indirectly damage the brain is to reduce the threshold at which hypoxia–ischemia is neurotoxic.[125] Eklind et al demonstrated that neither E. coli LPS (0.3 mg/kg) nor hypoxia–ischemia (unilateral carotid ligation and hypoxia 7.7% for 20 minutes) caused obvious brain injury in 7-day-old rats; however, LPS given 4 hours before the hypoxic-ischemic insult (HI) resulted in significant cerebral infarction.[126] This synergistic interaction is seen whether LPS is given intracisternally or systemically,[127,128] but is lost in mice with a loss of function mutation of the TLR4 receptor, which is necessary for LPS-induced microglial activation.[122] However, the nature of interaction between LPS and HI is very dependent on the time interval between the two insults; in a follow-up paper, Eklind et al showed enhanced vulnerability to HI in the acute (4–6 hours) and chronic phase (72 hours) but a protective effect at 24 hours.[129] These data are in keeping with experiments in adult rats where LPS priming 24–48 hours prior to HI has a preconditioning, neuroprotective effect.[130,131] The precise mechanisms underlying these different actions of LPS are unclear at present. LPS leads to widespread microglial activation,[116,120] and prevention of this blocks the sensitizing effect of LPS, presumably by decreasing the contribution of downstream mediators to cell death. Other potential mechanisms are nitric oxide-mediated mitochondrial dysfunction and hypoglycemia.[132] The preconditioning effect of LPS may relate to up-regulation of corticosteroids with the brain – LPS is known to increase levels of the stress hormone CRH (corticotropin-releasing hormone) in fetal brain, and treatment with RU486, a glucocorticoid receptor blocker, counteracts LPS-induced tolerance.[133,134] Another possible factor is the role of cytokines with an anti-inflammatory action, such as IL-10 and TGF-β (transforming growth factor-β). These cytokines, produced later in the inflammatory response to infection than pro-inflammatory cytokines such as TNF-α and IL-1β, which are observed within hours of LPS exposure, have neuroprotective actions. For instance, Pang et al show that IL-10 reduces the white matter damage (WMD) observed in rat pups following maternal *E. coli* inoculation during pregnancy, by suppressing microglial activation.[135] This would be consistent with the diminished cellular inflammatory response to middle cerebral artery occlusion observed with LPS preconditioning in adult rats.[131]

Overall, there is now a wealth of animal experimentation to support the role of infection-induced inflammation, observed in clinical epidemiological studies, in perinatal brain injury. However, there are many unanswered questions, including the role of more clinically relevant bacterial endotoxins and the mechanisms underlying the interaction between LPS and HI. It will also be important to investigate whether neuroprotective strategies, shown to be of benefit following HI, such as hypothermia, have the same effects following these multifactorial insults. Of particular interest is the role of progesterone; this steroid has anti-inflammatory properties, reduces the risk of preterm delivery in a high-risk population, and reduces fetal mortality following LPS injection into the uterus of pregnant rats.[136] However, it is not yet known whether it protects the fetal brain from infection-related inflammation.

PRETERM INFANTS

INFECTION AND PRETERM BIRTH

Intrauterine infection is commonly acknowledged to play an important role in initiating premature rupture of membranes and preterm delivery,[137–139] but the infective ecology remains unclear, and a complex picture whereby bacteria can be present in large numbers in the fetal membranes without inducing preterm labor or fetal damage has also been described.[140] Although organisms such as group B streptococcus and *E. coli* are well recognized in association with adverse outcomes, these types of infection are relatively rare, and do not appear to be the cause of most preterm births. Current data suggest that the most common pathogens in preterm birth appear to be *Ureaplasma urealyticum*, *Mycoplasma hominis*, and *F. nucleatum*.[138,141]

There is interest in the potential of chronic conditions such as bacterial vaginosis[142–144] and periodontitis[145–148] to lead to preterm labor, and periodontal organisms have recently been demonstrated to cause preterm labor by hematagenous spread in a murine model.[149] The role of the inflammatory cascade causing preterm labor is well established, and a persistent intrauterine inflammatory state has been demonstrated in preterm birth.[108,138,150] This suggests that chronic exposure to bacteria may result in preterm birth and affect fetal brain damage in a variety of ways, as previously described.

INFLAMMATORY BRAIN INJURY

INFECTION AND ADVERSE OUTCOME

Intrauterine infection is related to adverse neonatal outcome, including brain injury, chronic lung disease, and susceptibility to sepsis, which have been linked to positive culture in the amniotic fluid.[108,151]

Likewise, some investigators have also reported a significant association between intrauterine infection and CP,[152–154] whereas this association did not reach statistical significance in other studies.[155–157] Prematurity and the complications of prematurity, including cerebral infarction, PVL, and sepsis, have been shown to increase the risk for CP.[132]

A relationship between infection and brain imaging abnormalities has been described. Neonates with documented sepsis have been found to be at higher risk of PVL,[158] and PVL or intraventricular hemorrhage as well as significantly elevated levels of amniotic fluid IL-6 have been associated with cultivable bacteria in amniotic fluid.[159] Spontaneous preterm birth, most probably infection-related, has been associated with a 20-fold risk of white matter damage compared with preterm birth not involving infection.[160]

It has further been suggested that the inflammatory response to infection may be chronic in nature, and may precede delivery by months or even be preconceptual, involving a prolonged period during which damage to the fetal brain is effected.[161] This would support the etiological potential of conditions such as bacterial vaginosis (BV) and periodontitis as a source of infection. In support of this theory, mothers of infants with PVL appear more likely to have prenatal positive bacterial cervical and vaginal cultures, suggesting that chronic exposure to infection or inflammation may increase the risk for perinatal brain injury.[162]

INFLAMMATION AND ADVERSE OUTCOME

Histological chorioamnionitis, accompanied by raised cytokine levels in the amniotic fluid, has been found to be associated with an increased risk of white matter injury,[157] and chorioamnionitis has been specifically associated with an increased incidence of PVL, periventricular hemorrhage, intraventicular hemorrhage, and antenatal PVL in preterm infants.[51] Numerous studies have now reported associations between chorioamnionitis and CP,[152–154,163,164] and long term follow-up of neonates has demonstrated that those with a higher rate of funisitis and with higher concentrations of IL-6, IL-8 and white cells in the amniotic fluid were at increased risk of cerebral palsy at the age of 3 years.[165]

The association of proinflammatory mediators with white matter lesions and CP in preterm neonates is also well-described, and interleukins, in

particular, appear to have an important role. Inflammatory mediators in the amniotic fluid have traditionally been attributed to the maternal inflammatory response, and those in fetal blood to a fetal response, but it has now been proposed that both may actually constitute a fetal inflammatory response syndrome, which is also characterized by funisitis.[52]

Preterm infants with raised proinflammatory cytokine concentrations in the blood or amniotic fluid are more likely to develop abnormal cerebral USS abnormalities and later neurodevelopmental impairment than infants with normal cytokine levels,[157,165] and umbilical cord plasma or amniotic fluid concentrations of IL have been shown to be a significant and independent predictor of brain injury, including PVL.[166] Raised levels of amniotic fluid IL-6 have also been demonstrated to be an independent risk factor for developing PVL,[159] and increased amniotic fluid matrix metalloproteinase-8, a protease associated with preterm ruptured membranes, has been associated with the subsequent development of cerebral palsy at 3 year assessment.[167]

FETAL INFLAMMATORY RESPONSE SYNDROME

As previously emphasized, it appears that fetal inflammation may be the most important mechanism for preterm birth[52,168,169] and to predict adverse neurological outcome.[65,170] Funisitis appears to have the stronger association with white matter disease and CP, demonstrating an odds ratio of ≥ 3 in various studies;[53,165,170] for instance, in one multicenter prospective study, fetal vasculitis was found to be associated with an 11-fold increase in the risk of PVL and was associated with ultrasonically detected echolucent white matter lesions, whereas placental membrane inflammation did not show a corresponding relationship.[53]

EVIDENCE AGAINST INFLAMMATORY BRAIN INJURY

However, not all studies have confirmed a role for systemic inflammation in preterm brain injury.

Two studies have not demonstrated associations between inflammation and brain damage: the first study found no association between CP and cytokines of preterm children born under 32 weeks' gestation;[171] another study, where sample size was very small, reported lower levels of amniotic fluid cytokines in infants with white matter damage, although results did not achieve significance.[172]

Moreover, although there was an association between raised cytokine levels and CP found in premature infants of 31 weeks' gestation compared with controls of 33 weeks' gestation in a previously quoted study, the differences in cytokine values were not sustained when adjusted for birth weight and gestational age.[157]

A number of studies have also described no association between intrauterine infection and CP in preterm infants,[170,173,174] and the overall evidence linking intrauterine infection and CP is less convincing in very preterm infants than in term infants.[1,170,175,176] Difficulties in assessing the strength of evidence linking preterm infection and inflammation to brain injury include confounding problems specific to prematurity, such as the powerful confounders of pre-eclampsia in very low birth weight infants and the differences in gestational age ranges, as well as the method of adjusting for gestational age.

TERM INFANTS

Brain injury in the term infant has traditionally been attributed to intrapartum events, including birth asphyxia, but studies have observed that less than 10% of CP and 15% of mental retardation seem linked to intrapartum events.[177] The importance of hypoxic-ischemic insult as a cause of CP has since been debated, and population studies have demonstrated that birth asphyxia may account for only 6–10% of perinatal brain injury.[178,179]

The fact that most term perinatal brain injury appears idiopathic, with no identifiable peripartal or genetic cause, emphasizes the potential importance of other prenatal factors such as maternal pyrexia, coagulation defects, maternal thyroid disease, and intrauterine infection/inflammation.

A recent study of term infants with encephalopathy has demonstrated that signs of recent insult were apparent on MRI, whereas evidence of chronic antenatal injury appeared rare,[46] suggesting that major insult may have occurred peri-delivery, possibly following priming by antenatal factors such as infection. A plausible assumption would be that the term infant may be sensitized to hypoxic-ischemic damage by preceding cerebral inflammation from factors that include infection. This is supported by evidence of a significant 78-fold increase in the risk of CP in infants of normal birth weight if more than one adverse risk factor is present at birth, such as combined exposure to infection and asphyxia, which appear to act in synergy.[47]

Although neonatal infection with group B streptococcus is well recognized to lead to brain injury in term infants, there are still significant gaps in our understanding of intrauterine bacterial infection.

There is also a paucity of studies on the role of infection and inflammation in term perinatal brain injury, but interestingly the association appears stronger in term infants than in preterm infants.[180,181]

In infants of normal birth weight, maternal antenatal infection evidenced by clinical and histological chorioamniotis was associated with a significant ninefold increase in the risk of CP. The association of CP with intrauterine infection remained strong even when potential confounding factors were considered, and most of the affected infants did not demonstrate signs of neonatal infection, sepsis, or prolonged rupture of membranes,[1,182] highlighting the probability of chronic infection with organisms of low-grade pathogenicity.

Histological chorioamnionitis has also been shown to be a significant risk factor in a meta-analysis of both term and preterm infants with CP and PVL,[181] and intrapartum maternal pyrexia, a sign of chorioamnionitis, has been associated with an increased incidence of immediate postnatal neonatal encephalopathy, including seizures.[86,183]

In retrospective studies of infants over 35 weeks' gestation, analysis of frozen neonatal screening blood spots has demonstrated significantly higher levels of neonatal cytokines and coagulative factors in children with CP than in controls, with the interleukins (IL-6, IL-3, and IL-13) in particular reported to have a sensitivity and specificity of more than 88% for CP.[54] The same group has also reported raised neonatal serum interferon levels compared with controls in children who later developed CP.[184]

CONCLUSIONS

Overall, epidemiological and experimental studies have indicated that intrauterine infection and inflammation constitute a risk factor for adverse neurological outcome in both preterm and term infants. Although there are few studies in term infants, the evidence associating infection with perinatal brain injury appears stronger in term than preterm infants. We do not have a precise mechanistic understanding of how systemic or local inflammation leads to brain damage, but current evidence suggests a complex interplay between inflammatory mechanisms and other insults such as hypoxia–ischemia and excitotoxic damage.

With the aid of increasingly sophisticated technologies such as MRI, and with bioinformatics and genomic investigation, there could be better understanding and potential amelioration of the inflammatory damage seen in perinatal brain injury. There is no current clinical strategy aimed at modifying the maternofetal inflammatory response, although neuro-cooling studies promise potential future intervention in term hypoxic-ischemic encephalopathy.

REFERENCES

1. Grether JK, Nelson KB. Maternal infection and cerebral palsy in infants of normal birth weight. JAMA 1997; 278:207–211.
2. Meberg A, Broch H. Etiology of cerebral palsy. J Perinat Med 2004; 32:434–439.
3. Nelson KB, Ellenberg JH. Antecedents of cerebral palsy. Multivariate analysis of risk. N Engl J Med 1986; 315:81–86.
4. Hagberg H, Mallard C. Antenatal brain injury: aetiology and possibilities of prevention. Semin Neonatol 2000; 5:41–51.
5. Felix JF, Badawi N, Kurinczuk JJ et al. Birth defects in children with newborn encephalopathy. Dev Med Child Neurol 2000; 42:803–808.
6. Hagberg H, Wennerholm UB, Savman K. Sequelae of chorioamnionitis. Curr Opin Infect Dis 2002; 15:301–306.
7. Badawi N, Keogh JM, Dixon G, Kurinczuk JJ. Developmental outcomes of newborn encephalopathy in the term infant. Indian J Pediatr 2001; 68:527–530.
8. Dixon G, Badawi N, Kurinczuk JJ et al. Early developmental outcomes after newborn encephalopathy. Pediatrics 2002; 109:26–33.
9. Hamrick SE, Miller SP, Leonard C et al. Trends in severe brain injury and neurodevelopmental outcome in premature newborn infants: the role of cystic periventricular leukomalacia. J Pediatr 2004; 145: 593–599.
10. Mercuri E, Barnett AL. Neonatal brain MRI and motor outcome at school age in children with neonatal encephalopathy: a review of personal experience. Neural Plast 2003; 10:51–57.
11. Stanley FJ. Prenatal determinants of motor disorders. Acta Paediatr Suppl 1997; 422:92–102.
12. Hagberg B, Hagberg G, Olow I, van Wendt L. The changing panorama of cerebral palsy in Sweden. VII. Prevalence and origin in the birth year period 1987–90. Acta Paediatr 1996; 85:954–960.
13. Hagberg B, Hagberg G. The changing panorama of cerebral palsy – bilateral spastic forms in particular. Acta Paediatr Suppl 1996; 416: 48–52.
14. Mercuri E, Anker S, Guzzetta A et al. Neonatal cerebral infarction and visual function at school age. Arch Dis Child Fetal Neonatal Ed 2003; 88:F487–F491.
15. Weinberger DR. From neuropathology to neurodevelopment. Lancet 1995; 346:552–557.
16. Cummins SK, Nelson KB, Grether JK, Velie EM. Cerebral palsy in four northern California counties, births 1983 through 1985. J Pediatr 1993; 123:230–237.
17. Hack M, Friedman H, Fanaroff AA. Outcomes of extremely low birth weight infants. Pediatrics 1996; 98:931–937.
18. Colver AF, Gibson M, Hey EN et al. Increasing rates of cerebral palsy across the severity spectrum in north-east England 1964–1993. The North of England Collaborative Cerebral Palsy Survey. Arch Dis Child Fetal Neonatal Ed 2000; 83:F7–F12.
19. Pharoah PO, Cooke T, Cooke RW, Rosenbloom L. Birthweight specific trends in cerebral palsy. Arch Dis Child 1990; 65:602–606.
20. Nelson KB, Dambrosia JM, Ting TY, Grether JK. Uncertain value of electronic fetal monitoring in predicting cerebral palsy. N Engl J Med 1996; 334:613–618.
21. Azzopardi D, Wyatt JS, Cady EB et al. Prognosis of newborn infants with hypoxic-ischemic brain injury assessed by phosphorus magnetic resonance spectroscopy. Pediatr Res 1989; 25:445–451.
22. Wyatt JS, Edwards AD, Azzopardi D, Reynolds EO. Magnetic resonance and near infrared spectroscopy for investigation of perinatal hypoxic-ischaemic brain injury. Arch Dis Child 1989; 64:953–963.
23. Badawi N, Kurinczuk JJ, Mackenzie CL et al. Maternal thyroid disease: a risk factor for newborn encephalopathy in term infants. BJOG 2000; 107:798–801.
24. Keogh JM, Badawi N, Kurinczuk JJ, Pemberton PJ, Stanley FJ. Group B streptococcus infection, not birth asphyxia. Aust N Z J Obstet Gynaecol 1999; 39:108–110.
25. Keogh JM, Badawi N. The origins of cerebral palsy. Curr Opin Neurol 2006; 19:129–134.

26. Ferriero DM. Neonatal brain injury. N Engl J Med 2004; 351: 1985–1995.

27. Miller SP, Latal B, Clark H et al. Clinical signs predict 30-month neurodevelopmental outcome after neonatal encephalopathy. Am J Obstet Gynecol 2004; 190:93–99.

28. Vexler ZS, Ferriero DM. Molecular and biochemical mechanisms of perinatal brain injury. Semin Neonatol 2001; 6:99–108.

29. Rivkin MJ. Hypoxic-ischemic brain injury in the term newborn. Neuropathology, clinical aspects, and neuroimaging. Clin Perinatol 1997; 24:607–625.

30. Baud O, Greene AE, Li J et al. Glutathione peroxidase-catalase cooperativity is required for resistance to hydrogen peroxide by mature rat oligodendrocytes. J Neurosci 2004; 24:1531–1540.

31. Maalouf EF, Duggan PJ, Rutherford MA et al. Magnetic resonance imaging of the brain in a cohort of extremely preterm infants. J Pediatr 1999; 135:351–357.

32. Inder TE, Huppi PS, Warfield S et al. Periventricular white matter injury in the premature infant is followed by reduced cerebral cortical gray matter volume at term. Ann Neurol 1999; 46:755–760.

33. Volpe JJ. Neurobiology of periventricular leukomalacia in the premature infant. Pediatr Res 2001; 50:553–562.

34. Zupan V, Gonzalez P, Lacaze-Masmonteil T et al. Periventricular leukomalacia: risk factors revisited. Dev Med Child Neurol 1996; 38: 1061–1067.

35. Back SA, Luo NL, Borenstein NS et al. Late oligodendrocyte progenitors coincide with the developmental window of vulnerability for human perinatal white matter injury. J Neurosci 2001; 21: 1302–1312.

36. Baud O, Li J, Zhang Y et al. Nitric oxide-induced cell death in developing oligodendrocytes is associated with mitochondrial dysfunction and apoptosis-inducing factor translocation. Eur J Neurosci 2004; 20:1713–1726.

37. Haynes RL, Folkerth RD, Keefe RJ et al. Nitrosative and oxidative injury to premyelinating oligodendrocytes in periventricular leukomalacia. J Neuropathol Exp Neurol 2003; 62:441–450.

38. McQuillen PS, Sheldon RA, Shatz CJ, Ferriero DM. Selective vulnerability of subplate neurons after early neonatal hypoxia-ischemia. J Neurosci 2003; 23:3308–3315.

39. Oka A, Belliveau MJ, Rosenberg PA, Volpe JJ. Vulnerability of oligodendroglia to glutamate: pharmacology, mechanisms, and prevention. J Neurosci 1993; 13:1441–1453.

40. Leviton A, Paneth N. White matter damage in preterm newborns – an epidemiologic perspective. Early Hum Dev 1990; 24:1–22.

41. de Vries LS, Eken P, Dubowitz LM. The spectrum of leukomalacia using cranial ultrasound. Behav Brain Res 1992; 49:1–6.

42. Guit GL, van de Bor M, den Ouden L, Wondergem JH. Prediction of neurodevelopmental outcome in the preterm infant: MR-staged myelination compared with cranial US. Radiology 1990; 175: 107–109.

43. Holling EE, Leviton A. Characteristics of cranial ultrasound white-matter echolucencies that predict disability: a review. Dev Med Child Neurol 1999; 41:136–139.

44. Hope PL, Gould SJ, Howard S et al. Precision of ultrasound diagnosis of pathologically verified lesions in the brains of very preterm infants. Dev Med Child Neurol 1988; 30:457–471.

45. Krageloh-Mann I, Hagberg G, Hagberg B, Michaelis R. Origin of brain abnormalities in bilateral spastic cerebral palsy. Dev Med Child Neurol 1995; 37:1031–1032.

46. Cowan F, Rutherford M, Groenendaal F et al. Origin and timing of brain lesions in term infants with neonatal encephalopathy. Lancet 2003; 361:736–742.

47. Nelson KB, Grether JK. Potentially asphyxiating conditions and spastic cerebral palsy in infants of normal birth weight. Am J Obstet Gynecol 1998; 179:507–513.

48. Hagberg H, Peebles D, Mallard C. Models of white matter injury: comparison of infectious, hypoxic-ischemic, and excitotoxic insults. Ment Retard Dev Disabil Res Rev 2002; 8:30–38.

49. Hagan P, Barks JD, Yabut M et al. Adenovirus-mediated overexpression of interleukin-1 receptor antagonist reduces susceptibility to excitotoxic brain injury in perinatal rats. Neuroscience 1996; 75: 1033–1045.

50. Dammann O, Durum S, Leviton A. Do white cells matter in white matter damage? Trends Neurosci 2001; 24:320–324.

51. Dammann O, Leviton A. Maternal intrauterine infection, cytokines, and brain damage in the preterm newborn. Pediatr Res 1997; 42: 1–8.

52. Dammann O, Leviton A. Role of the fetus in perinatal infection and neonatal brain damage. Curr Opin Pediatr 2000; 12:99–104.

53. Leviton A, Paneth N, Reuss ML et al. Maternal infection, fetal inflammatory response, and brain damage in very low birth weight infants. Developmental Epidemiology Network Investigators. Pediatr Res 1999; 46:566–575.

54. Nelson KB, Dambrosia JM, Grether JK, Phillips TM. Neonatal cytokines and coagulation factors in children with cerebral palsy. Ann Neurol 1998; 44:665–675.

55. Silverstein FS, Barks JD, Hagan P et al. Cytokines and perinatal brain injury. Neurochem Int 1997; 30:375–383.

56. Balasingam V, Yong VW. Attenuation of astroglial reactivity by interleukin-10. J Neurosci 1996; 16:2945–2955.

57. Van Landeghem FK, Felderhoff-Mueser U, Moysich A et al. Fas (CD95/Apo-1)/Fas ligand expression in neonates with pontosubicular neuron necrosis. Pediatr Res 2002; 51:129–135.

58. Kadhim H, Tabarki B, De Prez C, Rona AM, Sebire G. Interleukin-2 in the pathogenesis of perinatal white matter damage. Neurology 2002; 58:1125–1128.

59. Kadhim H, Tabarki B, De Prez C, Sebire G. Cytokine immunoreactivity in cortical and subcortical neurons in periventricular leukomalacia: are cytokines implicated in neuronal dysfunction in cerebral palsy? Acta Neuropathol (Berl) 2003; 105:209–216.

60. Yoon BH, Romero R, Kim CJ et al. High expression of tumor necrosis factor-alpha and interleukin-6 in periventricular leukomalacia. Am J Obstet Gynecol 1997; 177:406–411.

61. Kadhim H, Tabarki B, Verellen G et al. Inflammatory cytokines in the pathogenesis of periventricular leukomalacia. Neurology 2001; 56:1278–1284.

62. Kahn MA, De Vellis J. Regulation of an oligodendrocyte progenitor cell line by the interleukin-6 family of cytokines. Glia 1994; 12: 87–98.

63. Vartanian T, Li Y, Zhao M, Stefansson K. Interferon-gamma-induced oligodendrocyte cell death: implications for the pathogenesis of multiple sclerosis. Mol Med 1995; 1:732–743.

64. Merrill JE. Effects of interleukin-1 and tumor necrosis factor-alpha on astrocytes, microglia, oligodendrocytes, and glial precursors in vitro. Dev Neurosci 1991; 13:130–137.

65. Cornette L. Fetal and neonatal inflammatory response and adverse outcome. Semin Fetal Neonatal Med 2004; 9:459–470.

66. Bruce AJ, Boling W, Kindy MS et al. Altered neuronal and microglial responses to excitotoxic and ischemic brain injury in mice lacking TNF receptors. Nat Med 1996; 2:788–794.

67. Loddick SA, Turnbull AV, Rothwell NJ. Cerebral interleukin-6 is neuroprotective during permanent focal cerebral ischemia in the rat. J Cereb Blood Flow Metab 1998; 18:176–179.

68. Bona E, Andersson AL, Blomgren K et al. Chemokine and inflammatory cell response to hypoxia-ischemia in immature rats. Pediatr Res 1999; 45:500–509.

69. Hudome S, Palmer C, Roberts RL et al. The role of neutrophils in the production of hypoxic-ischemic brain injury in the neonatal rat. Pediatr Res 1997; 41:607–616.

70. Blomgren K, McRae A, Bona E et al. Degradation of fodrin and MAP 2 after neonatal cerebral hypoxic-ischemia. Brain Res 1995; 684:136–142.

71. Chaiworapongsa T, Espinoza J, Yoshimatsu J et al. Activation of coagulation system in preterm labor and preterm premature rupture of membranes. J Matern Fetal Neonatal Med 2002; 11:368–373.

72. Leviton A, Dammann O. Coagulation, inflammation, and the risk of neonatal white matter damage. Pediatr Res 2004; 55:541–545.

73. Duggan PJ, Maalouf EF, Watts TL et al. Intrauterine T-cell activation and increased proinflammatory cytokine concentrations in preterm infants with cerebral lesions. Lancet 2001; 358:1699–1700.

74. Yanowitz TD, Jordan JA, Gilmour CH et al. Hemodynamic disturbances in premature infants born after chorioamnionitis: association with cord blood cytokine concentrations. Pediatr Res 2002; 51: 310–316.

75. Bada HS, Korones SB, Perry EH et al. Mean arterial blood pressure changes in premature infants and those at risk for intraventricular hemorrhage. J Pediatr 1990; 117:607–614.

76. Garnier Y, Coumans AB, Jensen A, Hasaart TH, Berger R. Infection-related perinatal brain injury: the pathogenic role of impaired fetal cardiovascular control. J Soc Gynecol Investig 2003; 10: 450–459.

77. Jensen A, Garnier Y, Middelanis J, Berger R. Perinatal brain damage – from pathophysiology to prevention. Eur J Obstet Gynecol Reprod Biol 2003; 110(Suppl 1):S70–S79.

78. Peebles DM, Miller S, Newman JP, Scott R, Hanson MA. The effect of systemic administration of lipopolysaccharide on cerebral haemodynamics and oxygenation in the 0.65 gestation ovine fetus in utero. BJOG 2003; 110:735–743.

79. Dalitz P, Harding R, Rees SM, Cock ML. Prolonged reductions in placental blood flow and cerebral oxygen delivery in preterm fetal sheep exposed to endotoxin: possible factors in white matter injury after acute infection. J Soc Gynecol Investig 2003; 10: 283–290.

80. Edwards AD, Wyatt JS, Richardson C et al. Effects of indomethacin on cerebral haemodynamics in very preterm infants. Lancet 1990; 335: 1491–1495.

81. McDonnell M, Ives NK, Hope PL. Intravenous aminophylline and cerebral blood flow in preterm infants. Arch Dis Child 1992; 67: 416–418.

82. Laburn HP, Mitchell D, Goelst K. Fetal and maternal body temperatures measured by radiotelemetry in near-term sheep during thermal stress. J Appl Physiol 1992; 72:894–900.

83. Minamisawa H, Smith ML, Siesjo BK. The effect of mild hyperthermia and hypothermia on brain damage following 5, 10, and 15 minutes of forebrain ischemia. Ann Neurol 1990; 28:26–33.

84. Bona E, Hagberg H, Loberg EM, Bagenholm R, Thoresen M. Protective effects of moderate hypothermia after neonatal hypoxia-ischemia: short- and long-term outcome. Pediatr Res 1998; 43: 738–745.

85. Dietrich WD, Busto R, Valdes I, Loor Y. Effects of normothermic versus mild hyperthermic forebrain ischemia in rats. Stroke 1990; 21:1318–1325.

86. Lieberman E, Eichenwald E, Mathur G et al. Intrapartum fever and unexplained seizures in term infants. Pediatrics 2000; 106:983–988.

87. Perlman JM. Maternal fever and neonatal depression: preliminary observations. Clin Pediatr (Phila) 1999; 38:287–291.

88. Shalak LF, Perlman JM, Jackson GL, Laptook AR. Depression at birth in term infants exposed to maternal chorioamnionitis: does neonatal fever play a role? J Perinatol 2005; 25:447–452.

89. Sfaello I, Daire JL, Husson I et al. Patterns of excitotoxin-induced brain lesions in the newborn rabbit: a neuropathological and MRI correlation. Dev Neurosci 2005; 27:160–168.

90. Sfaello I, Baud O, Arzimanoglou A, Gressens P. Topiramate prevents excitotoxic damage in the newborn rodent brain. Neurobiol Dis 2005; 20:837–848.

91. Tahraoui SL, Marret S, Bodenant C et al. Central role of microglia in neonatal excitotoxic lesions of the murine periventricular white matter. Brain Pathol 2001; 11:56–71.

92. Deng W, Wang H, Rosenberg PA, Volpe JJ, Jensen FE. Role of metabotropic glutamate receptors in oligodendrocyte excitotoxicity and oxidative stress. Proc Natl Acad Sci USA 2004; 101: 7751–7756.

93. Follett PL, Rosenberg PA, Volpe JJ, Jensen FE. NBQX attenuates excitotoxic injury in developing white matter. J Neurosci 2000; 20: 9235–9241.

94. Follett PL, Deng W, Dai W et al. Glutamate receptor-mediated oligodendrocyte toxicity in periventricular leukomalacia: a protective role for topiramate. J Neurosci 2004; 24:4412–4420.

95. Karadottir R, Cavelier P, Bergersen LH, Attwell D. NMDA receptors are expressed in oligodendrocytes and activated in ischaemia. Nature 2005; 438:1162–1166.

96. Salter MG, Fern R. NMDA receptors are expressed in developing oligodendrocyte processes and mediate injury. Nature 2005; 438: 1167–1171.

97. Cull-Candy SG, Leszkiewicz DN. Role of distinct NMDA receptor subtypes at central synapses. Sci STKE 2004; 255:re16.

98. Neyton J, Paoletti P. Relating NMDA receptor function to receptor subunit composition: limitations of the pharmacological approach. J Neurosci 2006; 26:1331–1333.

99. Guzick DS, Winn K. The association of chorioamnionitis with preterm delivery. Obstet Gynecol 1985; 65:11–16.

100. Jeffrey IJ. The critical role of perinatal pathology. BJOG 2003; 110(Suppl 20):128–130.

101. Naeye RL, Peters EC. Causes and consequences of premature rupture of fetal membranes. Lancet 1980; 1:192–194.

102. Khong TY, Bendon RW, Qureshi F et al. Chronic deciduitis in the placental basal plate: definition and interobserver reliability. Hum Pathol 2000; 31:292–295.

103. Keenan WJ, Steichen JJ, Mahmood K, Altshuler G. Placental pathology compared with clinical outcome: a retrospective blind review. Am J Dis Child 1977; 131:1224–1227.

104. Satosar A, Ramirez NC, Bartholomew D, Davis J, Nuovo GJ. Histologic correlates of viral and bacterial infection of the placenta associated with severe morbidity and mortality in the newborn. Hum Pathol 2004; 35:536–545.

105. Kim CJ, Yoon BH, Park SH, Chi JG. Histotopographic distribution of placental inflammation: analysis of 22 cases. J Korean Med Sci 1998; 13:519–524.

106. Wu YW. Systematic review of chorioamnionitis and cerebral palsy. Ment Retard Dev Disabil Res Rev 2002; 8:25–29.

107. Dollner H, Vatten L, Halgunset J, Rahimipoor S, Austgulen R. Histologic chorioamnionitis and umbilical serum levels of proinflammatory cytokines and cytokine inhibitors. BJOG 2002; 109: 534–539.

108. Gomez R, Romero R, Ghezzi F et al. The fetal inflammatory response syndrome. Am J Obstet Gynecol 1998; 179:194–202.

109. Romero R, Espinoza J, Chaiworapongsa T, Kalache K. Infection and prematurity and the role of preventive strategies. Semin Neonatol 2002; 7:259–274.

110. Yoon BH, Romero R, Moon J et al. Differences in the fetal inter-leukin-6 response to microbial invasion of the amniotic cavity between term and preterm gestation. J Matern Fetal Neonatal Med 2003; 13:32–38.

111. Gilles FH, Leviton A, Kerr CS. Endotoxin leucoencephalopathy in the telencephalon of the newborn kitten. J Neurol Sci 1976; 27: 183–191.

112. Field NT, Newton ER, Kagan-Hallet K, Peairs WA. Perinatal effects of Gardnerella vaginalis deciduitis in the rabbit. Am J Obstet Gynecol 2004; 168:988–994.

113. Yoon BH, Kim CJ, Romero R et al. Experimentally induced intra-uterine infection causes fetal brain white matter lesions in rabbits. Am J Obstet Gynecol 1997; 177:797–802.

114. Cai Z, Pan ZL, Pang Y, Evans OB, Rhodes PG. Cytokine induction in fetal rat brains and brain injury in neonatal rats after maternal lipopolysaccharide administration. Pediatr Res 2000; 47(1):64–72.

115. Duncan JR, Cock ML, Scheerlinck JP et al. White matter injury after repeated endotoxin exposure in the preterm ovine fetus. Pediatr Res 2002; 52(6):941–949.

116. Mallard C, Welin AK, Peebles D, Hagberg H, Kjellmer I. White matter injury following systemic endotoxemia or asphyxia in the fetal sheep. Neurochem Res 2003; 28:215–223.

117. Newnham JP, Shub A, Jobe AH et al. The effects of intra-amniotic injection of periodontopathic lipopolysaccharides in sheep. Am J Obstet Gynecol 2005; 193:313–321.

118. Collins JG, Smith MA, Arnold RR, Offenbacher S. Effects of Escherichia coli and Porphyromonas gingivalis lipopolysaccharide on pregnancy outcome in the golden hamster. Infect Immun 1994; 62:4652–4655.

119. Bell MJ, Hallenbeck JM. Effects of intrauterine inflammation on developing rat brain. J Neurosci Res 2002; 70:570–579.

120. Yan E, Castillo-Melendez M, Nicholls T, Hirst J, Walker D. Cerebrovascular responses in the fetal sheep brain to low-dose endotoxin. Pediatr Res 2004; 55:855–863.

121. Nadeau S, Rivest S. Role of microglial-derived tumor necrosis factor in mediating CD14 transcription and nuclear factor κB activity in the brain during endotoxemia. J Neurosci 2000; 20:3456–3468.

122. Lehnardt S, Massillon L, Follett P et al. Activation of innate immu-nity in the CNS triggers neurodegeneration through a Toll-like receptor 4-dependent pathway. Proc Natl Acad Sci USA 2003; 100(14): 8514–8519.

123. Cammer W. Effects of TNFα on immature and mature oligodendro-cytes and their progenitors in vitro. Brain Res 2000; 864:213–219.

124. Lehnardt S, Lachance C, Patriz S et al. The Toll-like receptor TLR4 is necessary for lipopolysaccharide induced oligodendrocyte injury in the CNS. J Neurosci 2002; 22:2476–2486.

125. Kendall G, Peebles D. Acute fetal hypoxia: the modulating effect of infection. Early Hum Dev 2005; 81: 27–34.

126. Eklind S, Mallard C Leverin AL et al. Bacterial endotoxin sensitizes the immature brain to hypoxic-ischaemic injury. Eur J Neurosci 2001; 13(6):1101–1106.

127. Coumans AB, Middelanis JS, Garnier Y et al. Intracisternal application of endotoxin enhances the susceptibility to subsequent hypoxic-ischemic brain damage in neonatal rats. Pediatr Res 2003; 53(5):770–775.

128. Yang L, Sameshima H, Ikeda T, Ikenoue T. Lipopolysaccharide administration enhances hypoxic-ischemic brain damage in newborn rats. J Obstet Gynaecol Res 2004; 30(2):142–147.

129. Eklind S, Mallard C, Arvidsson P, Hagberg H. Lipopolysaccharide induces both a primary and a secondary phase of sensitization in the developing rat brain. Pediatr Res 2005; 58:112–116.

130. Ahmed SH, He YY, Nassief A et al. Effects of lipopolysaccharide priming on acute ischemic brain injury. Stroke 2000; 31(1): 193–199.

131. Rosenzweig HL, Lessov NS, Henshall DC et al. Endotoxin precondi-tioning prevents cellular inflammatory response during ischemic neuroprotection in mice. Stroke 2004; 35:2576–2581.

132. Peebles DM, Wyatt JS. Synergy between antenatal exposure to infec-tion and intrapartum events in causation of perinatal brain injury at term. BJOG 2002; 109:737–739.

133. Gayle DA, Beloosesky R, Desai M et al. Maternal LPS induces cytokines in the amniotic fluid and corticotrophin releasing hormone in the fetal rat brain. Am J Physiol Regul Integr Comp Physiol 2004; 286:R1024–R1029.

134. Ikeda T, Yang L, Ikenoue T, Mallard C, Hagberg H. Endotoxin-induced hypoxic-ischemic tolerance is mediated by up-regulation of corticosterone in neonatal rat. Pediatr Res 2006; 59:56–60.

135. Pang Y, Rodts-Palenik S, Cai Z, Bennett WA, Rhodes PG. Suppression of glial activation is involved in the protection of IL-10 on maternal E. coli induced neonatal white matter injury. Dev Brain Res 2005; 157:141–149.

136. Elovitz M, Wang Z. Medroxyprogesterone acetate, but not progesterone, protects against inflammation-induced parturition and intrauterine fetal demise. Am J Obstet Gynecol 2004; 190: 693–701.

137. Goldenberg RL, Hauth JC, Andrews WW. Intrauterine infection and preterm delivery. N Engl J Med 2000; 342:1500–1507.

138. Goncalves LF, Chaiworapongsa T, Romero R. Intrauterine infection and prematurity. Ment Retard Dev Disabil Res Rev 2002; 8:3–13.

139. Yoon BH, Park CW, Chaiworapongsa T. Intrauterine infection and the development of cerebral palsy. BJOG 2003; 110(Suppl 20): 124–127.

140. Steel JH, Malatos S, Kennea N et al. Bacteria and inflammatory cells in fetal membranes do not always cause preterm labor. Pediatr Res 2005; 57:404–411.

141. Gerber S, Vial Y, Hohlfeld P, Witkin SS. Detection of Ureaplasma urealyticum in second-trimester amniotic fluid by polymerase chain reaction correlates with subsequent preterm labor and delivery. J Infect Dis 2003; 187:518–521.

142. Hillier SL, Nugent RP, Eschenbach DA et al. Association between bacterial vaginosis and preterm delivery of a low-birth-weight infant. The Vaginal Infections and Prematurity Study Group. N Engl J Med 1995; 333:1737–1742.

143. Holst E, Goffeng AR, Andersch B. Bacterial vaginosis and vaginal microorganisms in idiopathic premature labor and association with pregnancy outcome. J Clin Microbiol 1994; 32:176–186.

144. Krohn MA, Hillier SL, Lee ML, Rabe LK, Eschenbach DA. Vaginal Bacteroides species are associated with an increased rate of preterm delivery among women in preterm labor. J Infect Dis 1991; 164:88–93.

145. Bearfield C, Davenport ES, Sivapathasundaram V, Allaker RP. Possible association between amniotic fluid micro-organism infection and microflora in the mouth. BJOG 2002; 109:527–533.

146. Champagne CM, Madianos PN, Lieff S et al. Periodontal medicine: emerging concepts in pregnancy outcomes. J Int Acad Periodontol 2000; 2:9–13.

147. Dasanayake AP, Russell S, Boyd D et al. Preterm low birth weight and periodontal disease among African Americans. Dent Clin North Am 2003; 47:115–25, x–xi.

148. Offenbacher S, Lieff S, Boggess KA et al. Maternal periodontitis and prematurity. Part I: Obstetric outcome of prematurity and growth restriction. Ann Periodontol 2001; 6:164–174.

149. Han YW, Redline RW, Li M et al. *Fusobacterium nucleatum* induces premature and term stillbirths in pregnant mice: implication of oral bacteria in preterm birth. Infect Immun 2004; 72:2272–2279.

150. Gibbs RS, Romero R, Hillier SL, Eschenbach DA, Sweet RL. A review of premature birth and subclinical infection. Am J Obstet Gynecol 1992; 166:1515–1528.

151. Yoon BH, Romero R, Lim JH et al. The clinical significance of detecting *Ureaplasma urealyticum* by the polymerase chain reaction in the amniotic fluid of patients with preterm labor. Am J Obstet Gynecol 2003; 189:919–924.

152. Cooke RW. Cerebral palsy in very low birthweight infants. Arch Dis Child 1990; 65:201–206.

153. Murphy DJ, Sellers S, MacKenzie IZ, Yudkin PL, Johnson AM. Case-control study of antenatal and intrapartum risk factors for cerebral palsy in very preterm singleton babies. Lancet 1995; 346:1449–1454.

154. O'Shea TM, Klinepeter KL, Meis PJ, Dillard RG. Intrauterine infection and the risk of cerebral palsy in very low-birthweight infants. Paediatr Perinat Epidemiol 1998; 12:72–83.

155. Spinillo A, Capuzzo E, Orcesi S et al. Antenatal and delivery risk factors simultaneously associated with neonatal death and cerebral palsy in preterm infants. Early Hum Dev 1997; 48:81–91.

156. Wilson-Costello D, Borawski E, Friedman H et al. Perinatal correlates of cerebral palsy and other neurologic impairment among very low birth weight children. Pediatrics 1998; 102:315–322.

157. Yoon BH, Jun JK, Romero R et al. Amniotic fluid inflammatory cytokines (interleukin-6, interleukin-1beta, and tumor necrosis factor-alpha), neonatal brain white matter lesions, and cerebral palsy. Am J Obstet Gynecol 1997; 177:19–26.

158. Leviton A, Gilles F, Neff R, Yaney P. Multivariate analysis of risk of perinatal telencephalic leucoencephalopathy. Am J Epidemiol 1976; 104:621–626.

159. Martinez E, Figueroa R, Garry D et al. Elevated amniotic fluid interleukin-6 as a predictor of neonatal periventricular leukomalacia and intraventricular hemorrhage. J Matern Fetal Investig 1998; 8:101–107.

160. Verma U, Tejani N, Klein S et al. Obstetric antecedents of intraventricular hemorrhage and periventricular leukomalacia in the low-birth-weight neonate. Am J Obstet Gynecol 1997; 176:275–281.

161. Holzman C, Jetton J, Fisher R et al. Association of maternal IgM concentrations above the median at 15–19 weeks of gestation and early preterm delivery. Lancet 1999; 354:1095–1096.

162. Spinillo A, Capuzzo E, Stronati M et al. Obstetric risk factors for periventricular leukomalacia among preterm infants. Br J Obstet Gynaecol 1998; 105:865–871.

163. Dammann O, Allred EN, Veelken N. Increased risk of spastic diplegia among very low birth weight children after preterm labor or prelabor rupture of membranes. J Pediatr 1998; 132:531–535.

164. Nelson KB, Ellenberg JH. Epidemiology of cerebral palsy. Adv Neurol 1978; 19:421–435.

165. Yoon BH, Romero R, Park JS et al. Fetal exposure to an intra-amniotic inflammation and the development of cerebral palsy at the age of three years. Am J Obstet Gynecol 2000; 182:675–681.

166. Yoon BH, Romero R, Yang SH et al. Interleukin-6 concentrations in umbilical cord plasma are elevated in neonates with white matter lesions associated with periventricular leukomalacia. Am J Obstet Gynecol 1996; 174:1433–1440.

167. Moon JB, Kim JC, Yoon BH et al. Amniotic fluid matrix metalloproteinase-8 and the development of cerebral palsy. J Perinat Med 2002; 30:301–306.

168. Eschenbach DA. Amniotic fluid infection and cerebral palsy. Focus on the fetus. JAMA 1997; 278:247–248.

169. Salafia CM, Sherer DM, Spong CY et al. Fetal but not maternal serum cytokine levels correlate with histologic acute placental inflammation. Am J Perinatol 1997; 14:419–422.

170. Grether JK, Nelson KB, Walsh E, Willoughby RE, Redline RW. Intrauterine exposure to infection and risk of cerebral palsy in very preterm infants. Arch Pediatr Adolesc Med 2003; 157:26–32.

171. Nelson KB, Grether JK, Dambrosia JM et al. Neonatal cytokines and cerebral palsy in very preterm infants. Pediatr Res 2003; 53: 600–607.

172. Baud O, Emilie D, Pelletier E et al. Amniotic fluid concentrations of interleukin-1beta, interleukin-6 and TNF-alpha in chorioamnionitis before 32 weeks of gestation: histological associations and neonatal outcome. Br J Obstet Gynaecol 1999; 106:72–77.

173. Gray PH, Hurley TM, Rogers YM et al. Survival and neonatal and neurodevelopmental outcome of 24–29 week gestation infants according to primary cause of preterm delivery. Aust N Z J Obstet Gynaecol 1997; 37:161–168.

174. Grether JK, Nelson KB, Emery ES III, Cummins SK. Prenatal and perinatal factors and cerebral palsy in very low birth weight infants. J Pediatr 1996; 128:407–414.

175. Nelson KB. Can we prevent cerebral palsy? N Engl J Med 2003; 349:1765–1769.

176. Walstab J, Bell R, Reddihough D et al. Antenatal and intrapartum antecedents of cerebral palsy: a case-control study. Aust N Z J Obstet Gynaecol 2002; 42:138–146.

177. Paneth N, Stark RI. Cerebral palsy and mental retardation in relation to indicators of perinatal asphyxia. An epidemiologic overview. Am J Obstet Gynecol 1983; 147:960–966.

178. Nelson KB, Leviton A. How much of neonatal encephalopathy is due to birth asphyxia? Am J Dis Child 1991; 145:1325–1331.

179. Yudkin PL, Johnson A, Clover LM, Murphy KW. Assessing the contribution of birth asphyxia to cerebral palsy in term singletons. Paediatr Perinat Epidemiol 1995; 9:156–170.

180. Nelson KB, Willoughby RE. Infection, inflammation and the risk of cerebral palsy. Curr Opin Neurol 2000; 13:133–139.

181. Wu YW, Colford JM Jr. Chorioamnionitis as a risk factor for cerebral palsy: a meta-analysis. JAMA 2000; 284:1417–1424.

182. Shalak LF, Laptook AR, Jafri HS, Ramilo O, Perlman JM. Clinical chorioamnionitis, elevated cytokines, and brain injury in term infants. Pediatrics 2002; 110:673–680.

183. Impey L, Greenwood C, MacQuillan K, Reynolds M, Sheil O. Fever in labour and neonatal encephalopathy: a prospective cohort study. BJOG 2001; 108:594–597.

184. Grether JK, Nelson KB, Dambrosia JM, Phillips TM. Interferons and cerebral palsy. J Pediatr 1999; 134:324–332.

Index

Page numbers in *italics* refer to tables and figures.